THE GREAT HORSE FLU

THE GREAT HORSE FLU

A FORGOTTEN CONTAGION AND THE FATE OF RECONSTRUCTION AMERICA

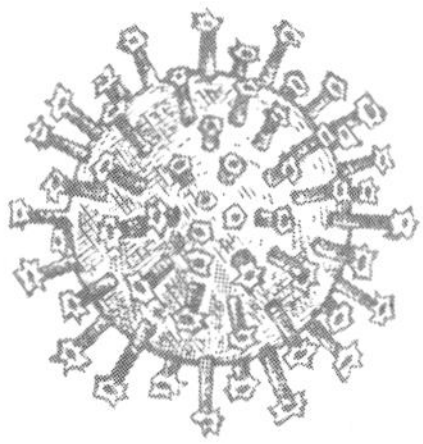

THOMAS G. ANDREWS

The University of North Carolina Press
CHAPEL HILL

This book was published with the assistance of the Anniversary Fund of the University of North Carolina Press.

Earlier versions of this work have appeared in Thomas G. Andrews, "Influenza's Progress: The Great Epizootic Flu of 1872–1873 in the North American West," *Utah Historical Quarterly* 89, no. 1 (2021): 4–30; and Thomas G. Andrews, "Remembering and Forgetting the Great Horse Flu of 1872–1873," *Modern American History* 8, no. 1 (2025): 108–14.

Designed by Lindsay Starr
Set in Quadraat Pro by codeMantra

Cover art: Horses drinking, photograph by John H. Tarbell, courtesy Museum of the City of New York. Coronavirus vaccine vector set © Adobe Stock / sketched-graphics. Newspaper pages © Adobe Stock / appl.

LIBRARY OF CONGRESS CATALOGING-IN-PUBLICATION DATA
Names: Andrews, Thomas G., 1972– author
Title: The Great Horse Flu : a forgotten contagion and the fate of Reconstruction America / Thomas G. Andrews.
Description: Chapel Hill : The University of North Carolina Press, [2026] | Includes bibliographical references and index.
Identifiers: LCCN 2026017557 | ISBN 9781469698434 cloth | ISBN 9781469696355 epub | ISBN 9781469698441 pdf
Subjects: LCSH: Equine influenza—United States—History—19th century | Horses—Diseases—Political aspects—United States | Reconstruction (U.S. history, 1865–1877) | BISAC: HISTORY / United States / 19th Century | MEDICAL / Veterinary Medicine / General
Classification: LCC SF959.I54 A63 2026 | DDC 636.1/0896203—dc23/eng/20260409
LC record available at https://lccn.loc.gov/2026017557

For product safety concerns under the European Union's General Product Safety Regulation (EU GPSR), please contact gpsr@mare-nostrum.co.uk or write to the University of North Carolina Press and Mare Nostrum Group B.V., Doelen 72, 4831 GR Breda, The Netherlands.

To Amy, the love of my life,

and in loving memory of

Martha Lee Andrews, née Tuthill (1938–2025)

and

Timothy Scott Lenaghen Kirkland (1969–2024)

CONTENTS

THE GREAT HORSE FLU

INTRODUCTION

A Pitiless Malady

This book tells the story of one of the strangest contagions ever recorded. More than a century and a half ago, what I call the Great Horse Flu began to ravage North America. In an outbreak that raged from fall 1872 to late 1873, a powerful new viral variant beset millions of horses, donkeys, and mules (collectively known as equines) throughout most of the present-day United States as well as large swaths of Canada, Mexico, Cuba, and Central America before dissipating into British Columbian forests and Nicaraguan jungles. Because people in all these places depended on equines to drive their lives and economies, the Great Horse Flu caused profound disruptions.

The ensuing chaos casts a more illuminating light on the societies this plague preyed upon. By depriving North American communities of motive power for weeks at a time, the outbreak exposed just how fully humans across the continent had grown to depend on the labors of illness-prone animals.

It also prompted searching discussions regarding the nature of infectious diseases as well as what, if anything, people might owe to the equines with whom they lived and labored.

As folks struggled to make do and get by without the work that ailing or recuperating equines could no longer do, they unwittingly sparked other problems. If history teaches us anything, it is that one crisis soon begets others. As those of us who lived through the COVID-19 pandemic know all too well, contagions, whether among humans or the animals we call our own, have the capacity to cause troubles that can go on to activate other calamities. In the early 1870s no less than in the present day, viruses and other scourges possessed the power to shunt individual and collective lives onto unexpected and often unwanted trajectories. The story of the Great Horse Flu thus offers an illustrative chapter in the ancient yet also all-too-present dynamics by which humans, the creatures we hold closest, and the pathogens that circulate between us and them continually make and remake what we call history.

This continent-conquering malady first entered human awareness in the countryside north of Toronto, Ontario, where farm horses pastured on late summer grasses started falling ill in September 1872 with fever and respiratory complaints. In the first widely disseminated account of the outbreak, Andrew Smith, a graduate of the world-famous Edinburgh veterinary college in his native Scotland and Ontario's leading authority on equine health, observed in the *Toronto Globe* that these horses' woes began with "a watery discharge from the nose, speedily followed by a severe hacking cough; the pulse is quickened, the mouth hot, the nasal membranes" reddened to a crimson hue, "and the ears and legs are unnaturally cold; the discharge from the nose increases, and becomes of a greenish-yellowish color; the breathing is increased and in some cases becomes labored and severe." Hundreds of other accounts penned in the ensuing year detailed similar or identical symptoms. In the worst cases, patients could muster neither the will nor the energy to do anything but stand in their stalls "as if benumbed or paralyzed."[1]

Days after farmers first noticed the illness running amok among horses outside Toronto, the Great Horse Flu began racing through Canada. Before long, Montreal's horse-powered street railways suspended operations, "farmers in the country" found themselves "unable to bring grain to market," and nearly every horse in Ottawa seemed to be ailing. "The progress of the disease since first heard of in Toronto," a newspaper in the Canadian capital declared, "has been so astonishingly rapid that from every town and village in Ontario, as well as many places in Quebec, the same cry is sent forth."[2]

In mid-October, the equine plague began pouring over the international border, invading New England and Upstate New York despite a US Treasury Department ban on importing Canadian horses who showed clear signs of illness. Just days later, with nearly all of Buffalo's equines on the sick list, a journalist observed that "the extent of mankind's dependence upon equine assistance is being vividly brought to view." In Rochester, two coroners "called upon to extricate the body of a drowned man" from the Erie Canal realized that with their horses ill, they had no way to cart off the deceased until "a bright idea struck one of them, and fastening a rope to the corpse they towed it, with the aid of a fishpole, a distance of several blocks." They then plucked the body from the water and carried it to "the dead house" under their own steam.[3]

A few weeks later, with the outbreak extending its reach throughout the Northeast, the *New York Herald* marveled at "the singular spectacle . . . of a great city almost at a standstill," with "thousands of persons, male and female, young and old," now "unable to reach their homes after a day of toil except on foot." In Lower Manhattan, "an ominous quiet" descended. Even Broadway, one of world's busiest thoroughfares, suddenly fell "motionless, dumb, paralyzed." On New York's piers and wharves, "goods of all descriptions" accumulated "promiscuously" in piles "reaching to the height of ten or fifteen feet, completely hiding the river from view." Hundreds of longshoremen, who could neither load nor empty ships without equine assistance, soon found themselves jobless and "penniless." Up the Hudson in Newburgh, masons, carpenters, and other tradesmen who relied on horses "to draw sand, brick, and other building material" also faced slowdowns and layoffs, while New York's "theatre and amusement managers" complained "of a perfect dearth of customers; and the playhouses, concert and lecture halls" all "reveal[ed] a disagreeable paucity of attendance."[4]

The pestilence ripped across vast stretches of North America with disquieting haste and thoroughness. "No sooner does one horse become affected," an agricultural magazine pronounced, "than within twenty-four hours three-fourths of all the horses in the place are down with it." The disease, another journalist marveled, "seemed to act by some malignant spell, prostrating equine victims by the thousand almost on the very instant of its appearance." The Great Horse Flu "apparently required no time for development," but instead was "born full-grown" with the capacity to sicken "the whole family" of equine creation all at once. In the face of this "pitiless malady," "the submissive, patient, hard-worked carthorse, the magnificent, sleek-coated, high mettled charger, and the blooded racer" had all "gone down together."[5]

With the outbreak expanding across a seven-hundred-mile front stretching from Maine to Ohio, traffic on Northeastern canals ground to a halt;

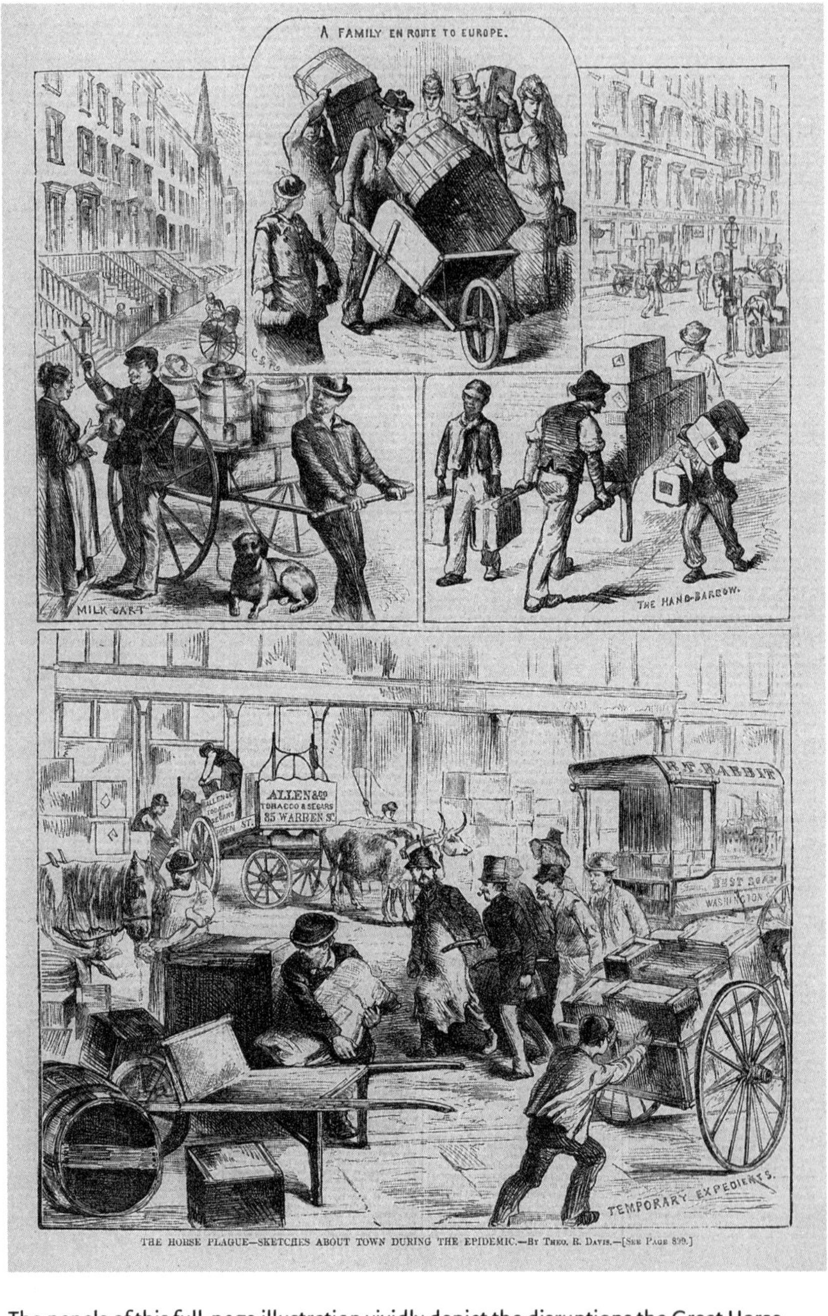

The panels of this full-page illustration vividly depict the disruptions the Great Horse Flu caused. Note the close focus on a succession of street scenes, with goods accumulating, onlookers gawking, and humans and oxen doing their best to provide the motive power that flu-stricken horses could no longer perform. Theodore R. Davis, "The Horse Plague," *Harper's Weekly*, November 16, 1872, 900. Courtesy of University of Colorado Libraries.

loggers in the "lumbering districts north of Saginaw" all but stopped their preparations for Michigan's upcoming logging season; and the *Hartford Courant* claimed that "a horse in the streets" had become "a rare sight." Farmers, meanwhile, complained that the flu was "greatly hindering the work of . . . harvesting" crops and throwing "a serious obstacle in the way of all kinds of business." Intent on isolating their equines from the fast-spreading plague, many countryfolk made the hard decision to put off their regular shopping trips to town until the malady relented.[6]

By early November, the Great Horse Flu had spread to Halifax; Quebec City; Concord, New Hampshire; Philadelphia; Baltimore; Washington, DC; Norfolk, Virginia; Pittsburgh; Cincinnati; and Chicago. "All the horses in the city are sick," complained the *Chicago Evening Post*, and had "disappeared from the streets." The disorder, the same article continued, "comes upon them with the suddenness of a flash of lightning. No sooner do they trot from the barn than they commence running at the nose." The only silver lining, the *Evening Post* concluded on November 2, was that "the poor beasts don't die." Subsequent events, though, disproved this hopeful prognosis. On November 6, the outbreak claimed the lives of ten Chicago horses. The next day, thirty more succumbed. By the time the plague finally moved on in early December, an estimated 561 of the city's roughly 24,000 equines had breathed their last. Although one paper reasoned that this was "a remarkably low death rate when it is borne in mind that nearly all the horses and mules in the city were affected," hundreds more horses would go on to die from the lingering effects of the malady and its complications.[7]

By hobbling equine-powered production and exchange throughout the continent, the outbreak augured deeper ills. Chicago's real estate market grew "dull." Realtors in Indianapolis griped that "suburban property" there was "selling slowly" because the flu outbreak made it harder to bring potential buyers to inspect empty lots on the city's outskirts. Railroads confronted "a general depression" as investors steered clear of their "securities, owing to the reduced business on account of the epizootic [a sweeping eruption of illness among other-than-human animals]." As the outbreak extended its reach to rural areas where farming, logging, mining, and stockraising predominated, some commentators even started to worry that flu-fueled disruptions might prompt additional contractions in the nation's already stringent money supply, with potentially disastrous consequences for the American economy.[8]

Fast forward to fall 1873, and the Great Horse Flu had permeated most of North America. It penetrated virtually every settled region in Canada, which had just confederated five years earlier (Prince Edward Island, which had joined that nation in July 1873, somehow eluded its ravages). It also attacked

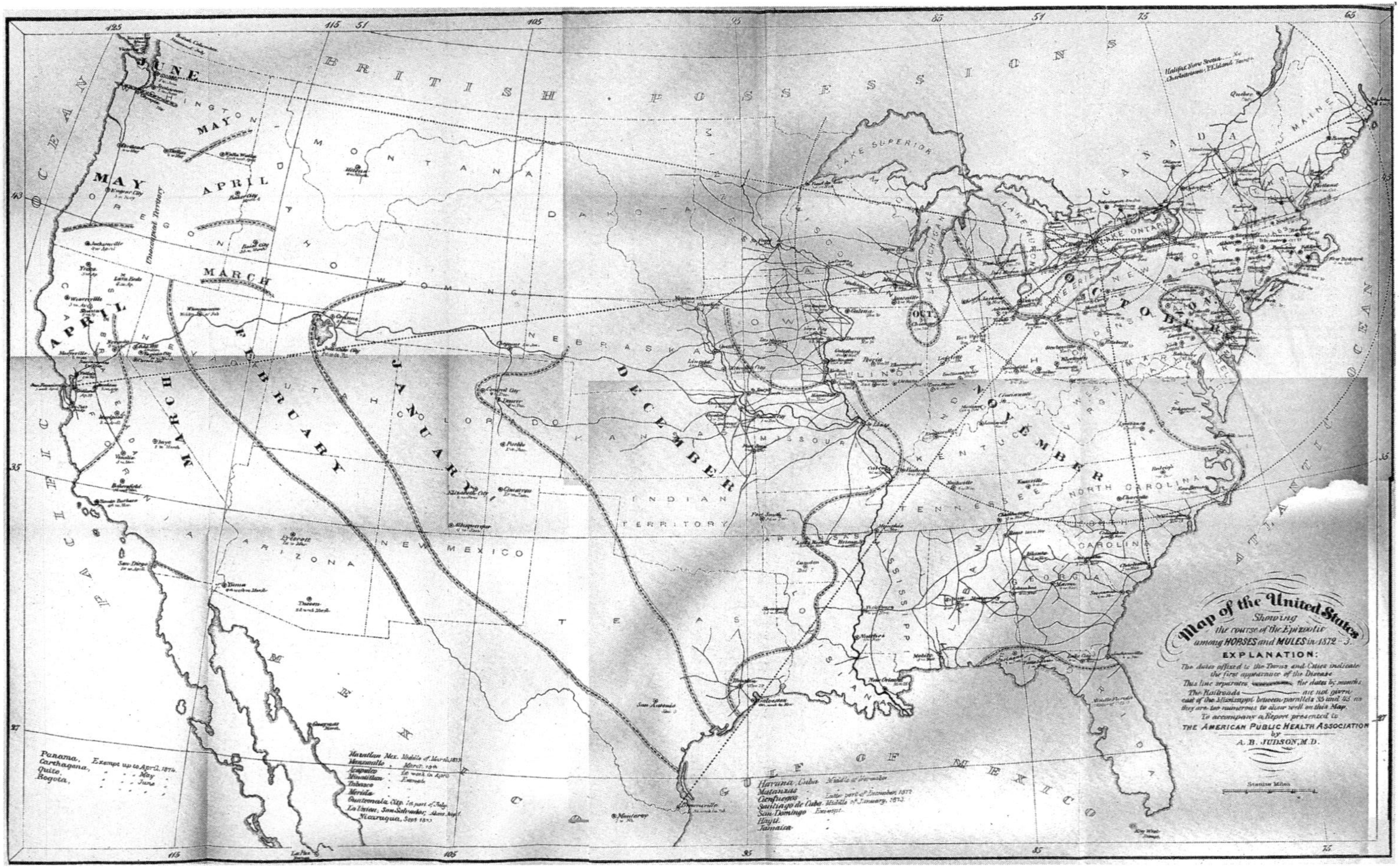
Map of the United States
Showing
the course of the Epizootic
among HORSES and MULES in 1872 - 3.
EXPLANATION:
The dates affixed to the Towns and Cities indicate the first appearance of the Disease
This line separates the dates by months
The Railroads are not given east of the Mississippi between parallels 35 and 43 as they are too numerous to show well on this Map.
To accompany a Report presented to
THE AMERICAN PUBLIC HEALTH ASSOCIATION
by
A. B. JUDSON, M.D.
Statute Miles
BRITISH POSSESSIONS
CANADA
MAINE
LAKE SUPERIOR
LAKE MICHIGAN
LAKE HURON
LAKE ONTARIO
LAKE ERIE
NEW YORK
OCTOBER
OCT.
NOVEMBER
DECEMBER
JANUARY
FEBRUARY
MARCH
APRIL
MAY
JUNE
MONTANA
DAKOTA
WYOMING
NEBRASKA
IOWA
ILLINOIS
MISSOURI
KANSAS
COLORADO
INDIAN TERRITORY
NEW MEXICO
ARIZONA
TEXAS
KENTUCKY
TENNESSEE
NORTH CAROLINA
SOUTH CAROLINA
GEORGIA
ALABAMA
MISSISSIPPI
LOUISIANA
ARKANSAS
WEST VIRGINIA
OREGON
CALIFORNIA
NEVADA
UTAH
IDAHO
WASHINGTON
PACIFIC OCEAN
ATLANTIC OCEAN
GULF OF MEXICO
MEXICO
Mazatlan Mex. Middle of March, 1873
Manzanillo . March 19th
Acapulco . 1st week in April
Minatitlan . Exempt
Tabasco
Merida
Guatemala City 1st part of July
La Union, San Salvador; About Aug 1.
Nicaragua, Sept 1873
Havana, Cuba Middle of December
Matanzas
Cienfuegos Latter part of December, 1872
Santiago de Cuba Middle of January, 1873
San Domingo Exempt
Hayti
Jamaica
Panama, Exempt up to April, 1874.
Carthagena,
Quito, May
Bogota, June

virtually all of the United States, from the nation's largest metropolitan regions to its least populated rural reaches. It hit the North as well as the recently defeated Confederacy, then struck the West's embattled Indigenous Nations as well as the US-Mexico borderlands.

While the Great Horse Flu moved across the United States and Canada like a wave, its movements proved more finicky in Latin America. The scourge reached most large towns and cities in Mexico but steered clear of the Yucatán, Baja California, and several other areas. In Cuba, where a coalition of planters, enslaved peoples, and others had been waging a desperate rebellion against Spanish colonial rule since 1868, the pestilence reserved its worst for Havana and scattered other locales. Few documents detail the outbreak's closing throes after it pushed from Mexico to Guatemala and Nicaragua, but the Great Horse Flu clearly had difficulty tracking down new hosts in Central America—probably because the region's rugged topography, tortuous transportation routes, and disjointed economies kept equine populations there more isolated than integrated.

In all these domains, the outbreak sometimes jumped to nonequine hosts. Newspapers from many parts of North America alleged that poultry, hogs, and other barnyard and household animals had contracted it. They also published hundreds of reports of humans falling ill with flu-like symptoms not long after the equine plague reached their communities, sparking localized infection hot spots and even occasional fatalities.[9]

Neither English nor any other North American language possessed any ready-made name for such a scourge. Terms for the Great Horse Flu soon popped up like mushrooms after spring rains. Some of the resulting labels—Canadian horse disease, horse plague, horse epidemic, equine distemper, or simply horse disease—were merely descriptive. Others—epibronquippomania,

Adoniram B. Judson, son of famous Baptist missionaries, Union army surgeon, and physician for New York City's Board of Health, mapped information on the outbreak's spread that he gathered from newspapers and correspondence. The result is a masterful example of the emerging techniques of epidemiological cartography. Note how Judson's map pinpoints the epizootic's initial emergence outside Toronto and plots its subsequent month-by-month spread. We know from press coverage that Judson presented versions of this map to at least two gatherings of public health experts, the first in New York City in January 1873 and the second in Cincinnati later that year. On both occasions, he used cartography to contest other authorities' assertions that the Great Horse Flu spread through atmospheric influences. Adoniram B. Judson, "History and Course of the Epizootic Among Horses upon the North American Continent," *American Public Health Association Reports* 1 (1873): 88. Courtesy of HathiTrust.

hiporhinophlegmatoblenocalastalagmus—turned equine tragedy into human comedy by mashing together Latin, Greek, and gobbledygook.[10]

Many folks, though, steered clear of name games and instead referred to the outbreak simply as the epizootic. By the time the Great Horse Flu ended its run, this animalized riff on "epidemic," which entered English from French in the late eighteenth century but had seen little use outside scientific circles, became a household word. In some corners of the American countryside, it even earned an enduring place in the folk lexicon as a catchall for colds and flu, especially among humans.

Healers, horse people, and dilettantes applied conflicting diagnoses to the epizootic. Some called it typhoid. Others linked it to cholera. And still others suspected that it was merely distemper. Most knowledgeable authorities, though, identified the disease as influenza, Italian for "the influence."

Past flu epidemics, they understood, had often coincided with widespread reports of horses and other nonhuman animals falling ill with similar or identical symptoms. Influenza's name reflected the long-standing supposition that this ailment's capacity to suddenly sicken huge numbers of individual organisms, often drawn from distinct branches of creation and invariably distributed across hundreds or thousands of square miles, could only result from atmospheric or astronomical influences. By the time the Great Horse Flu struck, though, a growing chorus of skeptics hypothesized that influenza spread not through air currents or the planet's passage through unhealthy quadrants of the cosmos but instead via contagion—the communication of a disease-causing agent from one host to the next. No one, though, could pinpoint the responsible agent with any certainty. Fungi, spores, insects, animalcules, and tiny plant seeds—"germs," people called them—all had their champions.[11]

A handful of observers even attributed the epizootic's brisk expansion to the interplay between contagionist and atmospheric dynamics. The germ responsible for causing influenza, a few eccentric but prescient thinkers speculated, might travel from victim to victim through the air—a synthesis not so different, as it happens, from our current understanding of influenza as an illness caused by a specific viral pathogen commonly communicated through aerosols as well as larger airborne particles. More likely than not, the epizootic resulted from an unknown variant of highly pathogenic avian influenza A, probably from the H7N7 strain.[12]

No flu tests yet existed, nor did local, state, or federal agencies gather reliable statistics on the Great Horse Flu. The available evidence, however, shows that the epizootic was astoundingly infectious. In some remote settings, only one-quarter to one-half of horses caught it. Nearly everywhere else, though, reputable authorities insisted that at least three-quarters of equines developed symptoms. James Law, founder of Cornell's veterinary school and a friend of Toronto's Andrew Smith, asserted on the basis of extensive research in daily newspapers as well as energetic correspondence with experts throughout the United States and Canada as well as with US consular officials in Latin America that "the percentage of horses attacked has been variously stated at from 80 to 99." Such estimates, Law hastened to add, were "mostly written before the disease ha[d] quite passed away," so he considered it "probable that the latter number is nearest the general average."[13]

A wealth of evidence supports Law's assertion that the Great Horse Flu reached near-total prevalence. Newspapers alleged that 90 percent of the equines in Cincinnati and 95 percent of those in Washington, DC, got sick; they also claimed that fully 100 percent of horses contracted the epizootic in places as small as Newport, Ohio, with a population of just over 2,000 people, and as large as Brooklyn, which bustled with more than 1.5 million. More granular—and perhaps more credible—figures documented infection rates of 96.2 percent in Cabot, Vermont; 96.7 percent in Minot Corner, Maine; 98.6 percent in the Baltimore's City Passenger Railroad's stables; and 99.4 percent of the animals employed by Connecticut's Westville and Fair Haven Horse Railroad. The Great Horse Flu's ability to sicken all or nearly all the equines everywhere it struck easily ranks it among the most transmissible outbreaks of mammalian disease ever recorded.[14]

The epizootic inflicted considerable misery on nearly every creature it infected. In a small but significant subset of cases, influenza and its complications even proved fatal. For reasons that remain unclear, as many as one-quarter of afflicted donkeys perished from the disease. The Great Horse Flu proved milder among horses and mules, killing 1 to 4 percent of affected animals from these species—slightly higher than human mortality rates in the Great Flu Pandemic of 1918–20 and the COVID-19 pandemic.[15]

Even though most victims survived the epizootic, the outbreak nonetheless left a harvest of death in its wake. Census takers enumerated some 8.69 million horses in the US countryside in 1870, supplemented by 1.1 million donkeys and mules. Large but unknown numbers of equines inhabited American towns and cities. The following year, Canada boasted more than 860,000 horses, most of them within a hundred miles or so of the US border. An 1873 US federal census of Native Americans counted 284,400 horses and mules among Indigenous Nations, while unrecorded but substantial numbers of equines plied farms and plantations as well as mountain trails, city streets, and country roads in Cuba, Mexico, and Central America.[16]

The total equine population of the realms the Great Horse Flu struck was at least 11 million and perhaps 15 million or more. By the time the horse plague finally burned out, then, it seems safe to estimate that it killed at least a few hundred thousand equines and possibly more than half a million. Although most victims survived, many struggled to wage full recoveries. An unfortunate minority even developed long-term debilities not unlike those suffered by many COVID survivors, including weakness, respiratory problems, and chronic exhaustion.

As the Great Horse Flu's rampage revealed, Americans, Canadians, Latin Americans, and Native Americans shared a common reliance on horses, donkeys, and mules—and thus a collective vulnerability to influenza, which had targeted equines for centuries and quite possibly millennia. North America's diverse peoples favored different species and breeds of equines, from the diminutive ponies cherished by Native Americans to the strapping draft horses that were becoming increasingly popular on farmsteads and in cities across the US and Canada, and from the dauntless burros who trod high mountain trails in the Southwest and Mexico to the hardy mules who plowed plantation soils in the US South and parts of Latin America.[17]

The labor North American equines performed knit them into a continuous population—an uninterrupted pool of potential hosts for influenza. The work that humans demanded of horses and their cousins kept the animals constantly on the go, bringing them into frequent, sometimes intimate contact with their fellow creatures. Influenza found favorable conditions through most of the continent because equines powered so many facets of human lifeways and livelihoods.

With the Great Horse Flu gripping New York City, *The Nation* reflected on the "position of the horse in modern society." The epizootic, this weighty journal of political commentary intoned, offered a "striking illustration . . . of the part which this animal has come to play in our commercial civilization, and of the close relation there exists between *his* physical condition and *our* material interests." Because "our talk has been for so many years of the railroad and steamboat and telegraph, as the great 'agents of progress,'" *The Nation* explained, "we have come almost totally to overlook the fact that our dependence on the horse has grown almost *pari passu* [Latin for "on an equal footing"] with our dependence on steam." Americans, like their Canadian and Latin American counterparts, had "opened up great lines of steam communication all over the country." Yet trains and riverboats, *The Nation* emphasized, still had "to be fed with goods and passengers by horses. We have covered the ocean with great steamers, but they can neither load nor discharge their cargoes without horses. We have collected at the mouths of our great rivers and at the intersections of our railroads vast bodies of people," assembled in cities "covering miles on miles of area with their dwellings and factories, but have left them wholly dependent for their intramural travel and for their regular supplies of food and clothing on horses."[18]

As the epizootic made plain, North Americans banked on equines to move goods and passengers over short and medium distances, not only on farms and ranches but also in cities as well as the spaces between steam-powered transportation routes. The advent of this "industrial and commercial dependence on the horse," *The Nation* proclaimed, had "been so gradual, so quiet, and . . . so completely overshadowed by the great applications of science to industry and locomotion, that little or no thought has been bestowed on its dangers. Indeed, most of us," it confessed, "have well-nigh forgotten that the horse was an animal like ourselves—liable to pains and aches and death." North Americans had largely come to mistake this living creature, in short, for "a machine, on whose endurance we could calculate as on that of an engine, and for whose mortality we could make ample allowance in our business under the head of 'wear and tear.'"

The epizootic showed that equines were just as vulnerable as humankind to the suffering that flu could inflict—and perhaps equally deserving of empathy and care, too. *The Nation* counseled readers "to be thankful . . . that the present epidemic has brought us face to face with the startling fact, that the sudden loss of horse labor would totally disorganize our industry and our commerce, and would plunge social life into disorder, would threaten the lives of hundreds of thousands of human beings, especially if it occurred in winter, and might expose our great cities to destruction by fire." The influenza outbreak had made it abundantly clear that equines were "not simply private property"; rather, they were "wheels in our great social machine, the stoppage of which means widespread injury to all classes and conditions of persons, injury to commerce, to agriculture, to trade, to social life."

Human existence as Americans and their neighbors knew it pivoted on equines—or at least it had before the Great Horse Flu attacked this vital interspecies partnership. Strip away man-made borders, peer beyond cultural differences, urban/rural divides, and sectional spats, and an oft-neglected reality becomes abundantly clear: The movements and labors of millions of equines wove together North America's diverse economies and societies. By disabling horses and their cousins and making it difficult or even impossible for these prime movers to continue laboring, the Great Horse Flu threatened the animal-powered ties that coursed both within and between the continent's political entities.

This book offers the first full-length account of the Great Horse Flu. Because the outbreak assumed continental proportions, this story necessarily adopts a continental perspective. The epizootic's travels across regional, national, political, and cultural borders raise questions akin to those humans have probably always asked when an infectious disease erupts to sow death and disruption: What caused this pestilence, and how did it expand its range? How did different individuals and groups—equine and human alike—respond to the sickness, suffering, and death that this disease meted out? How did encounters with this contagion upset people's sense of the world? What assumptions did this scourge test, what worldviews did it unsettle, and what innovations in thought and practice did it generate, empower, or suppress?[19]

The epizootic plagued an entire continent—yet it struck the United States hardest of all. The outbreak spent more of its short life there than anywhere else, presumably because the United States boasted North America's largest, most interconnected herds of equines. In contrast to Canada, Mexico, or Central America, horses and their cousins inhabited virtually every corner of the United States as well as the Indigenous homelands that Americans were intent on forcibly incorporating into the United States. Within the territories the nation claimed (but did not yet always control), the virus exploded because equines powered so many facets of economic, social, and cultural exchange. The work that humans demanded of horses and their cousins kept the animals on the go and brought them into regular contact with their fellow creatures, creating excellent conditions for viral transmission.[20]

This book focuses mostly on the United States not just because it boasted more equines than its neighbors but also because American media outlets covered the horse plague's ravages with greater thoroughness and depth than their counterparts in other parts of North America did. By the mid-1800s, the US press had become the envy of the world. As of 1872, the US boasted 6,432 newspapers and magazines—almost as many as all other nations combined. New York City alone had more than 150 papers; nearly 50 papers were published in Cincinnati, a city of around 225,000 people. American newspapers—roughly 10 percent of which were published daily—collectively printed over 1.5 billion total copies in 1872, four times more than were published in Great Britain, which had roughly 31.8 million people compared to a US population of about 38.5 million.[21]

Information flowed faster, more widely, and more smoothly in the United States than anywhere else on the continent because of the peerless scope, efficiency, and ubiquity of American telegraph systems, postal networks, express services, news agencies, and printing plants. Exchanges—arrangements whereby editors swapped copies of their respective publications—made it even easier for news to travel freely. "Any respectable paper received fifty to one hundred" other dailies and weeklies, one historian notes, "in exchange for copies of its own publication (and the New York *Tribune* got at least 2,500 on 'exchange')." No wonder newspapers, as one American journalist gushed on the eve of the Great Horse Flu in 1872, had become "the national teachers, every where in circulation, easily and cheaply obtained, and always clear to the comprehension of every one who can read."[22]

American journalists chronicled the Great Horse Flu tirelessly and in great detail. "The newspapers," one Boston correspondent quipped in late October 1872, "have had the disease as badly as the beasts themselves." "Our newspapers," the *Times of London*'s man in Philadelphia noted, "are full of the epizootic, discourse learnedly upon it, and print columns devoted to reports of its progress and mode of treatment." "The newspapers of the whole country for the last month," a South Carolina journal observed as the Great Horse Flu cantered into the Deep South, "have been fully occupied with the discussion of the horse disease." Like most major disease outbreaks, the Great Horse Flu made excellent copy, and editors throughout the country eagerly reprinted coverage of it from other publications. The recent digitization of a significant minority of US newspapers makes it easier than ever before to reconstruct the epizootic's American travels—and to do so in greater resolution than is possible for the scourge's Canadian, Mexican, Cuban, Native American, or Central American forays.[23]

The story that follows resembles other plague narratives because infectious disease outbreaks typically proceed through a familiar, mostly predictable sequence. "As a social phenomenon," the historian of medicine and disease Charles Rosenberg famously argued at the height of the AIDS crisis, "an epidemic has a dramaturgic form." Epizootics, like epidemics, "start at a moment in time, proceed on a stage limited in space and duration, follow a plot line of increasing and revelatory tension, move to a crisis of individual and collective character, then drift toward closure." This narrative of the Great Horse Flu adheres to Rosenberg's staging. The curtain rises on the virus's emergence outside Toronto in September 1872; the heart of the book proceeds to track the epizootic's rampage across North America and explores the many crises it unbridled; and the plot concludes with the epizootic's decline, its far-reaching legacies, and the important lessons it holds for us today.[24]

To adhere too rigidly to the conventions of the plague narrative by focusing exclusively on the Great Horse Flu itself, though, would be to ignore the fascinating, frequently unpredictable intersections and interactions between the outbreak and other historical events and processes. "As in flash of lightning," the historian Richard Evans observed in *Death in Hamburg*, which cast an 1892 cholera epidemic as an illuminating lens through which to reconsider the social and political history of imperial Germany, contagions can "illuminate a whole historical landscape, throwing even the obscurest

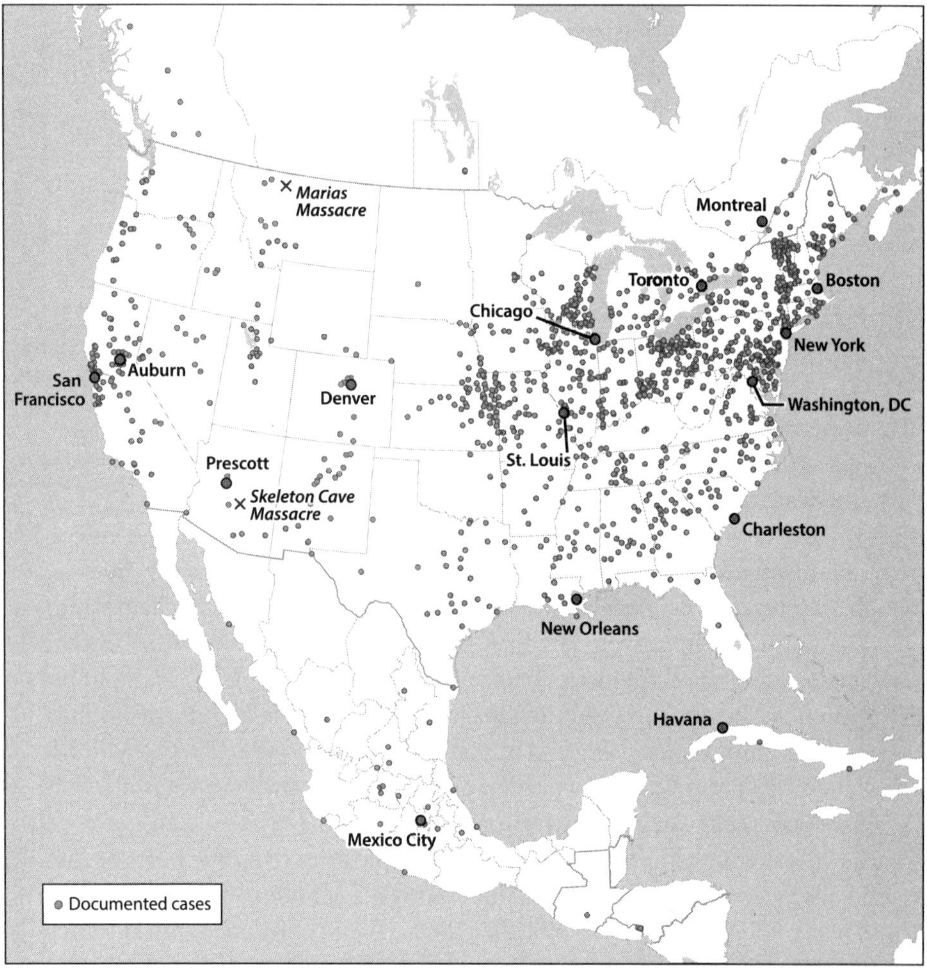

Each mark on this map represents a specific locale where newspapers or other sources reported the equine influenza outbreak. The Marias Massacre and Auburn, California, are covered in chapter 6. Chapter 7 centers on the Skeleton Cave Massacre and Prescott. For animations and other maps based on this data, see the companion website for this book. Cartography by Erin Greb.

features into sharp and dramatic relief." As Evans's study of Hamburg's cholera crisis showed, and as all of us who lived through the COVID pandemic will remember, infectious disease outbreaks hold the power to trigger latent vulnerabilities, heighten otherwise hidden tensions—and even alter history's course.[25]

When infectious diseases erupt, Evans explains, "the structures of social inequality, the operations of political power, the attitudes and habits of mind of different classes and groups in the population, come to light with a clarity of profile unimaginable in more normal times." By applying Evans's call to investigate how "the nature of the everyday lives out of which people" and the animals they called their own "were torn in the crisis," this book seeks to dispel "the historical obscurity that in other circumstances so often shrouds the ways in which those lives were structured." Although the equine influenza epizootic erupted twenty years before Hamburg's cholera crisis and concentrated its ravages on nonhumans, the story of the Great Horse Flu nonetheless shines a telling, if fleeting, light on a host of otherwise shadowy dynamics.[26]

The Great Horse Flu crossed into western New York and New England from Ontario and Quebec seven years after the guns of war between the Union and the Confederacy quieted. The virus found the United States deep in the throes of a tumultuous, transformative era that historians have struggled to corral into a coherent interpretation. Open practically any textbook or synthesis of American history, turn to the chapters addressing the late nineteenth century, and behold just how mightily scholars have labored to craft a narrative capable of drawing together the stories of the victorious North and the defeated South, the city and the country, the dozens of wars of conquest and extermination the United States waged against the West's Indigenous Nations, the rising immigration from Europe and Asia, the surge of US industry to global greatness, and the deepening discontent of the nation's working classes. Of all the eras of the American past, none seems more resistant to comprehensive understanding than the post–Civil War era.

This book does not presume to offer such a synthesis, but it does argue that the Great Horse Flu, the crises it unloosed, and the flashes of lightning the outbreak cast on other happenings and dynamics provide uniquely instructive opportunities to see a momentous juncture in national life more clearly and holistically. The epizootic lashed against a little-noticed but consequential vulnerability—the shared dependence of Americans on horses and their cousins—while striking at some of the most essential but mundane features of everyday life. In the process, the Great Horse Flu upended people's sense of themselves. By prostrating economic, social, and cultural life at a critical juncture in the nation's history, the scourge temporarily unmoored Americans, shook up their conceptions of themselves and the world around them, and eroded their confidence that they could build a shared future.

This process mattered in its own right, yet it also amplified the epizootic's material impact. The virus that propelled the Great Horse Flu resulted from an evolutionary accident but was ideally suited to parasitize American life. By temporarily disrupting Americans' ability to carry out their ordinary pursuits, the outbreak generated no shortage of headaches. Less than a decade after the Civil War and still in the thick of the centuries-long wars that settler colonists waged against Native nations, Americans of various sorts were fast in the throes of a nation-building project. The attending processes of reconstruction, modernization, and consolidation all required immense and ongoing inputs of equine labor. The Great Horse Flu simultaneously exploited and hampered these efforts by making it difficult or impossible for horses, mules, and donkeys to continue working. As the epizootic spread out across the United States like a vast, slow-churning wave, it disrupted life as people knew it. By slowing or even stopping the production and exchange of goods and services, the Great Horse Flu jeopardized the heady growth of the industrial capitalist economy that had propelled the Union to victory in the Civil War. That very same economy was also supposed to sustain enduring solutions to the many weighty problems that remained unresolved despite years of fractious efforts to reunite the nation, rebuild the South, redefine what freedom would mean for formerly enslaved persons, and revolutionize the federal government by charging it with releasing the nation's prodigious productive energies.

Influenza hardly ranked as the most decisive force driving Reconstruction's eclipse or the Gilded Age's advent. The recalcitrance of Southern white conservatives, bitter factionalism within the Republican Party, unchecked government corruption at all levels, widening cleavages between capitalists, workers, and farmers—these and other factors all carried more heft. As this book aims to show, though, the Great Horse Flu's American travels offer new vantage points from which to take stock of a pivotal time in the nation's messy history by thinking across the divides that have long prevented us from seeing this era whole. Hobbling the animals who powered human societies across the continent, a staggeringly aggressive form of influenza contributed to momentous changes that altered Americans' sense of who they were, the power they had to control their world, the constraints that animals and pathogens continued to place on that power, and what their still-healing country might become.

CHAPTER 1

EVOLUTION AND EMERGENCE

A Scourge Is Born

Where did the Great Horse Flu come from, and what factors shaped its emergence? People in the early 1870s had no way to isolate or identify the pathogen responsible for the equine plague. Present-day researchers, meanwhile, lack physical remains from the outbreak, which makes it difficult to pinpoint which flu variant caused the epizootic or trace its evolution. Firsthand accounts nonetheless provide valuable insights into the Great Horse Flu's origins.

Nearly everyone agreed that the malady first appeared outside Toronto, Ontario. Renowned veterinary surgeon James Law of Cornell declared in his 1872 report on the outbreak, written for the US commissioner of agriculture, that "unlike the majority of former epidemics whose origin has been obscure," the epizootic "appears to have sprung into existence in the center of the North American continent, and in a distinct locality, which can be definitely pointed out." Through his correspondence with Toronto veterinary surgeon Andrew Smith, Law learned that the Great Horse Flu made its debut "in the townships of York, Scarboro', and Markham, about fifteen miles north" of Toronto. Smith reported that locals first noticed the telltale signs of flu in late September "'among horses running at pasture.'" The illness took several days to spread to Toronto, where equines began falling ill around October 1, 1872.[1]

The remarkably high prevalence rates that characterized the Great Horse Flu from start to finish demonstrate that victims lacked the experience their immune systems needed to recognize the variant responsible for the outbreak—and thus to deploy antibodies to resist its incursions. This characteristic immediately limits possible explanations for the epizootic's initial appearance. Horses in Ontario, like their counterparts throughout North America, were no strangers to influenza. Over the preceding centuries, that disorder had caused seasonal cases and periodic outbreaks. A Vermont paper, for instance, reported that epizootic influenza "made its appearance in America about the middle of October" in 1733, "first in the New England States," while a New York journal noted that "a disease almost exactly the same prevailed to some extent in the city of Philadelphia in 1855." Yet even though equine influenza had long been "well known among the better class of veterinary surgeons," influenza's emergence in 1872 nonetheless marked "the first time," a Colorado newspaper insisted, that the disease "has attempted to conquer a whole nation of animals."[2]

The Great Horse Flu's tremendous infectiousness suggests that the outbreak must have been caused by a novel variant. Two other facts support this conclusion. First, no other part of the world suffered a major outbreak of equine influenza in the early 1870s. And second, veterinary experts and newspaper reports concurred that the epizootic originated not in Toronto or another Lake Ontario port but a dozen miles inland, in a landlocked agricultural district where the rivers no longer accommodated small craft, let alone the larger vessels that dominated the intercontinental livestock trade. Instead of a "virgin soil epidemic," a term coined by the historian Alfred Crosby to refer to outbreaks "in which the populations at risk have had no previous contact with the diseases that strike them and are therefore immunologically almost defenseless," the Great Horse Flu was almost certainly homegrown.[3]

How and why did a novel variant of influenza come to life in Toronto's market-farming outskirts, and what factors enabled it to spread from there to the rest of the northern Americas? Reading primary sources from the 1870s alongside recent scientific research on influenza's evolutionary ecology reveals a crucial insight: While chance played a role in creating the Great

Horse Flu, the scourge's emergence and spread were hardly random. Instead, the epizootic was made possible by longer-term political, social, and environmental changes in and around the horse plague's birthplace. Together, the settler colonial conquest of Indigenous lands, the replacement of Native lifeways with farms devoted to mixed husbandry, the enduring presence of wild waterbirds and the diverse influenza A variants they harbor, and the integration of Toronto and its immediate hinterlands into continental and international markets combined to create favorable conditions for a highly contagious new strain to develop and multiply.[4]

Making a New Flu

The variant that would soon convulse an entire continent almost certainly owed its infectious prowess to an unprecedented configuration of antigens, the result of viral evolution in the place where the outbreak first came to light. To understand how and why Greater Toronto became the venue for this landmark event in influenza's long, unruly history, we need to delve more deeply into the characteristics and processes that have empowered this pathogen to infect vast numbers of hosts across an array of species. Taken together, the structure of influenza viruses, the strategies they use to infect host cells, and the immune defenses that host organisms muster to protect themselves against influenza's incursions all hold valuable clues to the epizootic's origins. By reconstructing the evolutionary underpinnings of the Great Horse Flu's emergence, we can better grasp how an outbreak that began in a commonplace corner of rural Ontario became a continent-conquering scourge.[5]

An individual flu particle—called a *virion*—resembles a lopsided orange studded with golf tees. Eight segments of single-stranded ribonucleic acid (RNA) form the core of each influenza A virion. These "twisted, rod-like" RNA strands make up the virion's genome. This genome is surrounded, in turn, by a protein layer known as the capsid and encased within an envelope of lipids—fatty hydrocarbons—scavenged from the outer membranes of infected host cells.[6]

Each virion's octet of RNA strands encodes a total of eleven proteins. The most important of these for our purposes are the two that protrude from the surface of flu virions like so many spikes: hemagglutinin (traditionally abbreviated as H), which enables flu particles to latch on to host cells during the binding process; and neuraminidase (traditionally abbreviated as N), which "facilitate[es] the release of newly produced virus particles from the host cell" after virions invade their nuclei. H spikes outnumber N spikes by a ratio of roughly 4 to 1.[7]

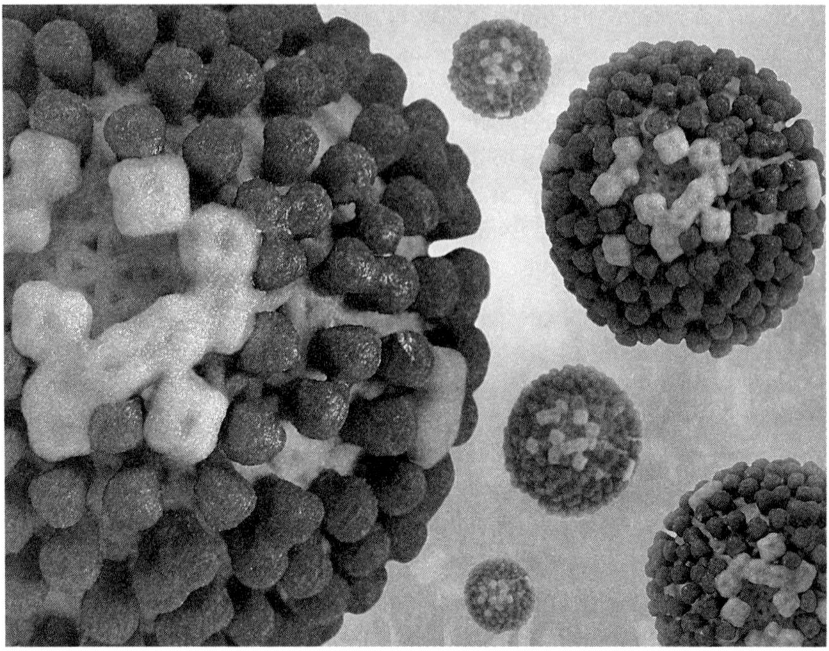

The spiky structures in this illustration of flu virions represent H and N antigens. 3-D illustration of influenza virus, courtesy of NIAID, Creative Commons Attribution 2.0 Generic License, https://commons.wikimedia.org/wiki/File:Influenza_Virus.jpg.

From the perspective of a host infected by influenza, the molecular structures that H and N form at a virion's extremities function as *antigens*—microbiological markers that trigger a suite of immune responses including the production of antibodies. Scientists have identified eighteen types of H and eleven of N in influenza A viruses. Numbered sequentially, these antigens offer a handy way for researchers to divide influenza into subtypes such as H1N1, H5N1, and H7N8.[8]

The flu virus's drastically stripped-down nature has important implications for reconstructing the Great Horse Flu's origins. Influenza virions are too small and simple to carry out even the most basic biological functions. Instead, they rely on the host cells they infect to obtain energy, reproduce, and move across space. This peculiarity has led biologists, philosophers, and others to debate whether viruses even qualify as living things.[9]

It has also led scientists to describe viral replication using a metaphor drawn from twentieth-century radical movements: hijacking. Rather than seeking to ransom hostages or sow terror, though, influenza viruses invade the cockpits of host cells—their nuclei—with an altogether different purpose. Unable to reproduce on their own, flu virions can only spawn a new generation by taking over host cells' reproductive machinery and reprogramming it to churn out large numbers of replicas and near-replicas of the hijacking virions. This next wave of virions then ventures outward from infection sites to access other cells and the external environment.[10]

Virions usually accomplish this through *budding*, a process by which replicants' N spikes enable them to exit a host cell and spread to other cells. On occasion, though, flu virions cause host cells to explode, suddenly releasing any replicants previously confined within these cells into surrounding tissues. For an infection to intensify, the H spikes on at least some next-generation virions must bind to receptor sites on the outer membranes of potential host cells, then invade their nuclei to begin the infection cycle anew.[11]

Flu virions can only invade a cell and appropriate its reproductive capacity if they avoid unleashing the immune defenses that potential hosts have developed to protect themselves against influenza's ravages. Before launching these responses, though, an organism must first recognize the pathogen involved. Creatures previously infected by influenza have little difficulty staving off any viral variants they have previously encountered, using the distinctive molecular structures that H and N form at the virion's extremities to identify invaders. When a host detects an attack by flu virions presenting a familiar antigenic structure, the organism immediately launches a full-bore immune response sufficient to prevent sustained or serious reinfection.[12]

Yet no such response is triggered when a potential host's immune system lacks previous experience with the antigenic configuration of attacking flu virions. For this reason, unfamiliar flu types can invade hosts and swiftly begin to spit out large numbers of replicants before facing significant opposition. Immunologically naive hosts—those who have no experience with a particular variant—are more likely to get sick when that variant attacks, and the symptoms they suffer are also likely to be more severe.

Influenza, like SARS-CoV-2, Ebola, and other single-stranded RNA viruses, owes much of its shape-shifting potency to its unreliability in carrying out a function that virologists often refer to as proofreading or copyediting. The stripped-down structure of flu virions makes it difficult for them to ensure that the replicants churned out by hijacked host cells are exact copies true to genomic type. Virologists refer to this type of evolutionary change as *antigenic drift*.

The subtle but incessant innovations that this process yields account for the frustrating, sometimes fatal, failure of seasonal flu vaccines to fully protect humans, horses, and other creatures. These incremental changes also help to explain why influenza A and other RNA viruses have proven so successful. As clinician and virologist Mark Denison notes, pathogens in this category "lack the ability to correct mistakes, so they generate mutant swarms of viruses that are ready for adaptation in different environments." Although the genetic differences introduced are minor, they often make it harder for hosts to identify attacking virions—and thus to stave off flu infections in their early stages.[13]

The effects of slapdash proofreading rapidly compound. This is because flu, like most microorganisms, reproduces so quickly. Each generation of virions requires just minutes or hours to replicate its genome—or, given the flu virus's lack of fidelity in proofreading, close approximations thereof. Taken together, short generation times and faulty proofreading make influenza notoriously shifty.

Although antigenic drift may have played some part in the Great Horse Flu's emergence, a second type of viral evolution—known as *reassortment*—offers a more plausible explanation for the epizootic's infectiousness. Whereas antigenic drift introduces relatively minor changes to influenza's antigens, reassortment causes more sweeping transformations. Reassortment can be likened to the output of an errant office printer. Imagine that at the exact same moment, two colleagues initiate an eight-page print job, one page for each of the RNA strands in an influenza A virus's genome. In a fit of apparent madness, the printer begins mixing and matching whole pages lifted from separate jobs to create a single discombobulated document. While antigenic drift produces the equivalent of a typo here or there, reassortment blends genomic material from two or more flu variants to generate entirely new combinations.

For a reassortment event to launch an outbreak of epidemic, pandemic, or epizootic proportions, two things must happen. First, virions from two or more distinct genomic lineages must invade a single host cell and attempt to replicate within its nucleus during the same short window of time. And second, the reassorted flu strain must succeed at replicating itself.

Nearly all novel viral mashups generated by reassortment soon vanish without a trace, either because the new strain is not viable or because it kills off its host before replicants can begin spreading to other victims. Every so often, though, a reassorted variant beats the odds and, once unbridled, extends its range to new hosts. Researchers have attributed every global flu pandemic since the mid-1900s to reassortment. Genomic material extracted from the bodies of Alaska Natives disinterred from permafrost, for instance, indicates that the H1N1 variant that drove the Great Pandemic of 1918–20 and killed more than 50 million people resulted from the combination of a human-adapted flu strain with one originating from wild bird populations.[14]

This foray into virology and immunology helps us to grasp an important insight regarding the Great Horse Flu: The variant responsible for the epizootic behaved like a novel pathogen. All signs point to reassortment as the trigger for the Great Horse Flu's emergence. That event presumably unfolded in the general vicinity of the area where the epizootic first came to light in September 1872, roughly fifteen miles north of Toronto, where Markham, Scarborough, and York Townships come together. At this remove, we cannot reconstruct the sequence of events that produced a novel flu strain there with precision or certainty. Still, by placing the outbreak's origins in a fuller historical and ecological context, we can better understand what made the area where the epizootic first erupted—a rural neighborhood I will call the Three Townships—a vibrant seedbed for influenza to evolve into new configurations.

Dedicated to mixed husbandry and crisscrossed by migratory flyways, the farms of Markham, Scarborough, and York afforded ample opportunities for close encounters between several flu-prone species: wild waterbirds, which have always comprised the main source of genomic diversity among influenza A viruses; humans and equines, two kinds of animals that had frequently suffered from simultaneous or near-simultaneous outbreaks of influenza dating back to antiquity; and domesticated creatures including poultry and hogs. For an evolutionary breakthrough to occur, two or more flu strains with distinctive antigenic arrangements had to infect the same cell within some equine patient zero. No specimens of the resulting influenza variants exist, so we will probably never be able to fully uncover how this came to pass. Yet by delving more deeply into the entangled histories of influenza, humans, horses and other animals, and the Ontario ecosystems these creatures together inhabited, we can better understand the circumstances that surrounded the Great Horse Flu's emergence.

Between the late eighteenth century and the summer of 1872, Indigenous dispossession, settler colonialism, agricultural intensification, and the eclipse of oxen by horses as prime movers throughout the Three Townships combined with the endurance of ducks, gulls, and other flu-bearing wild waterbirds to generate nearly ideal conditions for influenza A variants to circulate across species divides. Together with transportation improvements that linked this stretch of the countryside to Toronto, they also helped to speed a novel strain to new hosts throughout a fast-growing swath of North America, with disastrous consequences for horses and humans alike.

Wresting the Land

Indigenous peoples had made homes in the relatively flat, fertile lands stretching inland from Lake Ontario's northwestern shore for at least eleven thousand years and possibly much longer, but there is no evidence that influenza afflicted Native peoples in Ontario (or, for that matter, anywhere else in the Americas) before Europeans invaded. Instead, flu variants that had adapted to infect humans, horses, and other domesticated creatures first reached the area as an unintended consequence of European colonialism.[15]

Starting in the sixteenth century, imperial incursions and Indigenous initiatives combined to revolutionize politics, economy, and epidemiology throughout the Great Lakes. Archaeological evidence, colonial records, and First Nations traditions all show that disease, military conflict, and competition for beaver pelts, captives, and other commodified resources led a succession of Indigenous Nations to build villages on Lake Ontario's northwestern shore. Between the 1500s and the 1640s, members of the Wendat (also known as the Huron and Wyandot) and Petun confederacies inhabited what is now Greater Toronto, only to be displaced by Haudenosaunee (Iroquois) people after 1650. A third and final set of migrations brought Mississaugas and their Ojibwe kin into southern Ontario from the Upper Great Lakes starting in the mid-1690s.[16]

In addition to planting maize, squash, sunflowers, tobacco, and other crops, these First Nations peoples fished, hunted, and gathered a variety of plants on their sovereign territories. In his posthumously published *History of the Ojebway Indians* (1861), the Mississauga Methodist Kahkewaquonaby ("Sacred Feather," also known as the Reverend Peter Jones) described how "each tribe or body" of his people "has its own range of country." Mississaugas and other Ojibwes actively traded with Indigenous neighbors and Euro-Americans. Some of this commerce coursed along an ancient route known as the Toronto Carrying-Place. Connecting Lakes Ontario and Simcoe via the Holland and Humber Rivers, the Carrying-Place cut off more than a hundred miles of difficult, dangerous travel between the Upper Great Lakes and the St. Lawrence Valley. Early French maps identified the Carrying-Place's northern terminus as "Taranto." For reasons that remain unclear, that place-name soon drifted southward.[17]

In 1750, French imperial officials codified this curious migration by naming a new trading post at the Humber's mouth Fort Toronto. After the Seven Years' War impelled France to abandon the outpost, British forces rebuilt it and renewed its role as a vibrant center for commercial and cultural exchange between Mississaugas, other First Nations peoples, and Montreal- and Albany-based traders.[18]

When a baker's dozen of British colonies joined in rebellion, they initiated a chain of events that radically redirected the course of human and environmental history throughout North America and well beyond. The American Revolution triggered a wrenching six-year-long civil war that pitted self-declared Patriots against the roughly one-third of American colonists who remained loyal to the British Empire.[19]

After the rebels' ragtag alliance prevailed with crucial assistance from France, Spain, and several Indigenous allies, colonists who had cast their lot with Britain faced hard choices. Most Loyalists swallowed their pride, stayed in the United States, and tried to make their peace with the newly established American republic. Nearly one hundred thousand colonists, though, saw no viable future for themselves in the United States. As several Loyalist officers complained, "The personal animosities that arose from civil dissensions have been so heightened by the Blood that has been shed in the contest, that the Parties can never be reconciled." About half of these Loyalists sought refuge north of the uncertain boundary established by 1783's Treaty of Paris. They were joined by around two thousand Indigenous allies (mostly Haudenosaunees under Thayendanegea, also known as Joseph Brant) and perhaps four thousand African Americans (chiefly, formerly enslaved people who had escaped from Patriot enslavers, but also freeborn Black people intent on staying within the British Empire, as well as hundreds of men, women, and children who remained chattel to Loyalist enslavers). In the 1780s, American, Indigenous, and African American Loyalists intent on placing British North America on a sounder, safer footing began to set their sights on present-day Ontario.[20]

For settler colonialism—a form of colonialism, historian Nancy Shoemaker explains, in which "large numbers of settlers claim land" from Native populations, "become the majority," and "attempt to engineer the disappearance of the original inhabitants anywhere except in nostalgia"—to take root along the old Toronto Carrying-Place, though, British officials first had to wrest these lands away from First Nations. Crown negotiators plotted to finagle a series of land cessions from Mississaugas and some of their Ojibwe neighbors. British officials presumed that 1787's Toronto Purchase and 1788's Gunshot Purchase extinguished Indigenous title to the Carrying-Place corridor between Lakes Simcoe and Ontario, including nearly all of the area that government functionaries soon organized into Markham, Scarborough, and York Townships.

In 1797, though, Peter Russell, president of Upper Canada's Executive Council, confessed that because of the failure of British officials to follow basic record-making and -keeping protocols, both cessions were "totally invalid." Russell described his government as "exceedingly alarmed" at the mess that Sir John Johnson and other British negotiators had left for them. Indeed, he fretted that the rottenness of British claims to the Toronto area threatened to "shake the Tranquility of many respectable Persons, who have risked nearly their whole Property within its Limits." Rather than redressing the fundamental flaws that plagued these land grabs, though, Russell and other leaders continued to encourage Loyalists and other settlers to make the ancestral Mississauga and Ojibwe territories of the Carrying-Place a key beachhead for British colonialism.[21]

Thrusting Avenues of Aggression

Loyalist settlement in present-day Ontario had started slowly. By the early 1790s, though, government officials redoubled their efforts to reconstruct Britain's North American empire. To spearhead this important new departure, Prime Minister William Pitt the Younger's cabinet tapped Col. John Graves Simcoe, an Eton- and Oxford-educated veteran of the American Revolution who had fought determinedly from 1775's Battle of Concord through Cornwallis's 1781 humiliation at Yorktown. Although Simcoe remained in Canada for less than five years, he nonetheless played an outsized role in setting the stage for the Great Horse Flu's emergence. Together, he and his wife Elizabeth, a dauntless equestrian and skilled artist, documented the Toronto area's landscape and fauna and renamed the lands that the Crown had recently and illegitimately wrested away from Indigenous peoples. Simcoe also established the town of York near Fort Toronto's ruins and encouraged agricultural settlement in the town's hinterlands while planning a road designed to bind York and its countryside into an interconnected, self-sustaining region.[22]

Even before Simcoe reached Upper Canada, he had decided that British troops could never safely defend the province's two largest settlements, Niagara and Kingston, against American invaders because of these towns' exposed positions and lack of high ground. Simcoe and his subordinates thus began scouting sites for a new capital to replace Niagara as the province's main military base and governmental seat. After poring over maps of Upper Canada and interviewing Britons and Canadians with experience in the province, Simcoe identified Toronto as "the natural arsenal of Lake Ontario," adding that its Carrying-Place location "afford[ed] an easy access over land to Lake Huron."[23]

In late July 1793, Simcoe assumed personal responsibility for the construction of this new military outpost. Surveyors and troops were already hard at work by the time the Simcoes sailed to Toronto from Niagara. In the years that followed, Elizabeth and John explored the area by horseback, rowboat, and canoe. With pen and watercolor paints, Elizabeth documented their forays through thick forests of pine and hardwoods, broken occasionally by "some good natural meadows and several ponds." She found the area's bountiful bird populations particularly enthralling. She recounted, for instance, how she and John had "rowed some distance among low lands covered with rushes, abounding in wild ducks." A few months later, Elizabeth feasted on some of the same birds, shot at Lake Simcoe (which John had named to commemorate his father), and proclaimed them "so much better than any in England from their feeding on wild Rice."[24]

Unbeknownst to the Simcoes or their contemporaries, many of the Carrying-Place's wild birds harbored flu. Scientists now understand that geese, dabbling ducks, gulls, and several other migratory waterfowl species provide the primary natural reservoir for influenza A viruses. Upper Canada's prolific bird life greatly increased the odds that novel flu strains would evolve there—provided, of course, that wild waterbirds could survive the onslaught of settlers Simcoe and the British government were intent on drawing to southern Ontario.[25]

To realize his vision for a newer Britain along Lake Ontario's northwestern shore, John established several townships. In August 1793, he affixed the name Scarborough, which the Simcoes had initially planned to reserve for the estate Elizabeth wanted to build on the bluffs above the lake, to an entire cliff-topped stretch of shoreline. Three weeks later, he renamed the new town he was planning at Toronto in honor of the Duke of York. As for the township immediately north of Scarborough and York, the Simcoes named it after William Markham, archbishop of York, England.[26]

To attract settlers to these townships, John devised a three-pronged plan that united generous but rational land policies with town development and road construction. In the 1780s, the Crown had started distributing free parcels of Upper Canadian land to Loyalists as well as British and German veterans of the American Revolution, mostly in tracts known as "concessions" that typically spanned at least two hundred acres. Simcoe began extending British largesse to another group, too: "late Loyalists," colonists who fled the United States in the years following the 1783 Treaty of Paris. Upper Canada's future, Simcoe believed, depended on enticing migrants into settling there. From his wartime experiences, Simcoe understood that frontiersfolk from the former colonies possessed decided advantages as pioneers over former soldiers or other emigrant populations. Simcoe also recognized that many Americans—pushed by postindependence political quarrels and economic uncertainties as well as the high prices charged for western lands by the debt-ridden, cash-strapped US government—wanted to return to the British fold. Simcoe thus set rock-bottom prices for Upper Canadian lands (applicants paid only a filing fee of six pence an acre), then sweetened the deal by promising to provide settlers with tools, agricultural implements, and diplomatic and military safeguards against Indigenous foes and US forces. Simcoe understood that prospective American emigrants expected the rule of law and a modicum of self-government, but he also rightly suspected that former Yankees would want local and provincial governments to run on shoestring budgets.[27]

This recipe of "cheap land and low taxes," as the historian Alan Taylor notes, combined with the Crown's mostly cordial relations with Indigenous peoples to make Upper Canada a compelling draw. The province's white population exploded from fourteen thousand in 1791 to more than seventy-seven thousand in 1811; American-born settlers accounted for four-fifths of the influx. An Irish Moravian visitor accurately characterized these newcomers, who hailed largely from the mid-Atlantic states, as "mostly poorly people, who are chiefly concerned to manage, in the best manner, the farms which have been given them by the government."[28]

Simcoe embraced town-building as an essential complement to agricultural colonization. Farmers needed markets for their wheat and other crops, townsfolk required provisions, and British subjects throughout Upper Canada demanded protection from Americans, First Nations, and other potential enemies. Simcoe initially planned York to fulfill commercial and military purposes. He also intended another new settlement—London, in the Upper Canadian interior, safely distant from the American border—to serve as provincial capital. But Lord Dorchester, British North America's chief military officer, scuttled this proposal. Dorchester's obstinacy forced Simcoe to swallow his pride and throw his energies into making York a suitable seat for Upper Canada's government. Ironically, Dorchester's power play probably secured York's future, since the settlement's survival depended almost entirely on government expenditures well into the 1830s.[29]

The third and final component of Simcoe's plans—roads—would connect town and country. In addition to knitting together York and its hinterlands, surface transportation routes would integrate this embryonic British North American heartland into regional, continental, and global exchange networks. Simcoe ordered surveyors and soldiers to lay out roads leading north, east, and west from York, but for the purposes of this study, the most important of these routes was Yonge Street. Named for Sir George Yonge, Britain's secretary of war and a keen student of Roman roads, this route ran, as Simcoe described it, "due north, cut perfectly through the bush," from the provincial capital, through York Township, then along Markham's western border to the Holland River and Lake Simcoe.[30]

Simcoe intended Yonge Street to ease travel through the ancient Carrying-Place corridor, but numerous problems slowed its completion. In late September 1793, the lieutenant governor set out to blaze a route with the help of four Indigenous guides. On their return, though, "the Indians lost their way." Simcoe, his guides, and his men "were in danger of starving" until they "came on a Surveyor's line," which they followed to Lake Ontario and safety. Soon thereafter, Simcoe ordered the Welsh surveyor August Jones to lay out a "Military Street or Road," but Jones ran afoul of several Ojibwes who were understandably resistant to British roads, which one historian aptly describes as "thrusting avenues of aggression."[31]

Labor, which was scarce and costly on the Upper Canadian frontier, proved an even tougher nut for Simcoe to crack. Before establishing York, Simcoe had reconstituted the Queen's Rangers, asking his superiors to authorize their employment in advancing "the civil purposes of the Colony, in the construction of the various public works, of Buildings, Roads, Bridges, & communications by Land & on the Waters." In October 1794, though, border skirmishing between US forces under "Mad Anthony" Wayne and Britain's Indigenous allies diverted the Rangers from civil improvements. More than a year later, only the first four miles of a route that Elizabeth described as "33 Miles & 56 Chains" in length had been cleared.[32]

Simcoe realized that to finish Yonge Street, he had to find another workforce. With winter approaching in 1794, he arranged for a colony of German-speaking American émigrés to clear a route for wagon traffic from Toronto up through York Township and partway into Markham. Alas, construction languished because of short provisions and sickness among the colonists, who seemed more intent on carving homesteads from the area's unbroken forests than building roads through these dense woods. Yonge Street remained at a standstill until US-Canadian tensions began to ease in the wake of Jay's Treaty, which was signed in November 1794. With the Queen's Rangers no longer needed to keep watch over the international frontier, Simcoe redeployed the regiment to Yonge Street. At long last, he sent a boastful letter in early 1796 informing his superiors that "the Road from York to the Head Waters of Lake Huron has been opened by the Soldiers, & by these means, a very excellent Tract of Country is rendered accessible to future settlers & a ready communication afforded" to the Upper Great Lakes above. When Elizabeth took her maiden ride on the newly completed road later that winter, though, she decried it as "very bad," with "pools of water among roots of trees, & fallen logs in swampy spots." Many of these puddles, moreover, were "half frozen," making "them still more disagreeable when the horses plunge into them." For years to come, Yonge Street fell short of locals' and visitors' expectations even as it became the primary land route between York and the Three Townships.[33]

When the Simcoes returned to England later in 1796, their baggage included a Canadian sleigh and Ojibwe curiosities including "a canoe and paddles, bows and arrows, and Indian clothing." Simcoe fell ill and died in 1806 at the age of fifty-four. By the time Elizabeth followed her husband into the great hereafter in 1850 at the age of eighty-seven, Toronto, its Indigenous name restored in 1834, had grown into one of Canada's most important settlements. Meanwhile, beyond the town limits, the Three Townships were growing into a prosperous and increasingly progressive agricultural hinterland.[34]

Pioneers

In the three-quarters of a century that separated the Simcoes' Upper Canadian errand from the Great Horse Flu's emergence, settler colonialism remade southern Ontario's ecology in two overlapping stages. In the first, a pioneering phase that stretched from the 1790s through the 1830s, Three Townships settlers felled forests, targeted native fauna for consumption and destruction, built farms on which they cultivated a variety of plants and animals, and unwittingly introduced myriad flu varieties to Toronto and its hinterlands. During the second, a progressive phase that began in the 1820s and neared maturity by midcentury, farmers in Markham, Scarborough, and York intensified their operations and doubled down on their predecessors' commitment to mixed husbandry, particularly by importing so-called improved breeds of livestock and poultry that undoubtedly introduced additional flu strains to Greater Toronto from other parts of the Americas as well as Europe and Asia.

Pioneering hinged on multispecies collaborations. Just weeks after Simcoe first visited the Carrying-Place in the spring of 1793, the *Upper Canada Gazette* advertised the lease of "a farm on Yonge Street with team, cows, hogs, geese, poultry, farming utensils, five acres put in wheat, timothy and red clover, four acres of timothy and red clover, one year old, and one acre wheat stubble and potatoes." This notice tells us several important things about the initial stages of agricultural settlement in the Three Townships. First, settlers emigrated to Upper Canada with horses and a variety of other flu-prone creatures. Americans venturing into the Carrying-Place by land or lake sometimes brought stock and poultry with them from New York, Vermont, and other states, while others sent for animals from Quebec, other Canadian provinces, and the northern US after reaching Upper Canada. The *Gazette* advertisement also captures a second, subtler point: Pioneer farmers tended to view these animal companions as species or kinds ("cows," "hogs") rather than distinct breeds (Herefords, Berkshires). Last but hardly least, this lessor, like most area settlers, focused less on cash crops and more on establishing a broad-based agricultural ecosystem populated by a variety of plants and animals. Upper Canadian frontiersfolk, like their progressive successors, preferred multiculture to monoculture.[35]

Although just a handful of emigrants preceded the Simcoes into the York area, hundreds more pressed into the Carrying-Place before the couple returned to England. Riding through Markham Township, for instance, Elizabeth noted "some comfortable Log Houses inhabited by Germans & some by Pennsylvanians." Like the ten acres of cultivated land mentioned in the *Upper Canada Gazette* advertisement, these wooden buildings reflected the central role of forest clearing in agricultural settlement.[36]

Invading European Americans cut into Upper Canada's woodlands with such ferocity that one agricultural historian famously tarred the province's settlers as "land-butchers." Irish travel writer Anna Brownell Jameson presaged this view in the 1830s. "A Canadian settler," she griped, "*hates* a tree, regards it as his natural enemy, as something to be destroyed, eradicated, annihilated by all and many means." It goes without saying that the Three Townships' settlers hardly saw themselves as "land-butchers." Instead, they believed that necessity impelled them to fashion wild, Indigenous ecosystems into flourishing farms. Most pioneers aimed to prepare four or five acres for crops during their first year. Although the pace of clearing usually accelerated thereafter, it nonetheless took many years to cut down all the timber on each two-hundred-acre concession. As colonization picked up, though, the Carrying-Place's woodlands succumbed at a quickening rate.[37]

American emigration into the Three Townships slowed to a trickle by 1800, but Britons and, to a lesser extent, Germans, soon filled the void. As political and economic crises buffeted Great Britain and Ireland in the late 1820s and early 1830s, migration to Toronto and its hinterlands swelled. Ontario's population, which exceeded 150,000 in 1824, exploded to more than 432,000 by 1840. A growing proportion of newcomers arrived with little or no farming experience. Unlike the pioneers who preceded them, latter-day migrants rarely brought livestock or poultry, although some purchased farm animals after arriving on the Atlantic shore, then transported them to the Toronto area.[38]

These human and animal newcomers unwittingly introduced potent pathogens to the Carrying-Place. The first cholera epidemic to reach North America illustrated the epidemiological consequences of early nineteenth-century immigration. A Torontonian recorded the dreaded malady's arrival on June 19, 1832, a week before it struck New York. The first three cases in Toronto all involved recent steamship arrivals, and within three months, the outbreak had infected roughly 1,600 of the city's 6,000 residents, killing "about four hundred." The victims, "principally adults & more men than women," were reportedly "nearly all strangers who have

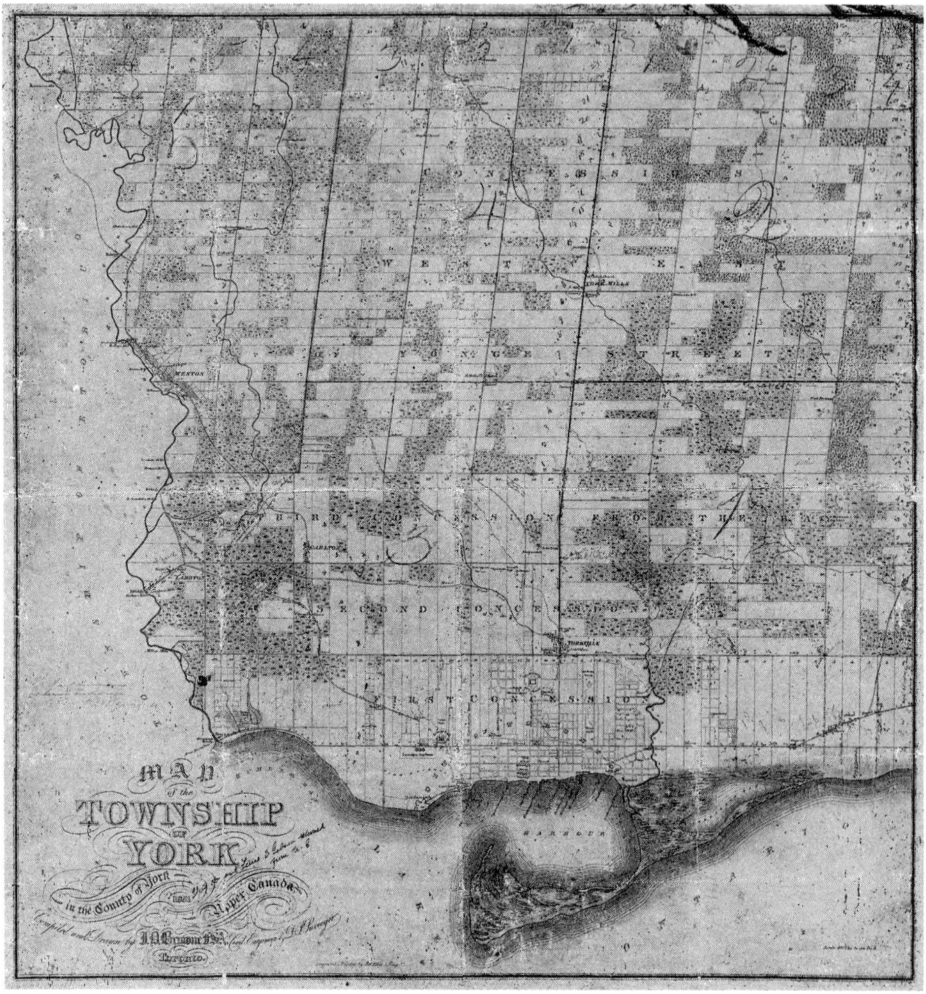

This map shows a portion of the Three Townships in 1851. Note the rectangular concessions into which the Ontario countryside was divided. Yonge Street leads from Toronto, which adjoins the sheltered harbor at the bottom center, northward through Yorkville and York Mills. Note, too, the remnant woodlands, shown as dark patches, that still cover scattered portions of the region. J. O. Browne, *Map of the Township of York in the County of York, Upper Canada* (Toronto: John Ellis, 1851). Courtesy of the City of Toronto Archives, series 443, file 40, Winearls, MUC no. 2215.

recently emigrated." The Society for the Relief of the Orphan, Widow and Fatherless later praised "the people of Markham" and a township to its north for "having given active and efficient assistance in . . . providing for many of the children" orphaned by cholera. Newly introduced plant diseases also ravaged settlers' crops; one historian noted that "the role of wheat had to be re-assessed" in the early 1800s "because infections and insect pests spread with settlement." Influenza, meanwhile, repeatedly beset southern Ontario. Months before cholera reached Toronto in 1832, an outbreak originating in China struck Upper Canada, reportedly afflicting "all organized beings," not just humans.[39]

In addition to battling forests and pathogens, settlers also took aim at southern Ontario's native fauna. Perceiving predators as existential threats, incoming Americans and Europeans set about eradicating wolves, bears, and other large carnivores. Local folklore cast colonization as a mortal struggle to expunge wild carnivores, as illustrated by a tale involving the Thomsons, a Scots family who ranked among Scarborough's earliest settlers. Worried by a nasty case of "ague" that his wife Mary had contracted in Toronto, David Thomson decided to move his clan from that malaria-prone town to a concession two and a half miles inland. "One day," according to a local history, "Mrs. Thomson heard a commotion among the domestic animals in the enclosure." She "ran out, and seeing a bear about the carry off a pig, she struck him with an axe and made him drop his prize." The wounded bear "made off to the woods, and one of the men followed, but failed to kill him." This ursine marauder was lucky to escape with its life. More commonly, agricultural colonists in the Carrying-Place exacted steep and mounting tolls on the Three Townships' apex predators. The unveiling of provincial bounties in 1793—"ten dollars for a bear's scalp and twenty dollars for that of a wolf"—drove several species to the brink of extirpation, as the capture of Scarborough's "last lynx" in 1801 or 1802 attests. Nor were predators the only beasts whose numbers dwindled alongside settler incursions. Pelts stripped from beavers, muskrats, and other furry creatures afforded pioneers a ready source of income, as did venison from white-tailed deer and kindred kinds. By 1856, provincial lawmakers attempted to check the rapid decline of ungulates and furbearers by instituting closed hunting seasons and other conservation regulations.[40]

Settlement even caused the prolific fish populations that had long sustained the area's Indigenous peoples to collapse. Salmon had once run so thickly up the Humber and Don that, as one historian asserts, "they could be speared by anyone with so much as a pitchfork." Settlers pulled in vast quantities of these toothsome, nutritious fish for their own consumption; they also marketed surplus salmon in Toronto and even shipped it salted or iced to New York City after the Erie Canal's 1825 completion. Dams and mills proved even more destructive than rods, nets, and traps. Sawdust and other mill waste choked the gravel beds where salmon had previously spawned while disrupting the life cycles of many of the invertebrates salmon ate. Dams, meanwhile, blocked fish from reaching spawning grounds and created impoundments filled with warmer, dirtier water than the free-flowing streams in which Atlantic salmon had evolved. Provincial laws intended to protect Upper Canada's fisheries—concisely dismissed by one historian as "half-measures that were generally ignored"—failed to reverse the combined effects of sawmilling, dam construction, overharvesting, and habitat loss. By the mid-1800s, the aquatic bounty that had sustained First Nations peoples since time immemorial had become a relic of the past—a nostalgic fixture of local lore alongside improbable tales of pillaging bears and axe-wielding frontierswomen.[41]

Settlers saw the elimination of indigenous species as a necessary precondition for transplanting plants, animals, and humans to the Carrying-Place from other parts of North America as well as the wider world. Yet from the pioneers' perspective, this process of faunal replacement unfolded with agonizing slowness. Ten years after the Simcoes named Scarborough, just over one hundred colonists had joined the Thomsons in a township that covered more than fifty thousand acres. As of 1803, these newcomers' farms sheltered a meager menagerie of five horses, eight oxen, fifteen hogs, and thirty-four head of cattle. Throughout Upper Canada's early decades, historian William Caniff later recalled, "beasts of burden were scarce." Shortages of oxen and horses meant that pioneers rarely used wagons or other conveyances. "There was but one here and there," Caniff claimed of early settlers, "who had occasion to make a vehicle of any kind, except what could be hauled by hand." During the early years of colonization, human muscle—especially family labor—continued to provide most of the motive power settlers required.[42]

As new emigrants poured into the countryside and pioneering families grew, though, Caniff recounted that "stock began to accumulate, and the future brightened up before them." By 1845, Scarborough's human population had increased to 3,816. The township's enclosures, fields, and stables witnessed even headier growth; that same year, Scarborough boasted 1,835 sheep, 1,958 hogs, 2,013 horses, and 3,615 cattle. By the 1840s, Markham, York, and adjoining townships teemed with similarly expansive livestock populations.[43]

The hard days of pioneering, in short, were passing away. Together, settlers and a multitude of other invading organisms had changed the land—and, with it, the Three Townships' disease ecology.

All Settled

Progressive farming, the second phase of settler colonialism in Toronto's hinterlands, built on pioneering foundations. Three Townships farmers remained devoted to mixed husbandry, but starting in the 1830s, they also became increasingly caught up in a broader transatlantic enthusiasm for so-called improved or pure breeds of livestock and poultry. With the area's farms coming of age, and the woebegone provincial capital growing into a vibrant, forward-looking city, horses became increasingly integral to settler colonial lifeways. As prime drivers of exchange and circulation, horses encountered an array of flu strains adapted to infect other farm animals, humans, and the wild waterfowl species that progressive settlers began protecting through provincial conservation laws.[44]

William Brown's *America: A Four Years' Residence in the United States and Canada* (1849) offered an especially insightful portrait of midcentury agricultural developments outside Toronto. "The names of the townships," gushed Brown, a former clothier from Leeds, England, "sounded very welcome to a Yorkshireman's ears." The area's "great resemblance" to Brown's home shire extended from the names the Simcoes had bestowed on Mississauga and Ojibwe lands to the farming methods the area's settlers embraced. Brown praised the "good ploughing and general management" he observed as equal to that practiced "in the best parts of England." He was especially impressed by the property of a Mr. Gates, one of Scarborough's many British emigrants. While pioneer settlers had generally permitted cattle and hogs to range freely, Gates and a growing proportion of his neighbors pursued more intensive farming techniques. To constrain livestock and poultry, Three Townships cultivators erected fences, stables, barns, and other wooden structures. Such enclosures enabled settlers to better protect their growing and increasingly valuable herds and flocks against bad weather, theft, and remnant predator populations. They also made it easier to collect these animals' manure, which settlers then worked back into the soil to restore nutrients stripped away by wheat, potatoes, and other heavy feeding crops. Gates's farm, like those of other area growers, was an inextricably modern operation guided by the scientific methods that agricultural reformers in Europe and North America had long touted.[45]

In addition to enriching the soil with composted dung, potash, and other amendments, progressive farmers began investing some of their growing profits in improved livestock and newfangled agricultural implements. Brown credited British emigrants with introducing creaturely kinds from their home counties. "The bulk of the farmers" in Scarborough and nearby townships, he explained, came "from Yorkshire, Lincolnshire, and

Cumberland. They carry out with them the knowledge they have acquired in their native counties, and with them are to be found the choicest breed of oxen, sheep, and horses."[46]

Around 1840, Three Townships settlers began "devot[ing] themselves" to the importation of "thoroughbreds," which was then a general term applicable to all types of livestock. Archibald Ward, proprietor of the Wellington Hotel Stables, helped to bring this trend to Markham. In 1841, Ward purchased a Clydesdale named Grey Clyde on Glasgow's coal docks, then shipped him to Ontario. Not long after Ward sold this strapping stallion to a fellow settler, Ward's wife "imported another famous Clydesdale, Merry Farmer." Soon after, progressive farmers in Scarborough and York began introducing these hardy Scottish draft horses. Rising populations of renowned British breeds—not just Clydesdales but also Shire horses; Ayrshire, Galloway, Durham, Devonshire, and Hereford cattle; Leicester and Cotswold sheep; and Berkshire and Suffolk hogs—led William Brown to declare that "everything you see and hear" in the Three Townships "reminds you strongly of your English home." Like human travelers and migrants, imported animals sometimes bore invisible burdens of influenza and other pathogens.[47]

Progressive farmers embraced improved stock breeds, but some dabbled in poultry, too. Just months before the Great Horse Flu erupted, the *Canadian Poultry Chronicle* bemoaned the tendency of most Ontario farmers to "look upon fowls as worthless in a commercial or pecuniary point of view; they are tolerated upon the farm to act as scavengers only and allowed to live as best they can, rather than being kept with an idea that profit may be realized by them." Yet as the *Chronicle*'s very existence made clear, Ontarians' enthusiasm for chickens was on the rise. Three Townships farmers, like their counterparts throughout the province, turned first to British, then to continental and Far Eastern varieties. An 1871 article in the *Canadian Poultry Chronicle* celebrated this shift by equating it with settler colonialism itself: "As the red man of the forest had to recede before the pale faces, so have the Dorking, Black Spanish and Polish fowls" seemed destined "to make way" for chickens "of the larger or Asiatic breeds, and among these the Buff and Partridge Cochins and Dark Brahma varieties were most in demand."[48]

Though their names connoted Indian or Indochinese origins, Brahmas and Cochins in fact descended from chickens exported from Shanghai and nearby treaty ports as a sidelight in the highly lucrative China trade. The forebears of these breeds initially reached Europe and North America in the first decade after 1842, when Britain's ambassador to the Celestial Empire gave three Chinese chickens to Queen Victoria and Prince Albert, the British Empire's two most famous poultry lovers. These royal birds' "monstrous proportions . . . astonished the people of England vastly," the Massachusetts breeder George Burnham exclaimed in *The China Fowl* (1874). The "pictures and accounts of these giant chickens" published in several popular magazines made these birds "a huge novelty." In the late 1840s and 1850s, Burnham and other American poultry enthusiasts began interbreeding chickens obtained from Shanghai and other southern Chinese ports with other breeds to produce Cochins and Brahmas; these hybrids, which Burnham extolled as "unequalled" in both "quietness" and "laying," soon found eager markets in the United States and Canada. Such birds, Burnham added, were also "hardy, easy to raise, and less liable to be affected by disease than those of many other breeds." By importing chickens whose ancestry stretched back to southern China, Three Townships farmers unwittingly fostered still greater diversity among the area's flu varieties. Viewed in this context, the title of Burnham's wry account of the furor China fowl had incited—*The History of the Hen Fever, a Humorous Record* (1855)—seems more than a little ironic.[49]

Taken together, Canada's 1871 census and an 1881 report by the Ontario Agricultural Commission offered telling portraits of agricultural colonization in the Three Townships around the time of the Great Horse Flu's emergence. The commission's local informants described this stretch of countryside as having been "all settled" by the close of the 1830s. With the exception of parcels that remained too wet or hilly to cultivate and small woodlots from which settlers drew fuelwood and building materials, the Three Townships' thick forests had succumbed to settlers' axes. Progressive farmers, like the pioneers who preceded them, remained dedicated to mixed agriculture. They raised a variety of crops and livestock for their own consumption as well as for exchange in local and Toronto markets and export to other parts of Canada, the United States, and Britain. In a column describing each township's "chief products," representatives from Markham, Scarborough, and York respectively listed "grain growing and stock raising," "hay, grain, dairy and stock," and "grain and hay." York's southern reaches also produced "large quantities of vegetables . . . for Toronto markets." No less important, these reports documented the prevalence of Clydesdale and other "heavy draught" horses, Durham and Ayrshire cattle, Cotswold sheep, Berkshire and Suffolk pigs, and "all kinds" of poultry. Unsurprisingly for an area populated by more than thirty thousand head of livestock, Markham, Scarborough, and York were all well fenced.[50]

The focus of Three Townships farmers on livestock, dairy, and hay reflected the area's growing importance in supplying Toronto with food and feed. The commission's report described the "market facilities" of Markham as "very fair," and those of both Scarborough and York as "good." Railway lines and roads bound the Three Townships to the province's most populous city and richest market; together with ports at Toronto and Scarborough, these routes also connected the Carrying-Place to trade networks that rippled outward to Montreal, Chicago, New York, London, and beyond. The high quality of the area's dwellings—settlers overwhelmingly lived in homes of brick, stone, or "first-class frame" construction—indicates that most Three Townships farmers had leveraged their proximity to fast-growing Toronto into at least a modicum of prosperity by the 1870s.[51]

The novel pathogen that emerged in the Three Townships in September 1872 preyed on animals who had established themselves over the previous decades as prime movers throughout southern Ontario's towns and rural neighborhoods. Nearly eight thousand horses populated the Three Townships by 1880. Mississaugas, Ojibwes, and Euro-American traders in the Carrying-Place all started drawing on equine labor in the early 1700s. Pioneer settlers also brought horses into the area, though they continued for several decades to rely on oxen. Slow but strong, these bovines excelled at the hard labor of clearing forests, grubbing stumps, and plowing unbroken soil. Yet starting in the early 1800s, oxen, as one local historian explained, "became despised as aids on the farm," and "horses came into general use."[52]

In place of crude hand tools and ox-drawn plows, midcentury farmers hitched their growing fleets of horses to an ever-expanding assortment of contraptions. "The demand grew for implements and machinery," the same local historian recounted, "as the clearings increased in size and the stumps disappeared." Scarborough's "day of machinery dawned" in 1851, when local farmer Martin Snider imported a Hussey reaper from Albany, New York. Three years later, other Scarborough settlers brought in self-rakers from Rochester, celebrating "the occasion of their introduction" by parading "a procession of seventeen wagons," each of them drawn by a horse and "carrying a reaper," down King Street from Toronto to Scarborough. Blacksmiths, mechanics, and manufacturers in Toronto, Markham, and the countryside beyond all "vie[d] with each other" to imitate and improve on American and British designs. By the early 1870s, Carrying-Place settlers had redesigned plows, reapers, and other horse-powered implements to suit local conditions. "Improved farm machinery," like improved livestock breeds, became nearly universal.[53]

Progressive farmers restricted other domesticated creatures to pastures, barns, and smaller outbuildings, but horses led more expansive lives. The work of pulling plows, reapers, binders, wagons, carts, sleighs, and a range of other machines and vehicles brought them into close contact with nearly the full spectrum of southern Ontario's flu-prone creatures, humans most of all. Farming families and their horses forged what one scholar calls "a negotiated relationship." Settlers "anticipated the horses' needs" in planning out

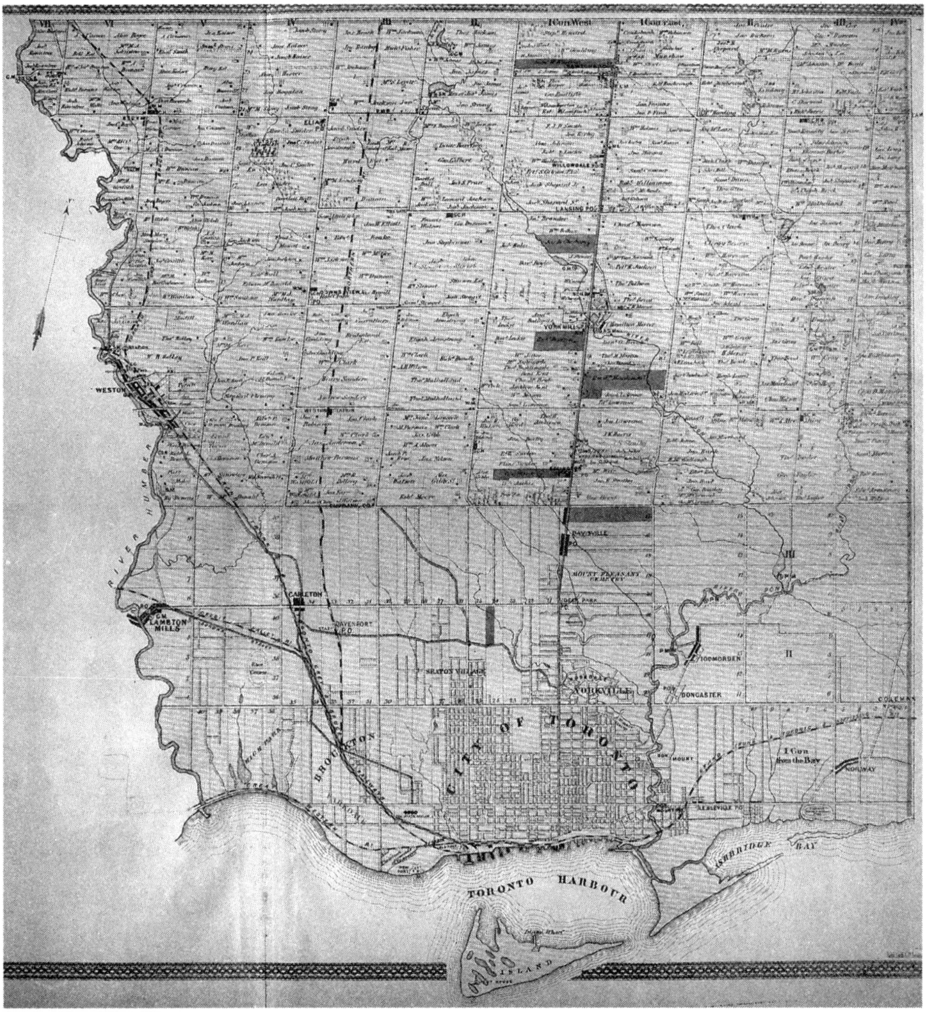

By the 1870s, the Three Townships had filled up. Note the roads and railroads that run throughout this map, as well as evidence of Toronto's expanding reach inland. "South West Part of York," in *Illustrated Historical Atlas of the County of York and the Township of West Gwillimbury & Town of Bradford in the County of Simcoe, Ont.* (Toronto: Miles & Co., 1878). Courtesy of Toronto Public Library.

the day's work, taking into consideration the creatures' "endurance given weather conditions" as well as their "need for periodic rest and nourishment." Rising "before sunrise to feed and groom" their horses, ready their tack, and "harness up," agriculturists typically "set off for the fields at first light." When the day ended and darkness descended, farmers drove their horses back from the fields and "stabled, watered, rubbed down, and fed" them. Close daily collaboration fostered intimacy between humans and horses. It also gave flu virions ample opportunity to circulate between the two species.[54]

Although railroad lines reached parts of the Three Townships in the 1850s, horses continued to dominate short-distance haulage in the area for decades to come. The work equines performed on behalf of their humans took them to virtually every part of their home farms. From time to time, they also ventured into the neighboring countryside atop a grid of local roads, as well as to Toronto and the world beyond via Yonge Street and other major thoroughfares. No other nonhuman creature covered so much ground, worked so closely with humans, or came into such frequent proximity to other creaturely kinds. As horses made the settlers' world go 'round, their movements generated unparalleled opportunities for two or more distinct flu strains to infect a single cell of the same host at the same instant—a precondition for viral reassortment.

Agricultural modernization expanded the Three Townships' viral mix between the 1840s and the early 1870s, yet the bodies of migratory wild waterbirds continued to provide far and away the biggest reservoirs of genomically diverse flu variants. Many of the flu strains that infected the region's ducks, geese, gulls, and other winged creatures likely possessed antigenic arrangements unlike any previously encountered by Ontario settlers or the animals they kept on their farms. The persistence of native waterfowl in Toronto and the Three Townships represented one of the clearest ecological throughlines between the eighteenth-century apogee of Mississauga power, the Simcoes' Carrying-Place endeavors of the 1790s, and the Great Horse Flu's emergence. Although overhunting, habitat loss, and other factors caused rapid declines in many bird populations during the early 1800s, sportsmen responded by successfully lobbying Ontario's legislature to enact closed seasons on "a number of game bird species" in 1839.[55]

Four years later, a resident of Bradford, Ontario, roughly a dozen miles north of the Three Townships and just southeast of Lake Simcoe, regaled *Globe* readers with the heartening success of local settlers' efforts "to aid the preservation of game." In addition to complying with game statutes, people in and around Bradford also refrained from collecting or selling ducks' eggs. "The supply of game," reported the *Toronto Globe* in 1871, had subsequently rebounded to levels "equal to any within the memory of the oldest inhabitant."[56]

Although the *Globe* may have overstated conservation's successes, the area's flyways and wetlands nonetheless continued to host prodigious populations of wild waterbirds—and thus also a teeming array of flu strains. In addition to splattering the Carrying-Place's lands and waters with a steady stream of flu-bearing excrement, free-ranging avifauna also came into more direct contact with the area's growing populations of livestock and poultry. Everyday occurrences—a raft of mallards landing to frolic among the snow-white ducks that pioneer settlers had introduced to Ontario, a farm dog stalking and killing a ring-billed gull, a gaggle of Canada geese grazing on pastures alongside Hereford cattle, Berkshire hogs, and Clydesdale horses—opened up new vectors for highly pathogenic flu strains to spread from wild waterbird populations to other creatures—and hence for a novel variant of the virus to evolve through reassortment.

No one observed the great leap forward in influenza's evolution that gave rise to the Great Horse Flu. With the benefit of hindsight, though, we can discern how the settler colonial transformation of the countryside north of Toronto laid the groundwork for a novel viral variant to emerge. Starting in the late 1700s, Loyalists and British imperial officials dispossessed Indigenous peoples and laid plans for agricultural colonization, town-building, and road construction. Pioneer farmers subsequently dismantled forest ecosystems and replaced them with mixed farms populated by horses, other livestock, and poultry. Various flu strains hitchhiked into the Carrying-Place within the bodies of human settlers and the animals they claimed as their own.

As progressive settlers embraced farm mechanization, breed improvement, and other innovations, they introduced still more flu varieties. The persistence of wild waterfowl, meanwhile, ensured a vast natural reserve of diverse viral variants. By midcentury, Three Townships farms were at once heavily commercialized *and* dedicated to systems of mixed husbandry. This combination brought relatively dense populations of humans, horses, and other flu-prone species into close and abiding contact. Influenza virions could hardly have found a better setting for circulating across species divides. The resulting reassortment event enabled influenza to take another giant step in its age-old struggle to evade host immune systems, producing a novel strain that would go on to infect vast populations of equines throughout North America as well as smaller numbers of humans and other creatures.

The conditions that enabled a new flu variant to emerge in this place and time were hardly inevitable, nor were they unique to the Three Townships.

Their commonality holds important clues for understanding how an outbreak first restricted to a bucolic rural neighborhood could rapidly expand to other parts of Canada, then to the United States. Following the roads that John Simcoe and his underlings had projected through the ancient Carrying-Place corridor, the Great Horse Flu soon raced toward Toronto, Montreal, and the northeastern United States, sickening horses and seeding havoc everywhere it reached.

CHAPTER 2

CAPITALISM'S CREATURES

The Great Horse Flu as Parasite

The Great Horse Flu would soon burst from Greater Toronto like a rodeo bronc busting out of a starting chute. At first, though, the malady's metastasis into a continent-wide outbreak eluded human perception. In the countryside north of Toronto, a viral variant evolved within a single cell of a single creature—presumably a horse—then hijacked that cell's reproductive machinery and began churning out copies and near-copies of itself. Those copies next began to invade ever more of its host's epithelial cells. Within a day or so, this horse would have started to shed the novel strain into their surroundings with every outward breath.

Some of the virus-bearing droplets and aerosols this first victim produced subsequently entered other creatures' respiratory systems. These particles' never-before-seen arrangement of spiky antigens made it easy for them to dodge these horses' immune defenses. Even before victims began showing symptoms, the novel influenza virus, which probably had an incubation period of one to three days, began to generate immense swarms of replicants. Within a week, half or more of the horses, mules, and donkeys in a widening radius would develop clear signs of flu, including fever, coughing, and running at the nose; within two weeks, 80 percent or more of the equines in any given city, town, village, or rural neighborhood would contract the disease. A snowballing cycle of viral invasion, replication, and viral shredding soon caused equines in widening expanses of Canada and the United States to fall ill. Within just a month of its initial appearance in the Three Townships, the epizootic infected millions of equines, paralyzing cities, towns, villages, and rural neighborhoods in Ontario, Quebec, New York, New England, and beyond.[1]

The speed and thoroughness of the epizootic's expansion raise intriguing questions. How could a virus lacking any capacity for self-propulsion expand its range so rapidly? How could a pathogen so minuscule—it would take eight thousand influenza virions to span the head of a single pin—manage to travel in less than three weeks from Toronto to Manhattan, a journey roughly proportional to a six-foot-tall earthling rocketing 2.5 billion miles to Pluto? And how could the Great Horse Flu infect nearly every equine in community after community within just weeks of the first cases coming to light?

Canadians, Americans, and Latin Americans would go on to debate the Great Horse Flu's epidemiology at great length but with no clear resolution. A strange brew of old chestnuts, new hypotheses, and misguided theories circulated alongside the novel influenza virus. Veterinary surgeon James Law, though, had scrutinized the epizootic more closely than nearly anyone else. Just four years after arriving in Ithaca, the Edinburgh-trained Law was already well on his way toward establishing Cornell as what one historian aptly describes as "the most widely emulated model of . . . veterinary education" in the United States. Unlike some of his colleagues, Law touted a clear-cut explanation for the disease's course. In an exhaustive December 1872 report on the outbreak for the US commissioner of agriculture, Law argued that the epizootic "has shown an unmistakable tendency to progress most rapidly along the great lines of commerce and travel."[2]

Most historians have leaned into Law's portrayal of railroads and shipping lines as the main vectors for the Great Horse Flu's expansion. Yet the epizootic also ventured from infected animals to new hosts via more prosaic routes. People in the city, the country, and everywhere in between employed equines to draw wagons, carts, plows, and other vehicles and conveyances, as well as to drag logs, pull boats, and power economic production, exchange, and consumption in myriad other ways. The movement of both people and goods thus hinged on the continued capacity of horses and their kin to toil—to apply their strength, power, intelligence, and collaborative abilities toward human purposes. The novel influenza virus inflicted sudden and debilitating illness on the animals who powered the North American economy. Almost overnight, regular life ground to a halt. Imagine if all the vehicles we depend on today—cars, trucks, buses, tractors, and the like—stopped working tomorrow, and you can readily grasp just how disruptive the Great Horse Flu became.[3]

Canadians and Americans designed their infrastructure in no small part around equines and equine labors, so the shape of farms, towns, and cities all reflected the central roles that animals played in human lifeways. The vital, mobile work that horses performed in all these places brought them into frequent proximity with their fellow equines. This dynamic, in turn, helps to account for two crucial features of the outbreak's expansion: first, the slow-moving but all-encompassing pattern by which the Great Horse Flu engulfed virtually every corner of the Northeast (and then the rest of North America); and, second, the speed with which the novel influenza virus achieved community spread, often reaching prevalence rates approaching 100 percent within two or three weeks of its initial introduction to any given locale.

The Great Horse Flu accomplished these feats by yoking equines and humans to spirit it from host to host and place to place. The outbreak exploded by taking maximum advantage of equine social behaviors as well as the deepening dependence of Canadians and Americans on equine energy. Political differences, a troubled history, and one of the world's longest international boundaries divided the United States and Canada, but the two nations also formed a common market—one in which horses and other equines played vital roles. By the early 1870s, immense inputs of equine labor had turned northeastern North America into a global industrial and commercial powerhouse. A shared commitment to capitalist development fueled speedy, constant, and voluminous exchanges of information, people, animals, and goods between the two countries.

As the epizootic's expansion would demonstrate, the novel influenza virus had evolved to prey on the horse-powered economies that Americans, Canadians, and other North American peoples had forged over the preceding decades. Even as it harnessed human exertions to race from the shores of Lake Ontario to the Atlantic coast, though, the novel influenza virus also exposed and exacerbated inequalities of wealth, status, and power, especially in urban areas. In these and other respects, the Great Horse Flu revealed itself to be capitalism's creature.

Social Animals

The rapidity and thoroughness of the epizootic's expansion resulted from the interplay between two dynamics: the long-distance transportation of infected animals by rail and ship, and the transmission of the novel influenza virus from equine to equine over shorter distances. The first process explains how the Great Horse Flu leapt across huge expanses with apparent ease. The second reveals how the epizootic permeated nearly every nook and cranny of North America. Although these modes of transmission differed in significant ways, both took advantage of the behaviors equines used to make and maintain bonds of affinity and community.

Recent research shows that horses typically prefer to form groups that vary in size, composition, and character due to contingent combinations of circumstance and choice. Donkeys, for their part, tend to be less social and more aggressive (although bachelor males often form relatively large groupings known as paces). Any form of "group living," as one team of wild horse researchers notes, "requires careful communication between members." Equines are social animals who navigate the complexities of collective life through interactions requiring direct physical contact or proximity. These exchanges gave the highly transmissible novel influenza virus easy ways to reach new hosts.[4]

Equine vocalizations communicated influenza alongside information. As science writer Wendy Williams explains, horses "talk to each other a lot"—so much, in fact, that Williams complains that they "never shut up." Individual horses, a team of equine-behavior experts notes, employ "characteristic contact calls, or whinnies, and they use different whinnies for negative situations, such as social separation from other group members, and positive situations, such as social reunions with group members." Donkeys and mules can be equally chatty. Individuals from these species issue warnings, call to friends, vent stress, or express other needs or desires by making distinctive cries that can be heard as far as three kilometers away. The whinnies, brays, and other "call types" equines employ to "talk" to each other also propel virus-containing aerosols and fluids into their immediate surroundings. The vocalizations that horse people usually refer to as snorts, blows, and nickers, for instance, can thrust virions into the air and onto nearby surfaces. Thus, when animals infected with the Great Horse Flu raised their voices to express an emotion, state of mind, or warning, they unwittingly hurled the novel influenza virus toward other equines.[5]

The epizootic also accessed new hosts through nonvocal communication. Horses constantly scan the air and ground in search of odoriferous clues. When a horse detects another animal's urine on the ground, it will often lower its head, then inhale deeply in hopes of unlocking whatever information this scent might disclose. Donkeys, for their part, have a habit of sniffing each other's dung piles, which serve "as communication posts and landmarks." Because equines infected by the epizootic shed steady streams of influenza virions onto their surroundings, previously healthy animals could easily have snorted or huffed disease-bearing particles off the ground. Whenever horses or their cousins shared information by smell or sound, in short, they could easily transmit influenza virions.[6]

Equines' fondness for touch offered still other opportunities for the Great Horse Flu to spread. Horses, for instance, frequently bite other horses—most often when combatting rivals or keeping foals in line, but also when mating. Donkeys and mules also interact by nipping at each other. In addition, all three species use their mouths to engage in mutual grooming, a behavior that helps equines to build, sustain, and even repair the all-important relationships that individual animals usually forge with one or two others (horses frequently form herds, but pairs and triads seem to endure even as larger groupings fuse, split apart, and re-form). When equines clean their companions with mouths and muzzles, they inevitably slather them with saliva and mucus.[7]

Engaging with other animals through touch, smell, and sound, flu-stricken horses, donkeys, and mules readily exposed previously healthy creatures to spit, snot, and other virus-bearing fluids, solids, and aerosols. From there, it took just a lick, huff, bray, or nicker for the epizootic to enter a potential host's respiratory system.

As If a Part of the City's Life Were Gone

Though the novel influenza managed to gain a foothold among "horses running at pasture" near the intersection of York, Markham, and Scarborough Townships, it nonetheless could have burned through the area's relatively small population of equines, then disappeared from history without a trace. Instead, the Three Townships' integration into Toronto's economy and ecology made the city a crucial stepping-stone in the Great Horse Flu's growth from a localized outbreak into a border-storming calamity.

The epizootic invaded Ontario's capital not long after Three Townships horses began falling ill in late September 1872. "Within the last few days," the *Toronto Mail* reported on October 5, "the disease has attacked hundreds of animals." The scourge, it continued, was "not confined to any particular stable, but has appeared in all the large ones in the city." That same day's *Globe* reported that "within the past week," Andrew Smith of the Ontario Veterinary College had cared for 660 horses. By October 8, less than a week after the malady hit Toronto, the *Mail* declared that "scarcely a horse in the city has escaped."[8]

This first leg of the Great Horse Flu's expansion hinged on many of the same circumstances that had facilitated the novel variant's evolution. Most households in Markham, Scarborough, and York owned horses. Ontarians, like people in much of the Northern Americas, commonly worked their equines in teams, hitching the animals just feet apart from one another and housing them in stables where the creatures shared air, water, feed, and bedding. Horses, moreover, typically spent many hours a day in motion. While other farm animals usually remained confined within outbuildings and fences, horses crisscrossed farmsteads to drag logs, tow vehicles, pull plows, and do other work; horses also routinely traveled beyond their owners' property to market goods and take people to shops, churches, neighboring farmsteads, agricultural fairs, and other destinations. All these horse-powered journeys gave the novel influenza virus ample opportunity to reach new hosts.[9]

The epizootic made its way from the Three Townships to Toronto via multiple routes. Property lines divided each township into blocks of roughly one thousand acres, subdivided into parcels of about two hundred acres. Between every other block, surveyors left a "road allowance" that was one chain (sixty-six feet) wide. So-called concession roads hugged the property boundaries that British surveyors had imposed upon Ontario's Indigenous homelands and woodland ecosystems, with narrower side roads, also numbered, running perpendicular to these country byways. Throughout the early years of settlement, writes geographer Thomas McIlwraith, "roadways straggled from side to side along the allowances set out for them, following the path of least resistance." Over time, though, considerable inputs of equine labor enabled settlers to build bridges and culverts while clearing, grading, and straightening concession and side roads. By the 1870s, artists invariably depicted southern Ontario as a land of tidy lanes passing through a prosperous countryside.[10]

Several larger, more heavily trafficked, and less bucolic arteries also linked the Three Townships to Toronto. Yonge Street remained the most important ligature connecting the city to its northern hinterlands. Although the road never realized John Simcoe's dream of diverting the Upper Great Lakes fur trade away from Montreal, its slow but steady improvement nonetheless pulled the Three Townships into Toronto's orbit. In 1822, a gentleman farmer named Robert Gourlay approvingly noted that "a noble chain of agricultural improvements" extended along Yonge Street from Toronto into York and Markham Townships, forming what Gourlay called the "only connected settlement" to the city's north.[11]

As Three Townships farmers embraced horses and abandoned oxen, equines displaced bovines on Yonge Street. In 1825, Lewis Bapp began advertising passage in a "Light Covered Waggon [*sic*]" from York to Holland Landing on Lake Simcoe; by the early 1830s, daily stagecoach service debuted on the route. After twelve miles of Yonge Street heading north from Toronto were resurfaced with crushed stone in 1835, horses and horse-powered vehicles could cover the distance between the city and the Three Townships more quickly and with less effort than ever before. "The traffic along Yonge Street," a local cleric observed later that year, had become "amazingly great." On a busy day in 1836, two hundred teams bent their heads at watering troughs outside just one of several roadside inns in Markham. William Brown later described the corridor between Toronto and the Three Townships as "like one continued country town," with inns, taverns, churches, meetinghouses, schoolhouses, workshops, and stores lining the route. Traffic increased yet again after the Royal Mail Stage Line launched regularly scheduled service in sixteen-passenger Concord coaches pulled by four-horse teams. By the early 1870s, travelers could choose between several competing coach lines and an omnibus, the largest type of horse-drawn passenger vehicle ever introduced. Four railroads, all of them built since the 1850s, also hauled people as well as livestock (including horses) and other freight between the city and the Three Townships.[12]

At an 1871 meeting of Toronto pioneers, eminent historian Henry Scadding waxed eloquent about Yonge Street's "pre-eminent importance." With "its pavements and central roadway everywhere astir with life," the road constituted what Scadding called "a great highway leading into the interior of a busy populous country." Horse-powered traffic made the route not only "the heart of the town," Scadding declared, but also "the 'main street' from and to the great world beyond."[13]

After alighting in Toronto, the novel influenza virus spread like wildfire. Within days of its arrival, so many of the city's equines had fallen ill that one wire service item described "the interruption to business" as "very serious." The next day's *Mail* lamented that Toronto's equines—"poor brutes," it called them—were "not in a fit condition to work," with "many inhuman drivers cruelly urging along weak and suffering animals. To their own shame and disgrace," the *Mail* chided, "it has to be added that many of those were not of the class who have to look to the labours of their horses for a means of livelihood." Wealthier Torontonians, in other words, joined humbler folk in neglecting their horses' welfare. Street railways stopped running, "carriages, both public and private, cabs, trucks, and in fact all vehicles moved by horse power" vanished from the streets, and city dwellers complained that it was becoming "almost impossible to secure a horse for any purpose."[14]

Three weeks after the epizootic invaded, the *Mail* estimated that "probably nine out of every ten horses" in Toronto were "afflicted." An American journalist claimed that "an air of dullness" had consequently descended on "the whole town." It was, the author observed, "as if a part of the city's life were gone." Capitalist commerce and urban vitality, this journalist recognized, hinged on equine health—not only in Toronto, but throughout the realms the epizootic stood poised to unsettle.[15]

Especially Those Belonging to the Poor Class

Toronto's booming, horse-powered economy gave the novel flu variant ample opportunity to continue spreading its wings. It reached Angus, roughly sixty miles northeast of the city, on October 9. Two days later, the scourge erupted "among the horses in Hamilton and neighborhood," sixty miles southwest of the provincial capital. By mid-October, the *Ontario Workman* marveled at the "almost daily reports of its appearance" in "various parts of the Province." With "most of the horses" in an ever-widening circle of Canada "so affected as to unfit them for travel," the all-important supply chains between Toronto and its countryside began to fray. Farmers increasingly found themselves "unable to bring grain to market," butter and eggs in Toronto grew "scarce," and the "supply of Potatoes was light." Dwindling shipments of produce forced market stalls, grocery stores, and provision dealers to hike prices.[16]

Even as the sickness infiltrated ever more of Ontario through horse-to-horse transmission along the province's byways, it simultaneously leapt across the landscape in a manner most easily explained by the long-distance transportation of animals by rail and ship. Flu struck Montreal, which remained Canada's most populous and powerful city, on October 11, having taken roughly ten days to travel about 340 miles. The *Montreal Gazette* described the "progress" of the scourge, which was already widely referred to as "the epizootic" in English and "*l'épizootie*" in French, as "astonishingly rapid." Days later, with autumn's first snow dusting the St. Lawrence River Valley, several of Montreal's veterinary surgeons proclaimed that "the malady prevails to an equal, and, if all we hear is correct, to an even greater extent" than in Toronto.[17]

Already, the outbreak evinced a remarkable capacity to parasitize North America's capitalist economies, first by using equine-powered systems of production, extraction, and exchange to reach new hosts, then by hobbling those systems to the point of paralysis. The *Gazette* described "the effects of the epidemic" just days after the Great Horse Flu reached Montreal as "immediately apparent" in the city's "deserted cab stands and general Sunday appearance of the streets." Less than a week after the first horses

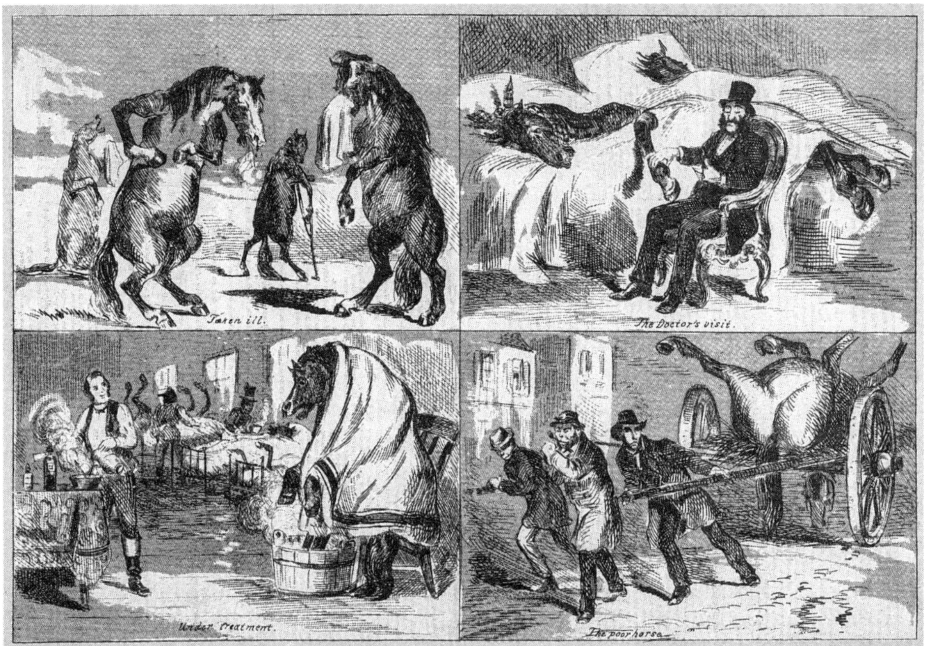

THE HORSE EPIDEMIC.—BY E. JUMP.

This is the first of several cartoons that poked fun at the ridiculousness the Great Horse Flu unleashed. Published in English in the *Canadian Illustrated News*, and in French in *L'opinion publique*, the illustration's four panels chart a sequence: "Taken Ill," "The Doctor's Visit," "Under Treatment," and "The Poor Horse." The first panel portrays horses as bipeds beset by symptoms all too familiar to readers who had tussled with the flu. In the second, a physician tends to a pair of bedridden beasts. The third frame depicts what some papers jokingly called "horse-pitals," with men dutifully nursing equines in a makeshift sick ward. While most Canadian horses survived the epizootic, some perished from flu or its complications. With nearly every equine in the Confederation too ill to keep laboring, men sometimes stepped in to do the work horses could no longer perform. As the last panel shows, this included straining to pull wagons containing the corpses of horses killed by the "Canadian horse disease." E. Jump, "The Horse Epidemic," *Canadian Illustrated News*, October 26, 1872. Courtesy of the American Antiquarian Society.

began showing clear flu symptoms, Montreal's horse railway monopoly, like Toronto's before it, "absolutely stopped" all service because of "the inability of horses, which are completely prostrated by the disease, to work any longer."[18]

Most carters, who drove freight through Montreal using two-wheeled vehicles pulled by one or two horses, stayed home to protect their animals' health—and, with it, their ability to continue earning a living. On Wednesday, October 16, though, "the few carters who were upon the streets," groused the *Montreal Herald and Commercial*, "raised their fares to an exorbitant figure." Back in 1864, Montreal's municipal government had allied with powerful business interests to quash a carters' strike. Victorious city officials then imposed a strictly enforced schedule limiting how much carters could charge. Having bristled against these regulations for years, Montreal's horse workers took advantage of the epizootic by "refus[ing] to engage at the old rates," instead charging whatever they thought the market could bear in defiance of "the law, and the tariff, and the exercise of policeman's authority." Cabbies, who drove lone or paired passengers in two-wheeled cabs, also found the public "comparatively at their mercy." With streetcars, hacks, and omnibuses all idled, they upped their tariffs by 200 percent or more.[19]

Cabbies and carters vowed to "resolutely maintain their new and extortionate prices," but the sudden deaths of four flu-stricken animals tested their determination. From the start of the outbreak, the Canadian press had downplayed the flu's deadliness. "The disease is not often fatal," one wire service report from Toronto assured readers, while a young veterinary surgeon from Goderich, Ontario, declared that "no danger need be apprehended."[20]

This perception of the epizootic as relatively benign began to waver, though, after the first of many horses to perish in Montreal died around 1:30 a.m. on October 17. The initial victim, a horse entrusted with pulling an omnibus, "showed signs of distress" minutes after stopping to pick up a crowd of passengers from a railway depot, then "dropped down exhausted. A few minutes more and it was dead." Later the same morning, an express company ordered "a fine iron-grey mare" back to its stable because it was "in a very weak condition," yet this precaution came too late to save the animal. A carter in the working-class, predominantly Irish Canadian neighborhood of Griffintown also "lost a valuable beast" to the flu. And in Beaudry Street, near downtown, "a hard worked horse, that had received little or no attention, suddenly became afflicted with a sore throat. This progressed rapidly," the *Montreal Witness* claimed, until "the poor beast died from sheer suffocation." News of these fatal flu cases circulated rapidly, unsettling Montrealers' expectation that the epizootic would remain relatively harmless. "No one," as the *Witness* exclaimed, had "believed the sickness could be fatal, until ocular demonstrations had proved to the contrary." After these four horses gave up the ghost within hours of each other, though, "fear and apprehension," the *Witness* exclaimed, "seized upon owners of horses still at work."[21]

This tragic turn exposed carters and cabbies, who were overwhelmingly drawn from the city's Irish and French Canadian working classes, to mounting criticism. On Friday, October 18, the *Witness*, a temperance publication that catered to the city's English-speaking upper crust, lashed out at carters, cabbies, and others who kept sick horses working. "Invariably," the *Witness* huffed in remarking on Montreal's mounting equine death toll, "the horses in question have had no rest from their labours, consequently the disease has been aggravated, and they are actually driven to death." The paper went on to complain that "as a natural consequence of this," Montreal's "business men," a group dominated by British Canadian Protestants, faced "great inconvenience, and a heavy loss."[22]

This framing reflected growing sympathy among some Montrealers for animal welfare. Yet it also spoke to the wrenching dilemma the Great Horse Flu thrust upon those who made their daily bread by the sweat of their horses' brows. In Montreal, as elsewhere, carters and cabbies were usually small proprietors who owned the animals they drove. The sudden slump in the supply of motive power enabled these and other horse workers to rake in sudden windfalls—but only if they were willing to risk their animals' health. A growing proportion of those who took this gamble lost, as *Le Nouveau Monde*, which served Montreal's sizable Francophone minority, indicated when it related "that a good number of horses have already died, especially those belonging to the poor class," depriving more and more families of their "means of existence when . . . most needed," with winter fast approaching.[23]

Little wonder, then, that nearly all of Montreal's "coachmen and the carters" decided on Monday, October 21, to eschew profit and instead prioritize their horses' survival by declaring, as *Le Constitutionel* reported, that they would "no longer dare to take their horses out." This decision undoubtedly saved many equine lives, yet it also compounded the costs the Great Horse Flu exacted from Montrealers. With horse-powered conveyances "few and far between," it became "almost impossible," newspapers complained, "to get carts to transport firewood," unload cargoes from boats and ships, or indeed to "move goods" of any sort. After the Grand Trunk Railway's draying contractor stabled all his horses, masses of "freight destined for the railroads" began "accumulating in the warehouses." Beside Montreal's rivers and canals, meanwhile, "thousands of tons of coal" and heaps of "bales, boxes, &c." piled up.[24]

With winter on the doorstep and the St. Lawrence River starting to ice over, a total "dead lock in all departments in the shipping trade" loomed. Only "the restoration of the horses' health," the *Witness* feared, could get business moving again. This deadening conjuncture of flu and frost confronted Montrealers with one of the stubbornest of capitalism's many contradictions. Most of the city's people equated industry and commerce with order and progress. Yet their pursuit of growth and wealth could afford them little protection against freezing seaways and fast-spreading flu. Having imagined themselves to have mastered the natural world, their enduring powerlessness in the face of seasonal cycles and viral intrusions unsettled their faith that their endeavors could deliver them from the uncertainties that had always bedeviled human existence amid a more-than-human world.[25]

Montreal's horses—and, with them, its economy—would not recover en masse until early November, roughly three weeks after the epizootic first struck Canada's greatest metropolis. By that time, the Great Horse Flu was already widening its assaults to other parts of Quebec, Canada's Atlantic Coast, and the northeastern United States. As it debilitated entire herds of equines throughout the continent's most populous and productive region, the epizootic pressed down on the wheels of commerce like some immense viral brake.

Sheets of Flame

On Friday, October 11—the same day the epizootic hit Montreal—William Somerville, a veterinary surgeon who headed the Buffalo Horse Infirmary, received a telegram calling him to Niagara Falls "to see several sick horses." The vet recounted in an October 15 letter to the *Buffalo Commercial* that he had ridden northward to examine animals afflicted by the illness, then "pronounced it the same disease as that by which the Canadian horses were afflicted." Somerville's diagnosis hinged on the close similarity between the signs he observed in these Niagara Falls horses and "the symptoms described by Prof. SMITH, V.S. of Toronto" in a letter to Somerville.[26]

Somerville's message to the *Commercial* also conveyed some scuttlebutt. A Buffalo physician named "Dr. CAREY," Somerville had been told, "drove his four-horse team to Niagara to meet the Governor General of Canada"—Lord Dufferin, an Anglo-Irish nobleman who represented Queen Victoria as Canada's head of state—"and a few days after [Carey's] return home the team were taken sick, and being called by him today to see his horses, I found every horse in his stable affected." Somerville concluded his letter, which the *Commercial* published under the headline "The Canada Horse Epidemic," by informing readers that this equine scourge had subsequently "got amongst our horses in Buffalo."[27]

As the novel influenza virus flooded across the international border, it aggravated already tense relationships between Americans and Canadians. North America's two largest nations shared a sprawling, sometimes ill-defined boundary as well as a tangled history of enmity and rivalry. Canadians took offense at accusations by Somerville and others that Lord Dufferin's recent visit had introduced the epizootic to the United States. The federal government's belated and ineffectual efforts to keep the outbreak at bay then added more fuel to the fire the American press had kindled by coining such objectionable handles for the scourge as the "Canadian horse disease," "Canadian horse distemper," "Canada consumption," and "Canadian horse plague."[28]

American and Canadian forces had not battled since the War of 1812, yet sixty years later, relations between the two nations were anything but tranquil. The succor Canada's British overlords provided to the Confederacy during the Civil War combined with Canadian outrage over the Fenian Raids, a series of attacks launched by American-based Irish nationalists, most of them Union veterans, against north-of-the-border targets, to push the United States and Canada toward open rupture. In 1869, Ontario historian William Caniff expressed the bellicosity that remained widespread among his countrymen. "The Americans ought to know, and remember," Caniff growled in reference to 1866 attacks against targets in Ontario and New Brunswick launched by American Fenians, "that no acts of cowardly villainy toward us will for ever go unpunished.... Let but one more attempt be made to secure a footing on our soil, and the Americans will learn that Canadians can, and will, retaliate." If their neighbors to the south insisted on threatening the recently formed Canadian confederation, Caniff warned, "*a sheet of flame will burst along their frontier.*" "We were then on the verge of war with Great Britain," US Treasury Secretary George Boutwell recalled of the late 1860s and early 1870s, "and demands were made in very responsible quarters which offered no alternative but war."[29]

This was the precarious situation that confronted Britain's minister to Washington, Sir Edward Thornton, when he disembarked in the American capital in 1871 at the head of a delegation that included Canadian Prime Minister Sir John A. Macdonald. The ensuing negotiations centered on American claims for compensation from the United Kingdom for damages inflicted by the CSS *Alabama* and four other British-built Confederate ships during the Civil War. But the talks also extended to long-running disputes over North Atlantic fishing grounds as well as the location of the international border through the San Juan Islands, between Washington Territory and British Columbia. After ten weeks of grueling negotiations, Thornton, Macdonald, and US Secretary of State Hamilton Fish unveiled a treaty that settled the *Alabama* claims in the Americans' favor, established a binational fisheries commission, and resolved every other major point of contention except the San Juan dispute, which the two sides agreed to submit to Germany's Wilhelm I for arbitration.[30]

The timing of the Great Horse Flu's American invasion could hardly have been worse. The very same day that Buffalo newspapers reported that the epizootic had become "general" throughout that city, Kaiser Wilhelm announced that his arbitrators had decided in the Americans' favor. This ruling added insult to the injury many Canadians felt after US Treasury Secretary George Boutwell ordered customs inspectors in Burlington, Vermont; Port Huron, Michigan; and numerous Upstate New York lakeports "to allow no horses to be brought into your port or district from [Canada] unless you are perfectly satisfied that they are free from contagious diseases." To make matters worse, newspapers on both sides of the border began amplifying allegations from William Somerville and others that the Canadian governor general's recent visit to Niagara Falls was responsible for bringing the Great Horse Flu onto American soil. The *Rochester Democrat and Chronicle* reported that "soon after" a team of horses driven by a "gentleman who drove over to attend" Lord Dufferin's reception at Queenstown "was attacked by the epidemic," the American's "whole stud" had fallen ill with flu-like symptoms. This rumor gained wider circulation the next day, after it was reprinted by the *New York Herald* and glossed by the *Montreal Witness*.[31]

Canadians, outraged by the arbitrators' adverse decision and incensed by American allegations that Canada's head of state had introduced the Great Horse Flu to western New York, immediately pushed back. "While our American cousins do not always show themselves willing to give us credit where credit is really due," the *Hamilton Times* huffed, "they are very anxious at times to credit us with what is not our due . . . . So, now they are pleased to dub the prevalent epizootic the 'Canada Horse Disease,' as though we had specially got it up, or it were a special out-growth of monarchical institutions." As Canadian newspapers smarted at American slights, the epizootic was already surging from the Great Lakes and St. Lawrence Valley toward the Atlantic Seaboard. "The rapid spread of the disease through all parts of the Northern States," the same *Hamilton Times* article went on to argue, "has made prevention impossible." "If the epizootic be really a Canadian development, as Yankee editors pronounced it," the same editor sarcastically concluded, "its prevalence in their cities shows how rapidly Canadian institutions are calculated to spread among our neighbours."[32]

The Great Horse Flu was already tightening its grip over Buffalo. By October 21, the *Commercial* estimated that "nine out of every ten horses in town are affected with it." The Buffalo Omnibus Company stopped running, street railways reduced service, "all branches of business in the city" contracted, and it became "almost impossible to secure a team of any kind," even for funerals. "The disease which at first was supposed to be merely a passing ailment," the next day's *Commercial* declared, "has demonstrated a degree of mischief which amounts to a positive public disaster." Travelers had "to walk to and from the depot with their trunks in a hand-cart, on their shoulders or perhaps in a wheel-barrow." With grocers and butchers also keeping their horses stabled, customers found themselves "obliged to engage small boys" for delivery duty. Meanwhile, a growing number of Buffalo's workmen faced unemployment; a local builder, to cite one of many examples, laid off "seventy-five men simply because he could not procure materials hauled."[33]

Superspreaders and Viral Clouds

Canadians sometimes attributed the epizootic's appearance at their doorsteps to recent arrivals of flu-stricken animals by rail or ship. How else, after all, could the malady have raced from Toronto to Montreal in just ten days? Americans likewise tended to blame the Great Horse Flu's onset in their communities on equines imported from their northern neighbors. The *Syracuse Journal*, for instance, claimed that the equine flu had been "noticed first in some Canadian horses shipped to this city," while Chicago officials traced the epizootic's appearance there to nine sick horses recently unloaded from Canada. As these observers understood, Ontario's farmers enjoyed brisk markets south of the border for the horses they raised—especially in fall, when harvest-related demand for draft power on farms overlapped with streetcar companies' preparations for the annual winter upswing in ridership.[34]

Once the Canadian horse disease became an American horse disease, too, the novel influenza virus still sometimes leapt from one city to another before infiltrating the intervening countryside. After a late October trip to Detroit to reconnoiter the Great Horse Flu, Chicago's sanitary superintendent reported that the epizootic "follows the lines of communication, and the general course of trade in horses." Veterinarian James Law, meanwhile, pegged railroad trunk lines for carrying the epizootic from Buffalo to New York City. Thereafter, the press continued to link the outbreak's growth to the shipment of sick horses by train. When the Great Horse Flu struck Pittsburgh at October's end, for example, the *Gazette* pointed an accusatory finger at a gang of horses recently arrived from Manhattan.[35]

Steamships and railroads helped to spirit the Great Horse Flu over long distances, enabling the outbreak to leapfrog in mere hours from one metropolis to the next. Yet horses, donkeys, and mules served not just as commodities and freight but also as prime movers. Even as the Great Horse Flu jumped from place to place via train and ship, it also swelled its range through the earthbound movements of hoofed superspreaders.

When the epizootic erupted, John O'Brien's Circus was touring Ontario. Several of O'Brien's two hundred steeds performed under the big top with trick riders, while the rest toiled offstage to pull circus wagons laden with tents, equipment, exotic animals, and human performers. By the time the circus reached Hamilton, Ontario, on October 12, many of its horses had contracted the flu, and two had died from it. When the caravan crossed the international border a few days later, sixteen horses were so ill that managers felt compelled to leave them behind. A Buffalo paper alleged on October 21 that "every horse attached to O'Brian's [*sic*] Circus, which came here from Canada yesterday, is sick." In addition to suffering "several" additional fatalities, "including some" among "their ring performers," fully "one-half" of O'Brien's horses remained "laid up" at Niagara Falls, too unwell to draw wagons or carry riders. But impresario John O'Brien, reckoning that time was money, refused to alter the circus's itinerary. By the time the company paraded through Rochester, its remaining "sixty or more" horses presented a sorry sight, with "all showing symptoms of the disease. Many were discharging freely from the nostrils and appeared as though they were well exhausted."[36]

When O'Brien's star-crossed outfit moved on again, it "met with a disaster while crossing Seneca River, by the breaking down of the bridge, before the vans had all succeeded in getting over." The circus's rhino, still locked in its cage, tumbled into the river, "while the elephant, after swimming this stream, got upon the rampage and finally had to be chained." O'Brien's horses presumably continued to carry the novel influenza virus, shedding virions pell-mell as they drew the circus through southeastern New York toward winter quarters outside Philadelphia. When a Port Jervis newspaper lamented just days after the circus departed the village that "epizoo' [one of many riffs on "epizootic"] reigns supreme in this village," it hinted at the role circus horses likely played in introducing the Great Horse Flu there.[37]

Circus horses were memorable creatures whose eye-catching processions drummed up media coverage and popular interest. Horses and mules laboring on canal towpaths drew less notice but were more numerous and widespread, making them ideal vectors for bearing the novel influenza virus into new territory. Even the largest artificial waterways of the early 1870s remained too shallow and narrow to accommodate steamboats, so equines continued to tow vessels loaded with raw materials and finished goods on canals throughout the Northeast.[38]

The novel influenza virus adeptly transformed these conduits of economic integration into disease transmission routes. Canal boats sometimes carried flu-stricken animals on deck or in their holds. "Many boats have tied up," reported an article describing the outbreak's "very discouraging" push along the Erie between Rochester and Buffalo, "and nearly every craft has sick horses, and some have arrived here with dead horses on board." Just a few days later, on October 28, three mules reached Ithaca from Buffalo via the Erie and Cayuga & Seneca Canals aboard the *Lucy* displaying unmistakable signs of "the horse disease." Within days, Ithaca became an epizootic hot spot.[39]

The towpaths and stables that lined most every canal, however, probably did even more to bring the Great Horse Flu to new hosts. As flu-stricken ponies and mules pulled boats and barges, recouped their energies with feed and water, and bedded down for the night in congested stables, they often came into contact with previously unaffected animals. "Reports received by the agents of different towing companies" on the Erie Canal, a wire service report declared on October 23, asserted that the epizootic was "commencing to sweep all along the entire" waterway, with canal ponies falling ill in "Rochester, Syracuse, Utica, and even as far east as West Troy."[40]

By late October, transportation on the Erie nearly stopped altogether because the epizootic's "prevalence and extensive fatality," as the *Missouri Republican* noted, made it nearly impossible to procure horses "to do the towing." Observers feared "that the canal will not only be seriously obstructed through to the close of navigation"—the yearly suspension of inland shipping as canals and rivers froze over—but could even be "entirely cut off." Shipping rates skyrocketed by 600 percent, sowing panic among "forwarders and shippers of canal freights to New York" and stoking "great depression" in Oswego and other upstate shipping centers. When news of the Erie's woes reached Chicago, the most important agricultural market in the North American interior, "a sensation in grain circles" erupted. The epizootic, Windy City brokers feared, "threatened [an] embargo" on grain, which often traveled by canal at least partway from the inland farms on which it was grown to New York, Philadelphia, Baltimore, and other Atlantic ports. As the epizootic convulsed the Erie Canal, horses and mules were also carrying the remarkably infectious virus along the towpaths of other equine-powered waterways, including the Champlain and Delaware & Hudson Canals.[41]

The Great Horse Flu harnessed both circuses and canals toward its own ends. It also spread through innumerable, unrecorded interactions between animals suffering from influenza and previously healthy animals as they crisscrossed turnpikes, country roads, and farmsteads. Passing from one creature to the next, the epizootic permeated the Northeastern countryside like an enormous viral fog. A variant that emerged in the agricultural context of the Three Townships found fertile ground in rural America. "Farmers in various parts of the county," the *Niagara Falls (NY) Gazette* remarked less than a week after the outbreak crossed over from Ontario, "are bitterly complaining of the pestilence among their horses."[42]

The Great Horse Flu's double-barreled epidemiology—its capacity to spring across large distances while simultaneously rolling in unbroken waves to inundate every corner of the countryside—helps us to understand why efforts to check the outbreak failed. No one in the early 1870s knew for certain what caused influenza, nor did anyone understand how it spread. Opinion about flu's epidemiology spanned a spectrum between two main positions: Influenza either traveled through the atmosphere, or it passed from one host to another more directly, through contact or proximity. Those who suspected the outbreak to be contagious sometimes tried to deploy government power or encourage private action in vain efforts to halt the Great Horse Flu's expansion. The US Treasury's mid-October order to restrict Canadian horse imports foreshadowed efforts by local officeholders and public health officials to enact quarantines and remove animals who displayed unmistakable flu symptoms from streets and other common spaces. Those who owned or worked with horses, meanwhile, often tried to isolate healthy animals from their ill counterparts. People in the country commonly steered clear of villages or towns where they knew the epizootic to be lurking. North Americans also implemented an array of sanitary measures, fumigating or applying lime and other chemical disinfectants to stables and horse gear. Attempts to combat flu through prophylaxis and isolation, however, overwhelmingly failed. The only clear exception was Prince Edward Island, which remained flu-free after banning equine imports from the mainland.[43]

Efforts to stop the outbreak in its tracks fell short for several reasons. First, flu virions can remain viable for days under favorable conditions, so the virus could be transmitted through contact with surfaces contaminated with the novel variant, including the floors and walls of railroad stock cars, holding pens at horse dealers and livestock markets, gear including bridles and harnesses, and the clothing, footwear, and skin of humans who came into close contact with traveling equines. No less important, government officials typically did not take decisive action until it was too late; the US government's quarantine on Canadian horse imports, for instance, began *after* the outbreak had already struck Niagara Falls and Buffalo. Finally, and probably most significantly, the outbreak's growth did not depend solely or even primarily on superspreading circus horses and canal ponies or the long-distance transportation of flu-stricken equines by rail or ship. Instead, the Great Horse Flu proved fully capable of subjugating the Northeast one victim at a time, passing from animal to animal, farm to farm, and village to village until it held the entire region tight in its maw.[44]

Motionless, Dumb, Paralyzed

New Yorkers had been reading wire service accounts of the epizootic for weeks before newspapers reported on Sunday, October 20, that the outbreak "was creating great havoc with the horses" in and around Albany, just 124 nautical miles north of New York Harbor. New Yorkers grew still more concerned as the epizootic "swiftly and surely . . . followed the course of the Hudson" from Albany toward Gotham, "leaving its traces in the towns and hamlets that stud the banks of that noble river." New York's street railway lines "at once consulted with the best veterinary surgeons in the city as to the best methods of resisting the inroads of the distemper, and immediate precautions were taken to guard against its appearance." Yet the next day, "symptoms of the disease were discovered among the horses of several of the railroad companies." By October 23, "the alarming spread of the disorder"—the Great Horse Flu had already "prostrated" seven thousand horses—led the *Evening Post* to warn "that a great public calamity may happen in the virtual stoppage of the different lines of travel." "There has been no time to take any necessary precautions," the *Herald* complained, "as the contagious qualities of the disease are so violent that within twenty-four hours from the time the first symptoms of sickness were noticed in one large stable in this city one thousand horses under the same roof were similarly affected . . . . It was the same story everywhere," the *Herald* continued: "Horses that were to all intents and purposes in perfect health on Monday night were coughing badly" when Tuesday dawned.[45]

The epizootic's metastasis, wire services reported, stopped "many branches of business" in their tracks, and transit companies slashed service. By Saturday, October 26, an estimated 27,684 of Greater New York's 42,516 horses had contracted the malady. Freight on Brooklyn's piers was "pil[ing] up for the want of horses to remove it," and bereaved New Yorkers lamented "the lack of horses for funerals." By Tuesday, October 29, the *Herald* declared that "the epizoot has struck business blind and severed its arteries. It is motionless, dumb, paralyzed, and the shock which it has received is greater than can be seen on the surface."[46]

Nearly identical disruptions convulsed Boston during these same late October days. Around noon on Sunday the twentieth, "fifteen or twenty horses" at a Northampton Street livery stable "appeared to be seized nearly simultaneously with spells of coughing." By nightfall, the *Evening Transcript* reported, "at least fifty" more had "joined in the chorus." Four days later, the *Globe* described the outbreak's spread as "so rapid" among Boston's eleven to twelve thousand equines "that at present there are over two thousand cases." Animals employed by horse railways, express companies, and trucking firms ranked as "the greatest sufferers," but the novel influenza virus even reached a horse who had been "kept constantly for seven years in the upper story of a warehouse in Congress street, for hoisting purposes." By Friday, October 25, the *Globe* pronounced that the outbreak's swift, unrelenting expansion meant "that it can now, without exaggeration, be regarded as a public misfortune," for, as the *Evening Transcript* reported, "two horses out of three on the street show plainly to the practiced eye the various indications of the distemper." People who worked downtown or did business there had little alternative but to walk, leading to the "almost complete desertion of the streets, while the sidewalks were positively crowded with umbrella-covered humanity." "In future years," the *Globe* mused, "when the children and grandchildren are told of the strange visitation which Boston received in the year 1872, and the extraordinary scenes and circumstances connected therewith, they will be hardly able to imagine the queer predicament in which we were placed. No horse-cars, no express wagons, no hacks, no coaches, nothing drawn by that most useful and docile animal, the horse." The novel influenza virus made Boston's reliance on equines plain for all to see. "What the horse does for the society, and what it accomplishes for the comfort, convenience and even necessity of mankind," intoned the *Evening Transcript*, "are now apparent to the least reflecting person." The epizootic, in short, was shaking horse-powered modernity to its core.[47]

Even as the Great Horse Flu was wreaking havoc on two of North America's greatest cities, it continued to enlarge its range. During the last two weeks of October, it invaded Brooklyn; Detroit; Providence; Newark; New Haven; Springfield, Massachusetts; Keene, New Hampshire; Lewiston and Augusta, Maine; and numerous other towns, cities, and rural neighborhoods. "A little cloud 'no bigger than a man's hand,'" the *Detroit Free Press* reported with palpable disbelief, "starting first from Toronto, Canada, has increased in magnitude until it covers and temporarily darkens nearly a whole continent."[48]

Although country-bred, the Great Horse Flu took full advantage of the ways that the physical layout, density, and dynamism of urban spaces concentrated equine encounters within close quarters. "The great tendency of the disease," as one journalist astutely observed, "is to crowds, where many horses are collected." In towns and cities throughout the Northeast, the everyday work that equines performed combined with the confined conditions in which these animals lived and labored to facilitate the epizootic's proliferation.[49]

The streets of New York, like those of Toronto, Montreal, and Buffalo before it, spurred viral transmission. Engravings, photographs, and paintings from the early 1870s almost invariably depicted these thoroughfares as swollen with equines. Images such as Currier & Ives's 1875 rendition of Manhattan's Broadway, probably the most heavily trafficked street in North America, showed horses straining behind conveyances ranging from buggies to drays to omnibuses. Under such circumstances, social distancing was impossible.[50]

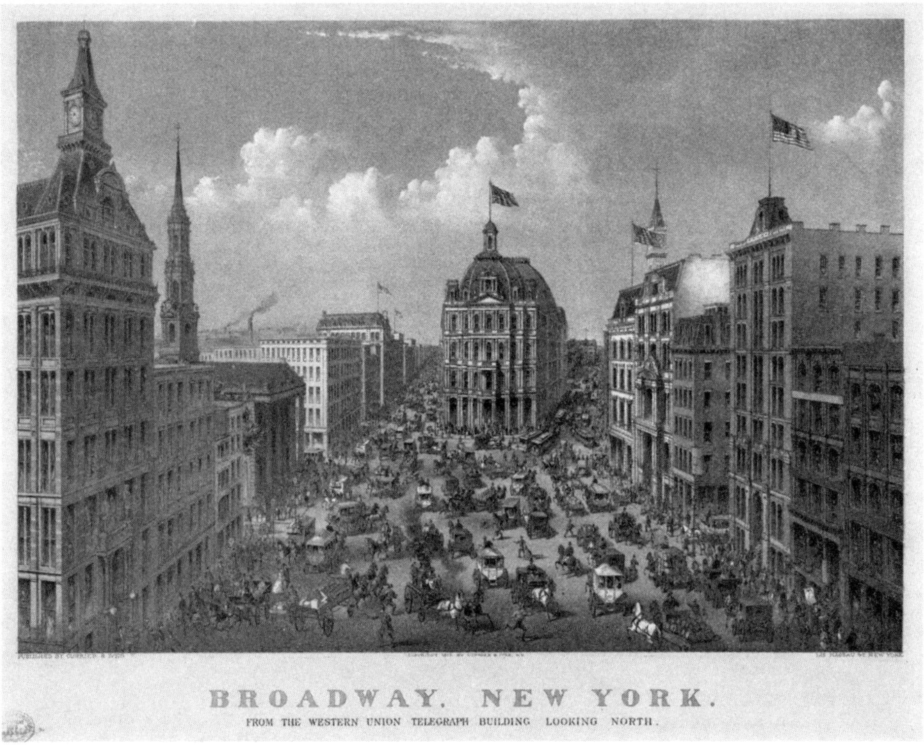

In New York as in other cities throughout North America, horses labored in chaotic, congested spaces where social distancing was utterly impossible. In this Currier & Ives print, equines—many of them in pairs or larger teams, but some of them working solo—draw vehicles of every size and description through crowded streets encased by soaring buildings. The novel influenza virus that evolved in Ontario's Three Townships could hardly have asked for better conditions in which to circulate and infect new hosts. Currier & Ives, *Broadway, New York: From the Western Union Telegraph Building Looking North* (1875). Courtesy of the Library of Congress Prints and Photographs Division, Washington, DC.

The English-born illustrator Horace Harral's *Sleighing at Harlem, New York* (1873) offers an intimate portrait of some of the circumstances that abetted the epizootic's rapid growth in New York and other cities. Harral's engraving pictured several well-heeled sleighing parties converging on a snowy Upper Manhattan thoroughfare. In the foreground, a jet-black steed lowers its head, digging deep as a driver and belle tucked beneath luxuriant bison robes hold on for dear life. In the midground, the top-hatted driver of a larger vehicle carrying two couples leans toward his team and cracks his whip. As all these horses jostle for space, condensation spirals out their nostrils to fill the air. As this engraving makes clear, Gotham's equines incessantly breathed in

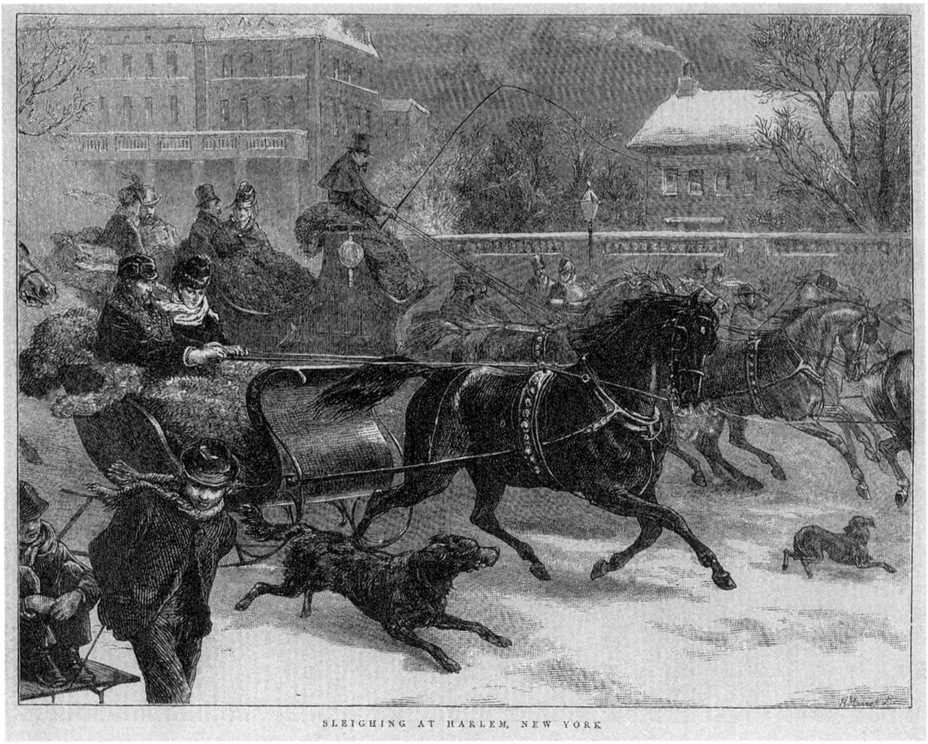

The English illustrator Horace Harral presented a vivid depiction of equines, canines, and humans dashing through Harlem's snow-covered streets. Horace Harral, "Sleighing at Harlem, New York," published in *The Survey Graphic* (London), February 8, 1873, from author's collection.

their fellow creatures' exhalations. Each inhalation thus held the possibility of introducing flu virions into their respiratory systems.

Watering troughs erected by well-meaning animal lovers provided the Great Horse Flu with another route to new hosts. Soon after the epizootic struck, the *Inquirer* complained that Philadelphia's "public fountains," which supposedly followed a design that was "the same in all large cities," held on to "all the scum or matter dropped from the mouth and nostrils of diseased horses." As an *Inquirer* reporter griped with overt disgust, this residue then "float[ed] upon the surface," where it could easily "be swallowed by the other horses drinking afterward." The scourge's ability to spread through shared drinking facilities, the same article concluded, meant trouble: Philadelphia's "sound horses must suffer from the diseased animals." Cincinnati's Board of Health responded to such reports just days before the epizootic arrived by "ordering the removal of all drinking troughs for horses along the street, alleging as a reason that they would be fruitful sources for the spread of the epizootic horse disease when it reached the city."[51]

While drinking fountains and congested streets enabled the Great Horse Flu to circulate among animals as they labored, stables compelled the same animals to share water, food, air, and space during off-work hours. Most stables in the Northeast were small, cheap structures housing just a few beasts. Contemporary observers frequently described the Northeast's smaller stables as resonant with whinnies, snorts, and other vocalizations as well as reeking of sweat, urine, and dung. An 1866 report by New York public health authorities, for example, lambasted stables in poorer neighborhoods as "crowded" into basements and alleyways and "frequently neglected and uncleanly." The "slovenly condition" of such stables led investigators to denounce them as "fever-nests," a role they undoubtedly reprised when the epizootic struck six years later.[52]

Livery stables, which were often midsize facilities, clustered near waterfronts, railroad depots, and affluent neighborhoods. Express companies, which specialized in delivering packages, business correspondence, and high-value goods, joined large firms in industries ranging from brewing to steelmaking in building stables that could accommodate several dozen equines. Such large stables were relatively uncommon in rural areas, although breeders and racing enthusiasts sometimes built sprawling housing for their animals in horsey districts of Long Island, New Jersey, and other upscale suburban areas. The biggest stables, though, usually belonged to steam railroads, which employed dozens or hundreds of equines to transfer freight and baggage at major stations, and street railway companies, private corporations that dominated transit within cities and towns across North America. Among the era's biggest investors in animal capital, street railways usually distributed their horses across multiple stables strategically dispersed across their track networks. The most densely populated of these buildings—equine counterparts to the tenements in which a fast-growing proportion of American urbanites lived—housed a thousand or more equines under a single five- or six-story roof.[53]

These cavernous stables may have proved even more conducive than humbler housing to spreading the Great Horse Flu. Many horsecar companies sought to rationalize operations and cut the steep cost of equine upkeep by investing in the 1860s and early 1870s in immense new stables that boasted what one sanitary expert praised as "superior ventilation, light, and cleanliness." These hulking structures of brick, stone, and iron streamlined how air, light, feed, water, vehicles, and—not least—human and equine laborers moved within their walls. The resulting efficiencies reduced the expense of horse care, but they also made it easier for influenza to spread from ailing animals to new hosts. Even stables that were hailed as sanitary models facilitated viral transmission, since the creatures they housed shared practically everything: feed, water, and the receptacles that held them; brushes, combs, bridles, harnesses, and other gear; the human workers who tended to equine needs; and, not least, interior surfaces including walls, floors, and partitions. Conditions in these facilities, moreover, often proved less than ideal. "In our large cities," *The Nation* lamented, "horses are exposed without let or hindrance on the part of sanitary authorities to just those conditions from which the great pestilences among human beings have sprung and do still occasionally spring. We take precautions in the public interest against overcrowding, filth, and absence of ventilation in tenement-houses," the author noted with dismay, "but we take no precautions against the overcrowding, filth, and want of light and ventilation of city stables; and yet every one of the large stables may fairly and properly be called a hot-bed of horse disease."[54]

Horses, mules, and donkeys, in short, hardly lived lives of isolation. The equines whose labors drove agriculture, industry, commerce, and much else sustained vibrant networks that bound every citizen and family, every structure and market, every district and neighborhood and suburb into a functioning whole that added up to far more than the sum of its parts. As horses and their cousins drank from the same fountains, touched the same surfaces, breathed the same air, and engaged their fellow equines in streets and stables through vocalization, touch, and other behaviors, they became essential if unwitting agents for the Great Horse Flu's explosive growth.

Vile Epizoot

The Great Horse Flu's expansion prompted a rolling transportation crisis. Within just a few days of arriving in any given place, the epizootic made it significantly more difficult and expensive to move people and goods. Flu-fueled shortfalls in motive power proved particularly intractable in the passenger sector.

Beefing up boat service offered one solution. As a journalist explained, New York boasted "enough unemployed steamers to form a sufficient fleet" to transport "our people to their homes with greater speed and comfort than can ever be secured on the horse railroads." Steam-powered railroad lines offered another alternative to equine-powered conveyances. Trains on routes connecting downtown districts to suburban neighborhoods saw big upturns in ridership; some also began making additional stops. "Snow blockades and the horse disease unitedly sing the paean of steam," the *Chicago Evening Post* declared as that city's steam railways became "almost wholly relied upon in lieu of the denuded horse railways." Although many rail lines even went so far as to add extra service on steam-powered trains, this recourse made little dent in the massive shortfall in passenger capacity the epizootic caused.[55]

Running coal-burning engines on street railways, which bore the lion's share of intra-urban traffic, held greater promise. Thanks to the horse flu, declared the *Brooklyn Union*, "the need of steam power, instead of horses," was "now universally admitted." The *Chicago Evening Mail* hailed fossil-fueled streetcars as "the Coming Horse—the horse that never tires, and whose nostrils never suffer from the epizootic." Known as "dummies," these small, boxy conveyances had been around for decades. Their adoption, though, had been shackled by municipal governments, which banned dummies because of concerns over air and noise pollution, as well as widespread fears that these little locomotives would exacerbate congestion and spark chaos by spooking horses. Several cities responded to the Great Horse Flu by temporarily easing restrictions on these coal-burning machines. Switching to steam on street railways, however, proved impractical. Most transit companies owned just a few such engines. Sealing these contraptions' fate, they underperformed. "The unintelligent dummies," the *Chicago Evening Post* jibed, "do not work as well as could be wished."[56]

Where steam failed, human muscle power prevailed, at least to a modest degree. When the epizootic forced Baltimore's horse railways to suspend service, one company permitted some of the employees it had just laid off "the use of the cars for their own benefit." The *Sun* detailed how "a line of man-railway cars was quickly improvised," with ten-man teams pulling passengers "at intervals of every hour, morning and afternoon." Even though the men charged twice the usual nickel-per-ride rate, "the novelty of the thing alone attracted many persons to patronize the cars, and the joviality of those hauling them tended to keep up a general good feeling among the patrons." Elsewhere, though, volunteers who stepped into horses' traces charged passengers as much as twenty-five cents. Together with infrequent service, high fares made human-powered streetcars a highly imperfect solution to epizootic disruptions.[57]

Pedestrianism served as the easiest, most popular alternative to horse-powered transportation during the epizootic, at least for the able-bodied. Many commentators hailed walking as a refreshing change of pace. A Buffalo newspaper, for instance, celebrated the "radical change" that had "taken place in the customs and habits of our city people." The same journalist declared it "almost marvelous that the custom of walking should have been so generally adopted in so short a time," wistfully concluding that there was "no knowing what a wonderful change of views . . . a raging horse epidemic will bring about." A week later, a Chicagoan urged his fellow citizens to embrace the health benefits of "this epizootic dispensation."

"By pedestrianism," he glimmered, "you are helping digestion, strengthening your lungs, and building up a nice pair of calves." Some city dwellers also embraced walking as an antidote to the growing stratification of urban society. "People who have not walked to any considerable extent for years," Akron's *Summit County Beacon* remarked, "are now compelled to 'boot it' just like poorer and healthier mortals."[58]

Others, though, viewed pedestrianism as a bane instead of a boon. "Walking is well enough," granted the *Raleigh News*, "but compulsion makes it rather a bore . . . , while on inclement evenings it is quite out of the question." Working-class Northeasterners, most of whom had to show up for work in any weather or risk losing their jobs, seemed especially frustrated at the prospect of hoofing it. Over the preceding decades, after all, many Americans of humbler means had left the region's cities to seek out more affordable housing in streetcar suburbs. After the epizootic struck Lansingburg, New York, for instance, the "large number of girls and workingmen" who commuted from this bedroom community to factories and shops in nearby Troy "suffered most." With streetcars shuttered, they had to walk four miles to work—and another four miles to get home at the end of the day. A Pennsylvania scribe set widely repeated complaints about pedestrianism to verse:

> Oh, epizoot, vile epizoot,
> You make me go too much on foot;
> You spoil our patent polished leather,
> By going in all kinds of weather.

"This horse distemper," as a correspondent from Boston summed it up, became "a singular trial of human legs and temper."[59]

Duly Thankful to the Ox

Equine labor proved only slightly easier to replace in the freighting sector. Neither water transport nor steam trains could satisfy the demand left unmet by the novel influenza virus's paralyzing impact on short-distance haulage. A few observers saw an opening for steam traction engines, but these ponderous juggernauts, which looked like tractors and rumbled atop roadways on enormous iron wheels, proved too rare and temperamental to make much impact. In the end, only muscle could remedy the shortfall in motive power the epizootic had caused. But whose muscles, and with what consequences?[60]

Manpower—together with childpower and womanpower—offered an obvious answer. "On every hand," a Kansan wrote from Chicago, "you see wheelbarrows, hand trucks, and every conceivable vehicle brought into requisition to meet the extraordinary emergency." As the epizootic entered its second week in Boston, postmen began hefting mailbags over their shoulders, sanitation workers stepped down from offal carts to drag stinking loads to rendering plants, and a quartet of policemen carried an injured man to the city hospital after no horse-drawn ambulance could be found. "Yankee ingenuity," the *Evening Transcript* noted, was "taxed to its utmost to perform the work usually assigned to horses." Business owners hastened to exploit the novel "mode of advertising" that human-powered hauling presented. The epizootic, the *Evening Transcript* mused, had "a ludicrous as well as a serious phase." One downtown factory owner, for instance, hired a brass band to parade a trio of wagons drawn by "nearly three hundred men" and loaded with "magnificent furniture" down the city's main commercial thoroughfare. "Instead of sitting down and sulking," Bostonians, as a *Globe* reporter smugly noted, "gayly harness themselves to the loaded wagons, and, with bands playing and colors flying, parade the principal streets."[61]

The *Sun* laid bare the economic calculus that drew many to take up horses' work. Because of the outbreak, it noted, "laboring men are enabled to make larger wages than usual in pulling vehicles." Workhands, blared the *Philadelphia Inquirer*, "were yesterday paid as much as TWENTY-FIVE DOLLARS FOR HAULING MERCHANDISE"—an astounding windfall for manual workers who considered themselves fortunate in ordinary times if they could earn three dollars for a full day's shift.[62]

Journalists offered few details regarding who stepped in to do the labor horses could no longer perform. Immigrants and African Americans, though, probably hefted more than their share of the burdens equines could no longer lug. A Chicago businessman boasted of having employed "a team for nearly two weeks that the 'epizootic' can't touch—an eight man power team of steady Dutchmen, steam made of 'zwei lager' [two beers]; very slow, but better than none." A Richmond scribe scoffed when he spied a wagon "loaded with flour, . . . with one stout darkey in the shafts, while the others pushed behind." A *Post* reporter, by contrast, praised the business acumen of several "stalwart colored men" who pulled "several 'muscular Express wagons'" through the Steel City. Evidently inspired by the twenty-one cents of "clear profit" these Pittsburghers raked in for every bushel of coal they delivered, "several women" huffily described by the *Post* as "well developed specimens of a class who can ill afford either to do without coal" or pay the epizootic-inflated price of thirty cents a bushel, soon began "hauling coal in an express wagon" of their own.[63]

Even with opportunity knocking, though, few people willingly took on such toil, especially when nonequine animals could be made to move the burdens equines could no longer draw. Some people initially hoped that the epizootic might spare mules from such ravages, but these creatures proved just as susceptible to the scourge as horses. Humans also hitched up dogs, goats, and even—if one newspaper is to be believed—a "pair of white stags." Yet oxen—castrated steers of at least two or three years of age trained since youth to follow a driver's verbal commands—quickly became the most popular stand-ins for sick equines. With the Great Horse Flu stupefying New York City, a Boston newspaper opined that "the introduction of oxen from the country" promised "the only solution" to Gotham's transportation woes. The sudden, wide-ranging experiment with bovine labor—not just in New York, but wherever the outbreak reached—marked a dramatic turnabout for a species of working animal that seemed well on its way to obsolescence. Over the preceding few decades, after all, townspeople and city dwellers alike had systematically replaced oxen with horses, leading the total US population of the former creatures to plummet from 2.2 million in 1860 to 1.3 million in 1870.[64]

Americans overwhelmingly associated oxen with a bygone era, so these bovines' sudden reappearance in Northeastern cities struck many onlookers as a quaint throwback. A Buffalo newspaper hailed the return of "this primeval method" of haulage. Less than a week later, with the Great Horse Flu pummeling Manhattan, the sight of a "multitude of ox-teams" on Broadway, with "bucolic drivers" piloting them, "caused a sensation." A reporter described how "an astonished and yet admiring crowd of people" accompanied "each caravan" of oxen as they lumbered off the boats that carried them to Manhattan's South Ferry and into the urban jungle beyond. "To judge from the amusing expressions of opinion and the general surprise at what seemed an innovation, or rather a retrogression," the same journalist wryly remarked of the time-warping spectacle that ensued, "one might almost have supposed that the majority of gazers had never beheld or known the existence of such an animal as the ox."[65]

The oxen who came to urbanites' rescue originated, of course, not in the past, but instead in rural areas where bovine labor remained a mainstay. Just days after the Great Horse Flu struck any given town or city, the cost to purchase or lease oxen shot upwards. Farmers with spare bovines sniffed opportunity, while Poughkeepsie mayor B. G. Eastman felt compelled to give the market a helping hand. In a letter published in the *New York Herald* on October 27, Eastman offered to send "a hundred, or many more, yoke of Dutchess county oxen, with drivers" to New York City by boat "on short notice." Dozens of Gothamites telegraphed responses to Eastman's proposition. "We want oxen by the week," one city dweller demanded; "supply us by tonight's boat," another urged. True to his word, Eastman dispatched an initial shipment of one hundred stout bovines down the Hudson on October 30.[66]

Oxen's initial success stoked further speculation. New York City's "large wholesale merchants, and those who were compelled to transmit goods in order to fulfill orders," began buying up yoke after yoke of the beasts from farms across New York and New Jersey. Manhattan's desperate retailers dished out as much as twelve dollars a day for every pair of oxen they could get, "with driver accompanying." Although one manufacturer grumbled at these "extortionate" rates, most businesspeople realized that they were at the market's mercy with demand for ox power becoming so "feverish" that, as the *Herald* declared, it became "impossible to supply it." As the epizootic fanned out, citizens of Boston, Newark, Burlington, Bridgeport, Chicago, Baltimore, Cincinnati, and other urban centers followed New Yorkers' lead and "sent to the interior," where livestock dealers began "rapidly collecting oxen." By mid-November, Vermonters and New Hampshirites were moaning that seaboard buyers were "carrying off all their oxen to play horse in the cities."[67]

Bovines possessed several advantages over the equines they replaced. They were often less expensive to buy or rent, not to mention hardier as well as easier and cheaper to feed, since oxen could subsist on grass or hay alone (urban equines typically required a mix of hay and grain). The wholesale return of oxen to city streets also had novelty value. In Boston, for example, the city's leading department store outfitted an ox-drawn wagon nicknamed the Bull Express to transport commuters downtown, while the Oriental Tea Company gilded its oxen's horns to match its golden delivery wagons. And in contrast to horses and other equines, whom Americans had long considered unsuitable for human consumption, oxen could be slaughtered and sold as beef once they could no longer earn their keep.[68]

Serious drawbacks, though, offset these advantages. Flu-fueled "demand for trained steers" swiftly pushed oxen prices through the roof. Prices hit $325 per yoke in Chicago, a markup of several hundred percent. Oxen were plodding as well as pricey. "We are duly thankful to the ox for service in this time of need," one New Yorker granted, before griping that "he is a little too slow for the bustling city." According to the *New York Turf*, oxen "travelled at the rate of about one mile in twenty-five minutes"—slower than the average human walked. Despite outweighing horses, oxen also proved unable to "draw such heavy loads" as equines did, or at least so the *Chicago Tribune* insisted.[69]

While oxen's pace and strength were essentially hard-wired, another physical disparity—oxen have softer feet than horses—became a problem only because Northeasterners had spent the previous few decades industriously paving over thousands of miles of city streets. "All our streets and avenues are primarily constructed for the horse," acknowledged the *Phrenological Journal* in an article that kept returning to a downcast refrain on human dependency: "We are hopelessly tied to the horse." As the epizootic brought oxen back to towns and cities, the mismatch between bovine requirements and roadways resurfaced to ease the passage of horse-powered vehicles became painfully obvious. A Boston newspaper reported, for instance, that "the feet of many" of the oxen shipped into that city from rural New England swiftly became "so sore that a bovine without a limp is the exception."[70]

Fitting oxen with iron shoes provided a ready solution. "Curious crowds" congregated in Chicago as "a corps of experienced ox-shoers from the plains" used "steam-driven blasts" fueled by ten raging coal fires to shoe forty oxen per day. As this mention of "ox-shoers from the plains" suggests, blacksmiths who had learned their trade in Northeastern cities usually had little or no experience in the peculiar art of ox-shoeing. Oxen's hoofs are not just cloven but also thinner than horses', so shoeing them required shorter nails. Furthermore, oxen, unlike horses, have difficulty balancing on three legs, which led many blacksmiths to suspend the hulking beasts in leather slings hooked to ceilings or roof beams. The *Boston Globe*'s Cincinnati correspondent noted that people there tried to avoid the difficulties shoeing presented by seeking out "light oxen," who seemed suited to "stand our boulder pavements better than beasts distinguished for avoirdupois [the system for measuring weight that Americans borrowed from Britain]."[71]

Oxen were not just soft-footed, slow, and ill shaped, but also hard to handle. Oxen brought to Albany to replace flu-addled horses showed an annoying tendency to "get balky and cause more trouble then [*sic*] a squadron of army mules." When an inexperienced truckman attempted to drive a pair of oxen through Philadelphia's busy center, mayhem ensued. After these restive bovines caused a traffic jam, the teamster unhitched the animals, then stood aghast as they sauntered off "to go into the Commonwealth National Bank" like proverbial bulls in a china shop. This tendency to "run away—with or without provocation—and smash things" led more than a few commentators to dismiss oxen as "entirely too firey [*sic*] for the city."[72]

Caricatures of oxen as unruly and stubborn, however, may tell us more about human limitations than bovine characteristics. Few inhabitants of Northeastern cities, after all, still knew how to manage the creatures. There was "as much science in driving oxen," insisted the *Nashville Union and American*, "as in running an engine or riding a two-wheel velocipede [a primitive bicycle that was legendarily hard to master]." Oxen were their own animals, and those who attempted to boss them using strategies calculated to bend equine wills usually met with failure.[73]

To avoid these issues, city slickers generally preferred to bring in experienced drivers, mostly adolescents or young men. Many urbanites, though, boasted rural roots, as reports from Chicago emphasized. An Ohio correspondent reported from the Windy City that a "good number of the prominent business men" there "ha[d] shown where they have passed their youthful days, by taking the whips and bringing the oxen around in." "The number of men who assert their ability, acquired by early education, to manage ox teams," gasped the *Chicago Evening Post*, "is astonishing." Not all who portrayed themselves as crack oxen drivers, however, could walk their talk. Even country boys who had grown into city men learned that it was not always easy to resuscitate skills they had not practiced for many years. Newspapers mocked "the rediclous [*sic*] failures of men with store clothes to manage the fiery beasts" and joked that the resulting standoffs and fracases "supplie[d] some fun" for onlookers intent on escaping the "melancholy" that circulated in the Great Horse Flu's slipstream. Meanwhile, the president of the Illinois Humane Society lashed out at drivers who "seem to think that oxen are incapable of pain or suffering, and consequently greatly overload them, besides treating them cruelly in various ways."[74]

Fortunately, such abuses seem not to have lasted. Oxen, observed the *Chicago Tribune*, "improve much by use," "and the difficulties in handling them that were at first experienced" were fast "disappearing." Even green drivers could begin to develop workable partnerships within just a week or two of taking up the bullwhip and learning to command oxen using voice prompts: "get up" or "come up" to start, "whoa" to stop, "gee" to turn right, "haw" to go left, and "back" to reverse course. The *Tribune* credited oxen for their growing spirit of cooperation, exclaiming that oxen "ha[d] become familiar with the city, and no longer refuse to turn street corners." Bovines who had returned to Chicago from its hinterlands in a "barefooted" condition, the same article quipped, not only began "wearing shoes," but also "acquired 'city airs.'"[75]

In early November, the *New York Herald* reflected on the cumulative impact of replacing epizootic-addled equines with oxen. Although "the idea" of "bringing the yoke and heavy wagons once more into use in the city" had been "derided at first," this bovine reappearing act helped New Yorkers to avoid total commercial paralysis. A Bostonian presented a similar perspective from Cincinnati, where, he claimed, the epizootic had "interfered comparatively little with trade and transportation" because of "the speedy and large importation of oxen into the city from the broad fields of Ohio, Indiana and Kentucky." As the Great Horse Flu swamped the countryside, oxen even began stepping in for flu-stricken canal ponies and mules to pull boats loaded with grain, coal, and other commodities.[76]

The *Chicago Tribune* expressed a common viewpoint when it celebrated the importation of trained bovines and skilled drivers from the country as "our salvation from general business stagnation." "The slow and stupid oxen," concluded the *Alton (IL) Telegraph*, "which, in all time, have been patient and uncomplaining workers" but "which have been so universally anathematized and abused by their drivers, are now on the topmost wave of popularity, and thousands are ready to appreciate their faithfulness and shout their praises."[77]

The epizootic's romp from the Three Townships to engulf the entire Northeast proved swift, thorough, and consequential. In less than a month, the new viral variant whose evolution had ignited the outbreak revealed itself to be a boundary-crashing superbug—a master parasite ideally designed to trouble the metabolic and replicative machinery of horses and the humans who depended on them at scales ranging from the cellular to the continental. The favorable disease ecology of southeastern Canada and the northeastern United States facilitated the Great Horse Flu's dramatic spread. Horses and their kin, as we have seen, were highly social creatures bound into immense, essentially continuous populations because of the central roles their brawn and brains played in a capitalist system that was inextricably equine-powered.

The novel influenza virus brought that system to its knees. The flu-fueled mayhem the outbreak unloosed laid bare, in turn, the social dynamics of urban societies on both sides of the international border—the push by immigrants and African American men and women to turn animal debility to their own economic advantage, the struggle of workers who depended on streetcars and other equine-powered transit technologies to journey from low-rent neighborhoods on urban peripheries to the downtown shops and factories where many of them labored, and the restiveness of carters in Montreal who had bristled for years against the humiliating settlement that city's business class had imposed after their unsuccessful 1864 strike for higher wages.

With the outbreak tightening its grip on the Northeast and human efforts to contain the outbreak failing miserably, veterinary experts, quacks, and animal welfare reformers all hastened to enter the fray. Whether they could do right by ailing horses, though, remained an open question.

CHAPTER 3

A HORSE'S LETTER

Sympathy, Healing, and the Limits of Humanitarianism

In early 1873, a few months after the epizootic brought New York to a standstill, the *Brooklyn Union* published "A Horse's Letter." This odd little article offered an arresting exploration of the outbreak's revolutionary potential as well as a touching testament to the kindness the Great Horse Flu momentarily kindled. Thomas DeWitt Talmage—an immensely popular Presbyterian minister whose five-thousand-seat Brooklyn Tabernacle had burned down just a few months earlier—credited himself as this missive's translator. Signed "Charley Bucephalus" and addressed from the "Brooklyn Livery Stables," the letter told a moving tale of suffering, interdependence, resistance, and care in the time of influenza.[1]

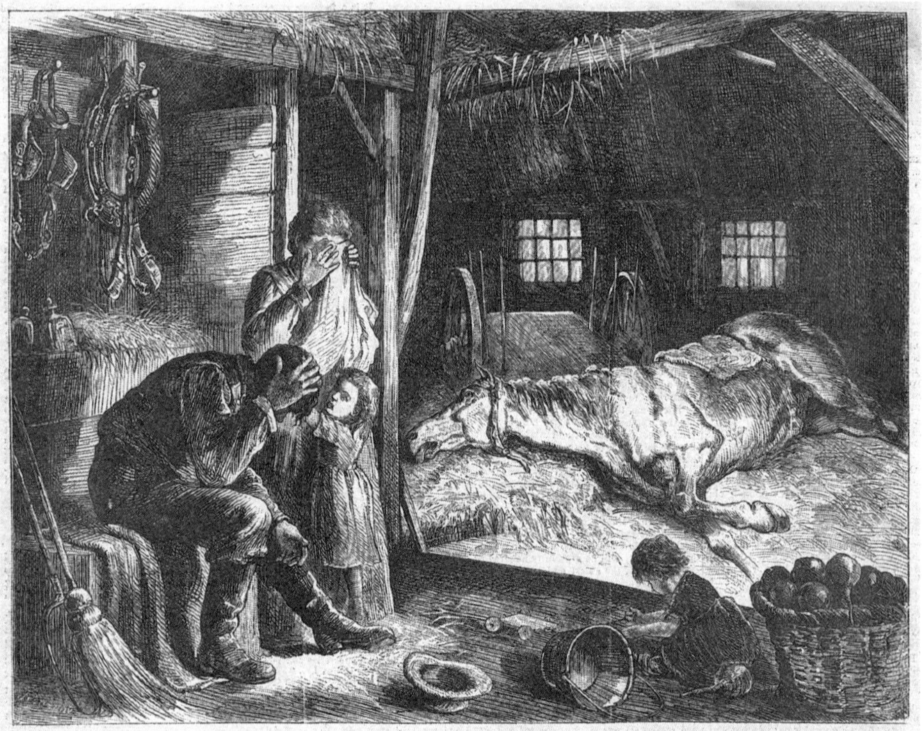

Paul Frenzeny's engraving poignantly illustrates both the suffering the epizootic inflicted on the horses it infected, and the devastation the outbreak often produced for working-class families. Paul Frenzeny, "Ruined, and Winter at the Door," *Harper's Weekly*, November 23, 1872, 908. Courtesy of HathiTrust, https://babel.hathitrust.org/cgi/pt?id=mdp.39015014703303&seq=865/.

"I am aware that this is the first time a horse has ever taken upon himself to address any member of the human family," Talmage's narrator intoned with a gravitas befitting the precedent he believed he was setting. And indeed, "A Horse's Letter" anticipated the two most famous works of equine ventriloquism in nineteenth-century literature, *Kholstomer* (*The Strider*, begun by Leo Tolstoy in the 1860s but not released until 1886) and *Black Beauty* (which Anna Sewell started in 1871 and published in 1877; its first American edition, released in Boston and subtitled *The "Uncle Tom's Cabin" of the Horse*, swiftly sold more than a million copies). Charley, who claimed direct paternal descent from Alexander the Great's beloved steed Bucephalus, declared that although he and his fellow equines had "endured in silence all the outrages of many thousands of years," the epizootic had convinced them that it was "now time to make remonstrance." The "recent attentions" that Brooklyn's horses had enjoyed during the outbreak's peak, Charley explained, "have made us aware of our worth."[2]

Back during the outbreak's peak, Charley recounted, "we had at our stables innumerable calls from doctors and judges and clergymen. Everybody asked about our health. Groomsmen bathed our throats, and sat up with us nights, and furnished us pocket handkerchiefs. For the first time in years we had quiet Sundays." Charley recounted how he and his stablemates had "overheard a conversation that made us think that the commerce and the fashion of the world [a]waited the news from the stable. Telegraphs announced our conditions across the land and under the sea," Charley reminisced, "and we came to believe that this world was originally made for the horse, and man his groom."

As Talmage's readers learned straight from the horse's mouth, the epizootic upended time-honored assumptions of human dominion. In Charley's telling, flu-related disruptions pulled back the curtain on a core paradox of horse-powered capitalism: Horses' labors became even more pivotal as the steam age intensified, but Americans' treatment of the equines they called their own seemed to deteriorate in inverse proportion to the animals' growing importance. Charley and his stablemates looked back on the Great Horse Flu with palpable nostalgia. By exposing this paradox for all to see, the outbreak, "A Horse's Letter" claimed, spurred Brooklynites and other Americans to mend their ways.[3]

Charley fondly remembered the turnabout the epizootic had conjured: "innumerable calls from doctors" and other community leaders to ailing animals, stablemen sitting vigil to nurse flu-stricken horses back to health, and round-the-clock reporting from newspapers and wire services. In Charley's telling, the epizootic had made the impossible seem attainable. The suffering the scourge had inflicted impelled people to come to their senses, acknowledge their deep reliance on equine labor, prioritize the commonalities between horses and humans over their differences, and extend consideration across species divides. With the horse plague paralyzing the continent's most populous and dynamic region for weeks on end, Charley and his fellow equines had dared to dream, in short, that a new ethic of care might be dawning.

The Great Horse Flu laid bare Americans' addiction to horsepower—and, with it, the profound vulnerabilities that stemmed from their utter dependence on flu-prone creatures. Wherever and whenever the epizootic struck, appreciation for equines surged. "Suddenly every horse-owner who has been accustomed to abuse his animal, now that there is a prospect of losing him," declared the *Chicago Tribune*, "discovers that he is a dear friend, a noble creature, deserving of the kindest consideration and most touching care."[4]

Unfortunately for Charley Bucephalus and his fellow equines, the heightened concern Americans expressed for their horses' welfare at the outbreak's height proved all too transitory. "Things," Talmage had Charley grumble, "are going back again where they were." After the outbreak relented its hold on the Northeast, Charley and his pals at the Brooklyn Livery Stables had once again been driven too far, fed too little, "jerked in the mouth, struck on the back," and left "unblanketed in the cold." And so "the other night," Charley informed *Union* readers, "after our owner had gone home, and the hostlers were asleep, we held an indignation meeting." When it came Charley's turn to address this equine assembly, he recounted his life story. Echoing a key trope in abolitionist literature, he recalled the day on which his "whole family was sold," his aunt's death from the flu, and the lifelong physical and emotional pain he had endured from "the saddles that gall, the spurs that prick, the snaffles that pinch, the loads that kill."

Charley's anguished recitation pushed one "vicious-looking nag" past her breaking point. Rearing up and taking the floor in a scene that was likely inspired by newspaper caricatures of shrill female radicals during the 1871 Paris Commune, the mare "squealed out the suggestion that it was time for a rebellion, and she moved that we take the field, and that all those who could kick should kick, and that all those who could bite should bite, and that all those who could bolt should bolt, and that all those who could run away should run away." By "fill[ing] the land with broken wagons, and smashed heads," she concluded, rebellious equines could "teach our oppressors that the day of retribution has come, and that our down-trodden race will no more be trifled with."[5]

The assembled horses decided to put the nag's proposal to a vote. "Not one said 'Aye,'" Charley approvingly reported, "but all cried 'Nay! nay!' And for the space of half an hour kept on neighing." Having shouted down the "harsh measure" of revolution, Charlie and his companions graciously resolved to give Brooklynites another chance. Favoring persuasion and patience over revolt and retribution, they "voted that . . . I should write this letter of remonstrance."

Charley concluded his plea by urging *Union* readers to "remember that we, like yourselves, have moods, and cannot always be frisky and cheerful." Talmage's narrator implored humans to get over themselves and mend their ways. "Care for us at some other time than during the epizootics [*sic*]," he begged, "so that we may see your kindness is not selfish. My dear friends," Charley entreated, "our interests are mutual. I am a silent partner in your business. Under my sound hoof is the diamond of national prosperity," and "beyond my nostril the world's progress may not go . . . . Be kind to me," he begged, "if you want me to be useful to you."

As equines in Brooklyn and throughout the Northeast learned, the epizootic brought no enduring salvation. Despite Talmage's playful efforts to remind readers of the prayers they had offered when their animals neared death's door and the promises they had uttered while nursing their steeds and nags back to health, Americans soon forgot the lessons the equine scourge imparted. The Great Horse Flu had highlighted the interreliance of humans and horses as well as their shared susceptibility to influenza and its complications. It also prompted a fleeting surge in Americans' capacity to sympathize with equines—to see them as fellow beings with whom they shared maladies, interests, and feelings. In all these ways, "A Horse's Letter" testified to both the heightened sympathy and care the epizootic fostered, and the deep-seated constraints in thought and practice that doomed American equines to disenchantment once the outbreak relented.

Brisk Business in Dead Horses

The Great Horse Flu confronted Northeasterners with a stomach-turning dilemma: What to do with the corpses the epizootic churned out? Different people devised disparate responses, variously casting deceased equines as beloved companions, broken-down machines, seedbeds of contagion, and storehouses of raw materials. Expert and amateur investigators alike, though, also saw the bodies of dead horses, mules, and donkeys as valuable repositories of scientific data. Postmortem examinations soon confirmed that the complications that traveled in the epizootic's wake posed even greater dangers than influenza itself. This finding served, in turn, to reinforce the emerging perception that the disease could circulate between equines, humans, and other hosts. It also underlined the wisdom of treating the epizootic by translating key principles of human flu care for equine patients.

A tiny fraction of flu victims received burial with honors. New York transportation mogul Cornelius Vanderbilt, whom one reporter described as "deeply depressed, as a parent at the loss of a child," interred Mountain Boy, a champion trotter he had purchased six years earlier for an estimated $14,000, in a four-thousand-square-foot plot that Vanderbilt vowed would forever remain "consecrated to the Commodore's favorite." In Evanston, Illinois, a donkey who "was the property of the children of Mr. O. French, and was of a very diminutive size," was given "a very elaborate and impressive ceremony," then "interred in shroud and coffin." And a valuable "bay stallion" named Star, whom the *Alexandria (VA) Gazette* characterized as a mix "of Black Hawk and Morgan stocks," was set in the ground following a funeral "attended by sixty-odd people" after succumbing to "the effects of the late epizootic" nearly a year after contracting the malady. "Most attendees" reportedly brought "home with them pieces" of Star's mane as mementos mori.[6]

Most of the equines killed by the epizootic, though, received no obsequies. Nineteenth-century North Americans often likened horses and their kin to living machines; once these machines ceased to function, many owners unceremoniously abandoned them like so much trash, leaving them to decompose where they had fallen. Canada's Gatineau Road, for instance, was lined with what the *Ottawa Citizen* called "a number of overworked and overdosed horses." In St. Louis's northern precincts, "numerous dead horses" littered "alleys and vacant lots." Others tossed dead equines into the nearest body of water. On one Pennsylvania waterway, "numbers" of canal ponies killed by the epizootic were described as having "been pitched over to the care of Davy's Locker," while the *Portland (ME) Press Herald* quipped that "lovers of eels," which many New Englanders of the time prized as delicacies, "may or may not be gratified to learn that numerous valiant steeds that succumbed to the epizootic have been cast into the briny deep at various points about the city."[7]

A few weeks later along the Ohio River, conflict erupted over the risks that equine corpses posed to human health. The trouble began, the *Pittsburgh Post* reported, after "quite a number of fatal cases occurred" in western Pennsylvania's largest metropolis and "nearly all" of the corpses were "dumped in the river. This will give our neighbors below," the *Post* teased, "sweet essence of 'epizoot' in their drinking water." Downstreamers, though, recoiled at the Pittsburghers' careless actions. "We see the carcasses of horses which have died of the epizooty in Pittsburgh floating past here every day or two," griped the *Wheeling Register*. A few days later, Cincinnatians raised a ruckus after a flotilla of equine cadavers washed up along the Ohio River. One wire service item reported, "The stomach of Porkopolis"—the nickname Cincinnati's illustrious slaughterhouses had earned the city—"squirms at the idea of imbibing horse tea." Such complaints led the *Pittsburgh Post* to change its tune. "There was and is no excuse," it conceded, "for thus poisoning the waters of our rivers as even during the crisis of the horse disease, it was much easier to bury the defunct equines in the suburbs than to haul them, as was done in many instances, several miles to the rivers."[8]

Not all dead equines, however, became refuse. Most, in fact, were turned into fertilizer, glue, and other products. In the early 1870s, most larger cities relied on so-called offal contractors to remove animal corpses from urban spaces. At the epizootic's height, though, these small proprietors struggled to keep up. A few weeks after the Great Horse Flu reached Brooklyn, that city's policemen began fielding "numerous complaints . . . about the non-removal of the carcases [*sic*] of horses that have died of the malady raging at present in the Redhook Point district." Around the same time, Philadelphia offal contractor A. W. Louth raised his fee for hauling away dead horses from two dollars to five and finally ten dollars a head. After influenza debilitated Louth's own steeds, though, the *Inquirer* contemplated the "unwelcome thought . . . that it may yet occur that dead bodies of the epizootic victims will have to remain where they fall." Fortunately for Philadelphians, Louth and his competitors soon pivoted to oxen, ensuring that the "bone yards at Bridesburg" outside the city could continue to do "brisk business in dead horses." Animal recycling industries on the outskirts of other towns and cities also boomed. A Mississippi paper described New Orleans's "bone factory" as "doing a good business, hauling off the dead epizootics," an Indianapolis newspaper griped that "the odors which are wafted over the north part of the city when the wind is from the west, give strong evidence that the dead animal man is trying up the horses and mules which have succumbed to the epizootic," and a *Free Press* reporter observed "quite a pile of bones . . . rapidly rising into monumental dignity" at a boneyard outside Detroit, "commemorative to the ravages of the malady."[9]

By the early 1870s, American industry had practically perfected the transmogrification of dead horses into salable goods. According to a *Scientific American* article, an expired equine's "blood is sought by the manufacturers of albumen, and by sugar refiners, and the burners of lamp black. Not a drop is allowed to go to waste." The horse's mane and tail provided "haircloth, sieves, bow-strings, and brushes." Its skin became "leather for cart harnesses, for boots and shoes, and strong collars. The hoofs are used for combs, horn work, [and] glue," while the teeth served "as substitutes for ivory." The animal's stomach and intestines could "make valuable strings and cords for musical instruments; and out of the bones so many useful articles are manufactured that it is almost impossible to make out a complete list of them," including "buttons, toys, tweezers, knife-handles, rulers, cups, dominoes, [and] balls." As for the animal's flesh, this was "boiled down in the rendering vat, and much oil and fat are obtained from it. Some of the choice bits may find their way into cheap restaurants," the reporter admitted, where they might "play the part of beefsteak, or help to enrich the hasty plates of soup" that cheaper eateries dished out to America's harried masses. Whatever remained of an equine's carcass "after all has been extracted from it that is of any service" would then be "burned" to make fertilizer; "worked up into nitrogenous compounds . . . to be used by the photographer in taking our pictures"; or "converted into phosphorus, for the manufacture of matches." A horse "must be a remarkably good one," *Scientific American*'s brisk but exhaustive recounting sardonically remarked, "if he is worth as much when alive as he is to the retorts and kettles of the chemist." With ghoulish ingenuity driven by market sensibilities, inventors, mechanics, and industrialists all scavenged profits from the corpses the Great Horse Flu offered up.[10]

These corpses held the potential not only to imperil other organisms but also to elucidate some of the scourge's many mysteries. Not surprisingly, amateurs and experts alike took up knives and scalpels and plunged them into dead horses in search of clues about the epizootic's pathology and epidemiology. Freeman C. Ham of South Berwick, Maine, for instance, sliced open a "valuable horse" he owned to reveal a chest cavity "full of matter"—incontrovertible evidence that pneumonia, one of the most common influenza sequelae, caused this animal's death. Veterinary surgeons and physicians often arrived at similar conclusions after autopsying the bodies of flu victims. A doctor with Cincinnati's Health Board, for instance, accompanied a druggist and an alderman to "the Fertilizing Company's stable." Having "asked for a fresh specimen," the group "were given the not yet cold carcass" of a coal deliveryman's horse. In Manhattan, a physician "attached to the Board of Health . . . made post-mortem examinations of a number of the bodies brought to the New York Rendering Company's dock." The "large quantity of viscid purulent secretion" he found in these animals' sinuses enabled him to pinpoint their cause of death as "capillary bronchitis, coupled in some instances with pneumonia."[11]

As autopsies often revealed, influenza rarely did its dirty work in isolation. An unknown but significant percentage of epizootic fatalities, in fact, resulted from the rogue's gallery of bacteria and other viruses that often attacked at the same time as the flu or soon after it set in. With the epizootic holding Buffalo tight in its thrall, the *Courier Express* reported in late October 1872 on the lessons local veterinary surgeon William Somerville had learned after he took a second journey of epizootic-related discovery to Ontario. Just days after returning from the Niagara borderlands and spreading rumors accusing Canadian governor-general Lord Dufferin of bringing the flu across the US border, Somerville interviewed Andrew Smith, founder of Ontario Veterinary College and Toronto's leading horse doctor. Smith told Somerville that it "took only four days" after the flu reached Ontario's capital for it to "spread throughout the whole country in that vicinity." The Canadian veterinary surgeon also told his American colleague that on dissecting one of the Great Horse Flu's first victims, he discovered the "mucous surfaces of the trachea" of the horse "to be highly inflamed," with the disease "extending to the lungs." Drawing on his interview with Smith as well as his own observations, Somerville warned western New Yorkers that "the disease now prevailing in this vicinity" appeared to be "more virulent in form than in

Canada," explaining that "symptoms of lung disease"—pneumonia, bronchitis, pleurisy, and other inner respiratory infections—seemed to be "more frequent" south of the border.[12]

Postmortems also highlighted the heavy toll that a second and rarer set of complications—the host of disorders North Americans of the early 1870s lumped together under the rubric of "dropsy" (*hydropsie* in French, Spanish *hidropesía*)—exacted on the animals it attacked. Derived from the Greek *hydrops* or "water," dropsy (widely referred to today as edema) involved excessive inflammation. It was correctly understood as "a sign," as one historian explains, "of underlying disease of the heart, liver, and kidney." As veterinary surgeons and physicians recognized, the odds that a flu-stricken horse would suffer serious debility or death skyrocketed once dropsy reared its head.[13]

Collectively, the many dissections conducted on epizootic victims confirmed that most fatal cases resulted from complications rather than unaided influenza infections. Some postmortem exams, though, also reinforced the perception that flu affected people and equines in common—a principle that soon became a lodestar for human efforts to combat the equine scourge. When "two practicing physicians" stood before "a large concourse of spectators" in Baltimore and sliced into the corpse of Buffalo Bill, a "diminutive" three-month-old donkey who "had died the previous evening from epizootic," they learned that Bill, whose skin was "preserved to be stuffed," had perished from "the same influenza which attacks the human family."[14]

The Baltimore doctors' conclusions aligned with mounting evidence that even as the Great Horse Flu was infecting ever more equines, it was also extending its reach to sicken humans and a growing array of other creatures. Although such cases of spillover did not ignite widespread outbreaks, they nonetheless pointed toward two crucial developments: first, an emergent belief that the best way to heal flu-stricken horses was by adapting best practices in human flu care for equine use; and, second, a strident crusade by humanitarian reformers and their allies to convince—and, when necessary, to compel—their fellow Americans into extending greater consideration to suffering equines.

The Human Family May Have Its Turn

In late October, after diagnosing the disease that had recently invaded New York from Ontario as "epiglottic catarrh or influenza of horses," veterinarian James Law added that this was a malady "which at irregular intervals sweeps over entire continents, prostrating the whole equine creation." Then, drawing on recent studies that documented dozens of historical instances in which equines, humans, and several other types of creatures had developed flu-like symptoms in roughly the same place and time, Law understatedly warned, "It is not impossible, therefore, that the human family may have its turn." After glossing Law's portrait of influenza as capable of jumping from equines to humans, a Rochester editor expressed fears that "the present epizootic may be followed by an epidemic."[15]

Already newspapers were asserting that influenza had jumped from horses to numerous humans, including a hostler and three stable workers in Buffalo, a Boston fireman, and several citizens of Albany. In the wake of Law's address, people in Manhattan, Brooklyn, Jersey City, Baltimore, and North Providence, Rhode Island, had all purportedly "taken the horse disease from horses." These claims motivated a Pennsylvania editor to advise readers not "to approach affected horses," while a New York physician implored that city's sanitary commission to "prevent all travel by horsepower for a few days" to protect passengers from contagion.[16]

Meanwhile, cows in New Jersey, hogs in Massachusetts, and poultry in several parts of the Northeast were also falling ill with flu-like symptoms. The *Scranton Republican*, for instance, noted that "the 'epizootic' or some other 'zootic' has attacked the chickens" in that hardscrabble coal-mining center, "and we learn that they are dying off in great numbers in this city." Rather than "applying any remedies" to their poultry, the *Chicago Tribune* reported, many farmers there were instead killing "the fowl as soon as it is attacked," and then "send[ing] it to market." With Thanksgiving just days away, it was hard to avoid the suspicion, the *Tribune* scoffed, that "we may be eating roast, fried, broiled, and fricasseed epizootic." Newspapers even alleged, usually without presenting any evidence, that the outbreak was rippling outward to other creatures including rabbits, deer, antelopes, elk, raccoons, opossums, prairie chickens, and even lions and tigers at the Central Park Zoo. After a recently imported rhinoceros owned by George Bailey's circus died, surgeons autopsied it before a crowd in the operating theater at Manhattan's Bellevue Hospital but could pinpoint "no traces of the epizootic disease." Instead, physicians attributed the rhino's death to its "very badly swollen" intestines.[17]

Although some reports of the epizootic spreading to other species seem fanciful at best, others strongly suggest that the Great Horse Flu was indeed transgressing species divides. Thomas Moffat of Galt, Ontario, told a local journalist that "several" of his cows had come "down with a disease which resembles the epizootic in many particulars. They have the same cough, the same running at the nose, and exhibit the same languor." Hogs in Northumberland County, Pennsylvania, meanwhile, "were first noticed running at the nose, then swelling along the jaws, and coughing." And two Michigan cats believed to have died from influenza supposedly "presented all the symptoms of the disease as found among horses."[18]

Public fears that the epizootic might mushroom into a multispecies plague deepened in early November when newspapers asserted that several humans had died from the malady. In contrast to most early reports of human epizootic, though, which were usually consistent with influenza as the pathogenic agent, these deadly cases most likely resulted from bacterial co-invaders rather than the virus itself. The first such fatality involved a man in Quarryville, New York. While mucking out the mangers of "a couple of horses that had the distemper," one account claimed, "the virus came into contact with a flesh wound on his hand. In a short time," the man's "hand and arm became so terribly inflamed and swollen, they had to be amputated." Desperate efforts to save the man failed, and he succumbed "soon after." A few weeks later, a physician briefed a gathering of colleagues in Saratoga Springs on another victim, "who received some of the discharge in his eye, from a horse, whilst in the act of sneezing." The "poisonous influence" of the phlegm from this flu-stricken steed, the physician alleged, "prov[ed] fatal in two or three days."[19]

A larger body of cases, hardly any of them fatal, strongly suggested that the novel influenza virus itself often afflicted human communities soon after striking local equines. By November, observers were blaming the epizootic for localized upswings of flu-like illness in several parts of the United States. Medical experts and laypeople alike linked stories of "human epizootic" to the equine version partly because of timing: With hardly any exceptions, cases of the human complaint seemed to spike soon after the equine scourge struck. Even more tellingly, observers listed symptoms matching those widely noted among equines at the time—and all too familiar to anyone who has ever hosted an influenza A infection: "coughing and running at the nose and ears"; "barking, expectorating at the nose, sore throat and general indisposition"; "enlargement of the glands, with inflamation [*sic*] of the mucous membrane of the trachea and bronchia" accompanied by "violent headache" and "fever for the first day or two"; loss of appetite, with some patients growing "painfully stiff"; "sudden prostration, and a disinclination to move"; "chills" and "pain in the limbs and back," heightened during the disease's first few days by "restlessness" during the day and "at night sleeplessness."[20]

Some skeptics cried foul. A Michigan newspaper, for instance, accused locals there of mistaking correlation for causation. "In the days of yore when Port Huron people had colds in their heads," that city's *Herald* argued, "they used to say frankly that they had 'a bad cold,'" but "now they disguise the naked fact by saying that they 'have an attack of the dreaded epizootic.'" Considerable evidence, though, indicates that within days or weeks of the epizootic's arrival, a significant percentage of people in many communities fell ill with complaints identical or very similar to those that were besetting North American equines. Media accounts portrayed flu as sickening "perhaps one-third of our people" in Monongahela, Pennsylvania; "whole families and villages around Windsor, Vermont; "every four persons out of five" in Seaford, Delaware; and "everybody" in Georgetown, Delaware. Human flu became so widespread and intense during the epizootic's American invasion as to leave enduring traces in vernacular speech. Even today, folks in some places refer to cold- or flu-like illnesses as "epizootic" or variants thereof, a clear linguistic callback to the Great Horse Flu's capacity to infect human victims.[21]

A few observers went so far as to explain epizootic spillover by invoking Charles Darwin, whose *Origin of Species* (1859) remained highly visible and controversial in the early 1870s. A writer in the *Minneapolis Star Tribune*, for instance, claimed that the "hundreds of cases of sore throat among our citizens which are accompanied by other symptoms similar to those shown in horses effected [*sic*] with epizooty . . . proves Darwin's theory." By positing that humans shared ancestors with nonhuman animals, the British scientist's work—especially his 1871 *On the Descent of Man*—showed why people and horses might suffer in common from the same complaint. Darwin observed that "man is liable to receive from the lower animals, and to communicate to them, certain diseases . . . and this fact proves the close similarity of their tissues and blood, both in minute structure and composition, far more plainly than does their comparison under the best microscope, or by the aid of the best chemical analysis." A Nevada newspaper applied such reasoning to the epizootic when it declared, "We believe these simultaneous attacks of human beings and brutes in different parts of the country by epidemical diseases of the same general type cannot be laughed away as mere coincidental circumstances of an ordinary character." It reasoned that "good natural philosophy sustains the assumption that these human and brute ailments are referable to the same general cause," even though debate over whether that cause was atmospheric or contagious remained heated and unresolved.[22]

The Great Horse Flu's spillover to humans and a host of other creatures prompted concern and even panic. Yet the supposition that "the same general cause" could explain both human influenza and "brute ailments" dovetailed with postmortem findings about the dangers of pneumonia, dropsy, and other complications to heighten concerns that bleeding, blistering, and other strenuous interventions were more likely to harm sick horses than to help them. The best way to ensure that equines would recover from the epizootic, Canadians and Americans were coming to discover, was to apply the Golden Rule: in other words, to minister to ailing equines in much the same way that human flu patients expected to be treated.

Turning Public Misery to Private Profit

As the Great Horse Flu sickened more and more equines in a fast-growing list of locales, Americans, like Canadians before them, enlisted a hodgepodge of practitioners who embraced various ideas about sickness, wellness, and healing. No orthodoxy on epizootic therapies ever took root. Broad agreement nonetheless emerged that minimalist approaches, those premised on the notion that what was good for humans suffering from influenza would also be beneficial for horses, ensured better outcomes than more aggressive regimens.

Many urbanites considered veterinary surgeons their go-to horse healers. The best-known of these equine health experts had trained at British and French veterinary colleges; several had subsequently emigrated to North America and established veterinary programs in the United States and Canada. By 1872, these institutions were credentialing a few dozen graduates yearly, nearly all of whom studied under Toronto's Andrew Smith or Montreal's Duncan MacEachern. The US Veterinary Medical Association dated to 1863, but this early effort at professionalization foundered. It took the organization several more decades before it could convince state legislatures to require veterinary practitioners to have earned a degree from accredited programs. When the Great Horse Flu struck, self-described veterinary surgeons ran the gamut from charlatans to savants. The most reputable suddenly had more business than they could handle. MacEachern and his students, to cite just one example, had "prescribed for and visited over 3,000 sick horses" within the outbreak's first two weeks in Montreal, "losing but eight."[23]

Yet there was nothing to prevent people who lacked advanced training in animal medicine from declaring themselves experts, then hawking their quackery to a desperate public. "The greater majority of the so-styled veterinary surgeons," griped Chicago physician G. A. Hall, "are very poorly qualified to discharge their duties, being uneducated, and possessing very little 'HORSE SENSE.'" "The great bulk of men, who profess to be veterinarians," one editor pointed out, "are those who have 'picked up' a small knowledge, if . . . they have any, of the domestic animals, and are about as well qualified to pursue their calling, as old wives, armed with their superstitial antidotes and harmless potions, are to be licensed as practicing physicians." Stable owners, hostlers, and others who drew their understandings of equine health and illness from practical experience instead of book learning probably saw at least as many flu patients as self-declared veterinarians and legitimately trained veterinary surgeons did.[24]

Physicians treated epizootic patients, too. "Some of our most intelligent physicians," the *Chicago Evening Post* approvingly noted, "are making the epizootic a special study, and are responding to all calls made upon them for medical attendance upon our afflicted equines." Human healers sometimes began treating flu-stricken horses because the animals they used to pull their buggies, carriages, and sleighs to the homes of their human clients fell ill. Yet physicians were also drawn to care for equines by the fundamental similarities they often noted between the epizootic and human flu. "The symptoms as detailed by the daily journals afford so strong an analogy to some epidemics of influenza among the human family," noted the *Scranton Republican*'s medical contributor, "that it should hardly be allowed to pass unnoticed, more especially when the treatment found most successful among men may afford an indication for treatment of the sick horses." Mounting evidence that the Great Horse Flu was spreading to human hosts presumably gave physicians added confidence in their methods. One appeal in the *Cincinnati Enquirer* implored junior physicians "with more time than patients on their hands" to "roll up their sleeves, and bring down to a focus the whole strength of their schooling, in order that we may find out something about the disease that is hourly making gaps in our stables." While it seems safe to presume that many doctors felt moved to make themselves useful as the crisis deepened, a mention in the *Herkimer (NY) Democrat and Little Falls Gazette* that "veterinary surgeons are too scarce to reap the rich harvest which is now ready for gathering" suggests that profit motives probably enticed more than a few physicians to repurpose their favorite flu therapies for equine rather than human patients.[25]

With healers of so many stripes bent on exploiting the bull market for veterinary care the Great Horse Flu stimulated, most people turned to their own devices. "Every farmer," a Pennsylvania journal astutely pronounced in early December, "is his own veterinary physician," and many city dwellers and suburbanites proved equally intent on taking charge of ailing animals' care. Intent on helping their horses survive the scourge, people who owned equines or owed their livelihoods to them picked and chose among potential treatments drawn from three overlapping sources: folk remedies, print media, and patent medicines.[26]

After reading a newspaper story on the "fearful calamity raging among the horses in your part of the country," a Pottsville, Pennsylvania, farmer wrote the mayor of Rochester, New York, and urged him to encourage his

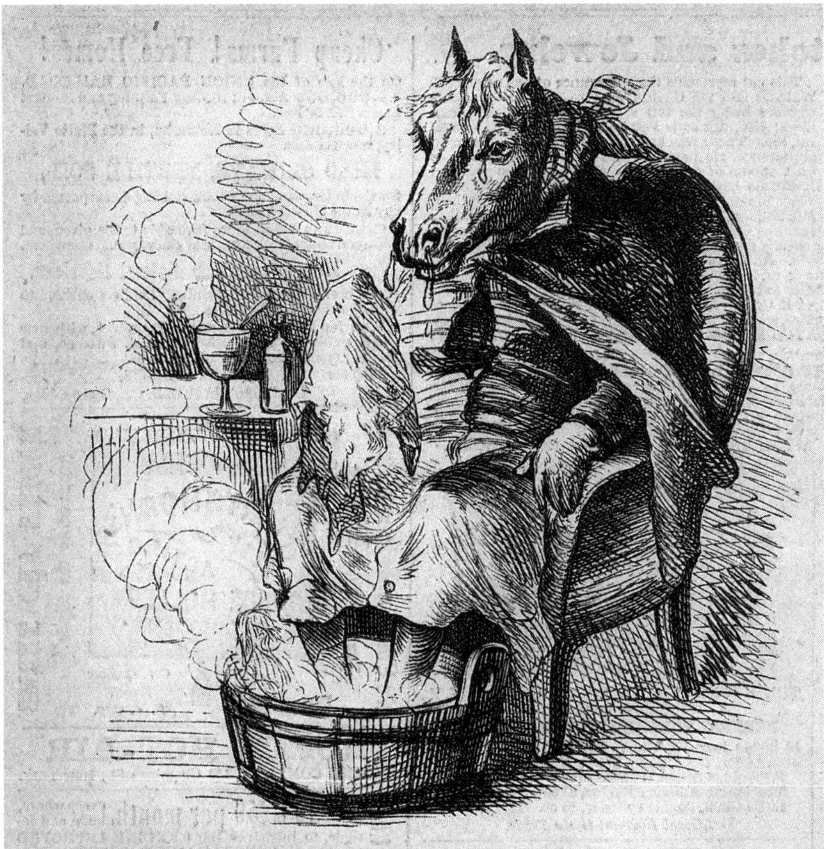

A CHEVAL-ROUS PATIENT.

"Ungrateful man never appreciated my faithful services until now. When I am convalescent I hope he will treat me with more consideration and kindness."

This *Harper's Weekly* cartoon portrays a flu-stricken horse in quasi-human form. His running nose and weeping eyes suggest the depths of his misery. The illustrator garbed the animal in a scarf; replaced his front hoofs with hands, one of which holds a handkerchief; and positioned the beast's hind legs in a steaming tub. The background, meanwhile, features a bottle of patent medicine beside a half-empty tumbler holding a straw or stirrer. The illustration's playful title riffs on the French word for "horse" to highlight this creature's virtue and commitment to duty—and, by extension, that of other equines afflicted by the epizootic. The caption, meanwhile, impugns Americans for their ingratitude toward horses but also speaks to the hopefulness some observers felt during the outbreak. By exposing the interspecies interdependence that people usually took for granted, the epizootic seemed poised to usher in a new era of human-equine sympathy. "A Cheval-rous Patient," *Harper's Weekly*, November 16, 1872, 904. Courtesy of University of Colorado Libraries.

citizenry to "try the following remedy. Let them burn a dead horse on a wood fire or log fire, burn it all up and then take the ashes of it and pulverized bones, and feed them to the other horses, and I will guarantee the epidemic to cease." This method, the farmer claimed, had helped to vanquish both a cattle "epidemic" and a "chicken sickness." Less bizarre folk cures included "steaming by putting vinegar on a hot brick in a bag," then "compelling" flu-stricken horses "to inhale the steam," as well as exposing sick horses to molten tar—a method that ended disastrously when a flu-addled horse belonging to a Delaware farmer "accidentally kicked over the pot and the tar caught and set fire to" a farmhouse and corncrib while also leaving the offending animal "pretty considerably singed."[27]

Like folk healers, newspapers and magazines—which the *Times*'s American correspondent reported were "full of the epizootic"—sought to do well from the epizootic by doing good. Several tidbits of therapeutic counsel drawn from correspondence or interviews with stablemen, physicians, veterinary surgeons, and US military officials soon entered such widespread circulation as to become memes. A regimen that veterinarian E. H. Mink supplied to a Rochester newspaper in mid-October 1872, for instance, subsequently appeared in the *New York Herald*, several upstate newspapers, *Moore's Rural New Yorker*, *American Farmers Advocate*, and the *American Farmer and Rural Register*. Thanks to the speed of telegraphic and postal communications, flu advice often reached readers weeks or months before the novel influenza virus struck.[28]

Editors and publishers sought to sell copies by providing plenty of guidance from supposed experts, but they also did brisk business selling flu-related advertisements. Patent medicine manufacturers, distributors, and vendors eagerly seized upon the Great Horse Flu to peddle powders, liniments, drenches, oils, and other treatments. Sherman Hall & Cook, for instance, marketed rosin-weed root in the *Chicago Tribune* as a "SURE CURE FOR THE EPIZOOTIC." The sellers of Renne's Pain-Killing Magic Cure—"BUY THE LARGE SIZE"—and James Welch, who plugged his compound as a "Certain Cure for the Epizootic," made nearly identical claims in the *Troy Weekly Times* and *Saratogian*, respectively.[29]

True to their reputation as "snake oil salesmen," many in the patent medicine trade eschewed transparency and instead marketed their products through advertisements masquerading as news stories. The makers of Centaur Liniment, which was manufactured by a Manhattan firm that one scholar describes as "a pioneer in mass marketing and advertising," placed copy in daily journals published in Buffalo, Chicago, New York City, and beyond. The liniment maker often plugged its advertisements into columns filled with real news articles, designing its ads to mimic these

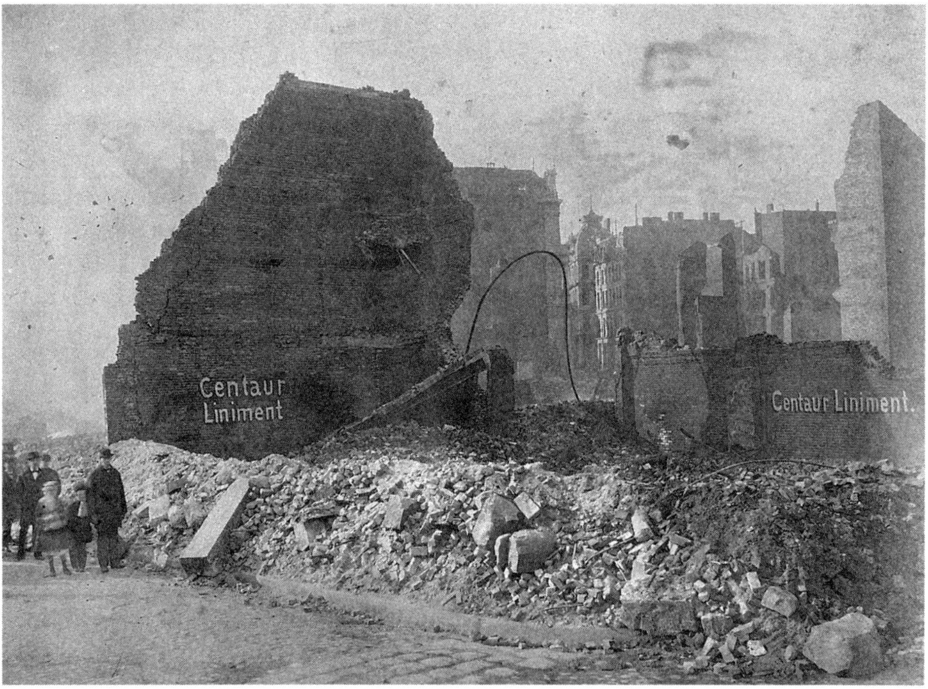

Centaur Liniment took advantage of the ruins created by the Great Boston Fire to advertise their product. James Wallace Black, *Ruins of Centaur Liniment near City Hall*, photograph (ca. 1872). Digital Commonwealth, https://ark.digitalcommonwealth.org/ark:/50959/2801pj89x.

items' layout and typography. Such ads began by triggering readers' anxieties: "The disease travels in the air," one plug for Centaur Liniment warned, "and seems to attack about one-third of the horses in a stable at the same instant"; "its treatment is not understood"; and "the disease seems to be without precedent." The marketers then turned to the hard sell: "When the throat, belly, and legs" of "well horses" were "rubbed with this Liniment," the animals "thus treated," they promised, "will not take the disease; and in stables where four-fifths of the horses have been attacked this treatment has cured the most of them in a few days." Centaur Liniment's "effects," in short, were "simply wonderful"—or so its makers professed.[30]

At least one popular medicine—asafetida, which is best known today as an ingredient in South Asian cuisine but has been used for millennia to treat pulmonary conditions—experienced an all-out "panic" after newspapers extolled it as "a sure remedy for the epizootic" when placed in a small bag and hung from "the halter directly under the animal's nose." A lone druggist in Chicago—an 1873 directory listed seventy-seven pharmacists in that city—sold three tons of this pungent gum resin at two dollars per pound, a 400 percent markup from pre-epizootic prices.[31]

"Turning public misery to private profit," the media, one Missouri critic carped, touted "everything from Godfrey's cordial to Costor's rat poison" as an epizootic cure. Wire services reported that by late November, "two hundred and eighty-five distinct remedies ha[d] appeared in the daily papers as warranted to cure the horse disease." One Wisconsin editor asserted that although "some" of the "hundreds of prescriptions" circulating in the press were "serviceable and good," far more, were, "without doubt, . . . mere quack nostrums, more injurious than beneficial." N. H. Paaren of Chicago, veterinary editor for that city's *Prairie Farmer*, urged readers to turn a wary eye to "the number of 'great epizootic remedies' . . . going under the name of condition powders, liniments and ointments" touted by manufacturers, retailers, traveling salesmen, and street criers. Paaren vented about one "enterprising concern," for instance, that "posted placards everywhere, even on my doorsteps," championing "a liniment . . . that 'will cure the disease inside three days.' Does any one," Paaren implored, "believe that within three days all the sick horses in this city can be restored to usefulness?"[32]

Laboratory analysis confirmed Paaren's distrust. One "of these great epizootic remedies," he found, consisted of "a large proportion of calomel [a mercury compound], a little laudanum [tincture of opium], oil of spike [a lavender extract often used to thin oil paints], and assafoetida [*sic*], made palatable and bulky by the addition of molasses and water." A second compound, meanwhile, contained only "syrup of ginger, syrup of squills [an extract made from the bulbs of a relative of the hyacinth], and water" in a "very deceiving panel bottle, nicely labeled." Although Paaren estimated that these ingredients were "sold to confiding dupes for 'only one dollar,'" the contents of each bottle were only "worth about fifteen cents." Paaren concluded that most epizootic "cures" were "absolutely dangerous"—too much calomel, for instance, could easily kill a horse—and nearly always "ineffectual," lending "the poor horse but little chance for his life."[33]

Northeasterners' eclectic responses to the Great Horse Flu had contradictory consequences for flu-stricken equines. The remedies Americans embraced sometimes proved deadlier than the epizootic itself. Unskillful, excessive, or venal care aggravated mortality and heightened horses' suffering. Over the longer run, though, growing awareness of these failings among experts and laypersons alike lent additional momentum to the eclipse of so-called heroic therapies. It also reinforced the growing consensus that abundant rest and watchful nursing comprised the most powerful stratagems Americans could wield against influenza and its complications. Yet it remained to be seen whether this pragmatic sense of interspecies commonality would foster greater sympathy across species divides—and, in turn, prompt meaningful steps to prioritize horses' well-being over corporate profits, workers' earnings, and public convenience.

Rest over Harm

Canadian horse healers overwhelmingly advised clients during the outbreak's early weeks to give sick horses a break from their customary labors while lavishing them with supportive care. Although some veterinarians hewed fast to traditional treatments—one Hamilton vet, for instance, prescribed "diuretics and stimulants for *internal*, and ammoniacal liniment for *external*, application"—most seemed intent on following guidance summed up in an 1868 *Canada Farmer* article: "If what has been called heroic treatment is resorted to, viz., bleeding and purging, influenza proves a very fatal disease. From the beginning the strength of the animal must be sustained." When William Somerville traveled to Toronto to interview Canadian colleagues about how best to manage the epizootic, Andrew Smith implored him to steer clear of any treatment that sapped the patient's vitality. "Owners of afflicted horses," Smith urged, must "on no account give cathartics, or nauseating medicine of any kind." People who kept their horses at work or doctored them too aggressively, Smith and most other Canadian experts advised, opened the door to dangerous complications.[34]

Bleeding, blistering, emetics, cathartics, and other "depletive" therapies, these healers insisted, generally did more harm than good. "There is no doubt," Montreal's *La Minerve* proclaimed, "that the generality of cases" of pneumonia and dropsy resulted from "the use of quack remedies . . . which, far from curing" horses, "increase their suffering." After consulting with "the most learned veterinarians" in the city, *La Minerve* counseled readers "that the less drugs are used, the better." Instead of besieging flu patients with perilous nostrums, Canadian veterinary authorities cast equines as innately capable of warding off and recovering from influenza—but only if they could focus their energies on healing rather than laboring. The *Bowmanville (ON) Merchant* summed up prevailing Canadian wisdom in upholding "warmth and rest" as "the two great essentials" of flu treatment.[35]

This regimen gained wide acceptance in the United States partly because of incontrovertible evidence that it had limited the outbreak's death toll in Canada. W. T. Boyd, the *Chicago Tribune*'s man in Toronto, touted Smith's "diagnosis and treatment" as so "entirely successful that the disease has nearly disappeared from the city." The *Ontario Workman* likewise reported that because of the "rational" therapies espoused by Canadian veterinary surgeons, "nearly all" Ontarians were "now congratulating themselves upon the saving of the lives of their animals during the trying ordeal of the epidemic."[36]

In the years before the Great Horse Flu emerged, most equine healers and horse owners in the United States had started to turn away from heroic practices, yet some of these risky therapies nonetheless remained in widespread use. After acknowledging that "bleeding cannot safely be trusted to ignorant hands," for instance, a Maryland doctor nonetheless insisted that trained practitioners could still fight flu to "good effect" by tapping into ill horses' veins and releasing "three or four pounds of blood." As the epizootic intensified, though, bleeding, blistering, and other similarly intensive treatments faced mounting scrutiny. One vet later recalled that during his "very large and extended experience" treating flu-stricken horses "in Chicago, Madison, and other places," he had "found whole stables full of horses" in which "nearly all were blistered in a most fearful and horrible manner, without in the least checking [influenza] or helping the patient, but, on the contrary, causing a greater amount of suffering." "In all cases where bleeding has been resorted to by the surgeons in attendance," a late October report from Rochester, New York, intoned, "the patient has died." "Do not bleed or give purgatives in this disease," Chicago veterinary surgeon J. S. McKenzie implored. Instead he advised the public to place "reliance . . . upon the curative powers that God has implanted in the constitution of all his creatures." An Ohio healer offered a more prosaic version of the same guidance: "There is no need of drugging a horse," an Ohio healer declared, "with every thing which Tom, Dick and Harry, may recommend and making use of every thing in the *materia medica*."[37]

The adoption of minimalist flu therapies built on Canadian precedents, but it also reflected the success of homeopathic veterinary medicine. The epizootic, the *Boston Globe* observed, had "brought about a war between veterinary surgeons of the Allopathic and Homœpathic schools over the relative efficiency of their respective systems for the treatment of horses." Although there was no clear victor, homeopaths seemed to gain the upper hand. The San Francisco homeopathic veterinary surgeon A. F. Cooper declared in an 1868 manual that "it is something to be emancipated from drugs, from lancets, leeches, blisters and poisons; but it is more," he continued, "to be relieved from the fear of them, and to be restored and preserved by forces mild as love, and gentle as the dews of heaven—forces unknown and unrevealed, until elicited by the genius of this system." Intent on supporting "the curative powers of God," Cooper and other veterinary homeopaths sought to cure flu-addled horses by giving them infinitesimal doses of a single medicine (they decried mixtures or compounds of medicines as ineffective and even dangerous) purported to cause or intensify telltale influenza symptoms like fever or coughing. Homeopaths believed that a wisely selected medication—aconite for fever, for instance, or arsenicum "should the animal appear weak and languid"—would stir the patient's "vital force" into action, reacting "with all its might against the impression which it receives" from the infinitesimal doses they had been prescribed. "*The effect of reaction*," declared Friedrich August Gunther's *New Manual of Homeopathic Veterinary Medicine*, a German treatise published in an English translation in Boston in the 1850s, "*is always to produce a change precisely the reverse of that which had been occasioned by the medicine*." While homeopathic and allopathic practitioners relied on many of the same remedies, homeopaths invariably prescribed "less frequent and bulky" doses. This approach, as the *New York Times* noted, led to their equine patients being "less worried by the treatment." Many American healers noticed during the outbreak's early weeks that patients treated homeopathically rarely developed life-threatening complications. Such observations reinforced longer-term trends toward more restrained flu therapies, as the counsel one allopathic physician provided to the *Troy Weekly Times* indicated: "Remember, the disease is *scarcely ever fatal*, except in aged or over-worked horses; that it must and will run a certain course; that nothing you can do will break it up."[38]

From the start of the epizootic, experts had emphasized the need to give unwell horses a rest. The *Chicago Evening Post* summed up the commonplace prescription soon after the epizootic reached that city: "Let the poor beast, 'that noble animal, the horse,' rest when he is sick." The first principle in treating equine influenza, as a traveling railroad agent wrote from Illinois in mid-November, was "*perfect ease from all labor*," which was precisely what most humans of the time wanted for themselves and their loved ones when they fell ill with flu. Yet because the livelihoods and even the fortunes of many Northeasterners hinged on the brains and brawn that horses and their kin placed at human disposal, giving equines a break proved a hard pill for many people to swallow.[39]

Questions of Humanity

By heightening both the risks and the rewards of keeping flu-stricken animals on the job, the outbreak sparked conflict between newly founded animal welfare organizations and those whose jobs and profits hinged on the labor horses performed. Humanitarians and their allies in the press often cast the epizootic as an opportunity to redress the pervasive neglect and abuse animals suffered in the Northeast's big cities. "If any domesticated animal in the whole range of brute creation has reason to complain, it is the horse," agreed the *Chicago Tribune* in criticizing the "frequent maltreatment" that was everywhere so apparent. Many folks, the *Tribune* alleged, felt that "any sort of stabling is good enough for him," and "no amount of work is too heavy." Yet despite such wrongs, the horse "must neither expect favor, mercy, or rest, but drudge along uncomplainingly, until he is incapacitated for further work, and then he is turned out to die, perhaps of starvation."[40]

When George Angell, founder and president of the Massachusetts Society for the Prevention of Cruelty to Animals (MSPCA), reflected on "the lessons of the malady," he detected an unmistakable moral behind this "public calamity": "Every man, woman, and child in the community," Angell professed, "has been affected by it; it has made people think about animals, and feel for them . . . . Now that so great an interest has been created through so much suffering to animals, and inconvenience and loss to men," Angell anticipated that support for the anticruelty crusade would finally move from the fringe of American politics to its center. The epizootic, Angell declared, did more "to awaken the public sense of justice to animals than years of pleading by all the societies in the land."[41]

Angell was hardly alone in seeing the Great Horse Flu as a defining moment. Editors, ministers, and agricultural societies all saw the outbreak as an opportunity for Americans to change their thinking and behavior. The epizootic, the *Hartford Courant* intoned, "ought to be a lesson to us that should lead to instant reform in our method of treating horses; for the manner in which he is worked and cared for now is liable at any time to induce an epidemic, a plague, as fatal as ever attacked the human race." This same editorial concluded "that the horse cannot bear the increasing burdens which our civilization is putting upon him unless we give him the benefit of our civilization. *We must either get some other machine to do his work or we must cease to treat him like a machine.*"[42]

By detailing the profound misery that influenza and its complications inflicted on equine victims, journalists cultivated readers' sympathies. Their maudlin accounts of epizootic woes were calibrated to convince readers that infirm horses deserved to be treated as living beings rather than unfeeling automatons. A week after the epizootic struck New York, for instance, an *Evening Post* journalist visited a street railway stable and found "over one hundred horses . . . shivering and coughing." More patients limped in every few minutes, "many of them seeming almost unable to move without the application of the whip." The same reporter then stopped at another transit company's makeshift "horsepital," which the article described as "filled with horses apparently dying . . . . Unable to stand," nearly all "of these unfortunate brutes" were instead lying down, "shivering and coughing."[43]

In Chicago, meanwhile, a *Prairie Farmer* scribe beheld "almost incessant" coughing that was "frequently so painful, as to occasion much impatience and violent stamping in the horse . . . . The great soreness of the throat," the reporter added with a gulp, "makes it difficult for the animal to swallow any thing." "No one seems to think much of the suffering the poor horses endure," lamented a Boston correspondent after visiting "a famous club stable" inhabited by "some twenty animals." Although he found it "pitiable to hear them cough" and alarming to "see their distressed condition," the correspondent nonetheless took solace in the fact that these ailing horses were "comfortably blanketed and tended like babies." Indeed, he continued, these creatures received "the same watchful care, the same regular medicines, as if they were wholly human . . . . You wonder," he mused, "what they thought about it all."[44]

Media eyewitnesses found the extreme distress inflicted by dropsy and respiratory complications to be especially relatable and poignant. A Cincinnati reporter, for instance, recounted the agonies of a horse he found gasping for breath because "the cells" of its lungs were "gradually filling with serum." This unfortunate creature's "efforts . . . to gain health" struck the reporter as indistinguishable from "those of a human in the throes of asthma." The horrid swelling that typified severe cases of dropsy, meanwhile, prompted compassion alongside disgust. A Saratoga Springs newspaper presented a gothic sketch of one horse's travails; "the disease," it alleged, "puffed the poor animal so that its head, neck and chest were almost unrecognizable." Another reporter, meanwhile, described how a "valuable young horse" in Portsmouth, Rhode Island, "swelled up in its nose and legs" with such force that blood began to "ooze from the under side of his eyelids, and also from his legs." This ill-fated beast "continued to swell" for several more days before finally succumbing to dropsy. "In some of the cases," grimaced the Cincinnati reporter who likened a horse suffering from respiratory distress to a human asthmatic, dropsical horses' "hind legs had swollen to the hocks," and their knees had assumed "an immense roundness." Edema even distended one horse's neck, engorging its head to such "a fearful size" that it "assumed the appearance of a hippopotamus."[45]

Such harrowing portrayals tugged at human heartstrings. With sympathy stretching across species divides, anticruelty organizations—Johnny-come-latelies to American reform—seized the opportunity the epizootic offered and leapt to the defense of ailing equines. A year after the Civil War ended, Henry Bergh, scion of a wealthy New York shipbuilding family, established the first such organization in the Western Hemisphere, the American Society for the Prevention of Cruelty to Animals (ASPCA). Horrified by the callous neglect and vicious abuse of horses that he had witnessed as secretary for the US legation to Russia, Bergh was inspired to create the

ASPCA along lines first laid out by the Royal Society for the Prevention of Cruelty to Animals, founded in 1824 by British clergymen, lawyers, and members of Parliament. Bergh pressured New York legislators into enacting an anticruelty statute in 1866 that empowered the ASPCA to arrest and prosecute violators. By 1872, humanitarian reformers in several other American and Canadian cities, including Boston's George Angell, followed Bergh's lead by organizing numerous Societies for the Prevention of Cruelty to Animals (SPCAs). After lobbying state and provincial legislatures to criminalize some of the most egregious forms of abuse and neglect, these crusaders moved to enforce these new laws via the police powers that legislators had delegated to them.[46]

As the epizootic intensified, animal welfare activists harnessed growing popular resentment of those who jeopardized sick horses' lives by refusing to rest them. Before the outbreak entered its second week in New York City, the *Herald* accused people who compelled ailing animals to continue working of "downright cruelty." Such charges initially dovetailed with popular sympathies. One New York street railway official described "the public" as "rich of pity for the horses," while the *Herald* noted that "public feeling . . . throughout the city" had grown "strongly derisive of the inhumanity of forcing sick steeds to work." Anticruelty organizations tried to leverage public opinion into meaningful action by targeting two main types of offenders: street railway corporations and common horse workers. The eventual failure of the ensuing campaigns, though, revealed Americans' ongoing unwillingness to place the needs of equines above those of humankind.[47]

Even after the epizootic had sickened nearly all of New York's fifteen thousand streetcar horses, the *Herald* claimed that transit companies, "with an eye to their profits," were "persist[ing] in keeping up the traffic over their routes as well as they could." In late October, as more and more animals became too sick to work, those perceived fit enough to continue laboring on street railways faced added burdens. Passenger demand hardly budged—indeed, with fewer cabs, stages, and omnibuses in service, it almost certainly increased. Once street railways reduced service, passengers packed into the remaining cars like sardines; some even clambered onto the roof to ride al fresco. "The horses who are left," the *Herald* lamented, "have about twice the ordinary work to do; and are consequently likely to be worked to death." The same author went on to describe the "coughing and straining" of the horses who were compelled to pull badly overloaded cars as "most painful to look at," especially after "complete exhaustion sets in, and the horse pants as if for life."[48]

Transit corporations initially responded to New Yorkers' mounting sympathy and outrage by blaming riders. Thomas Sullivan, president of the

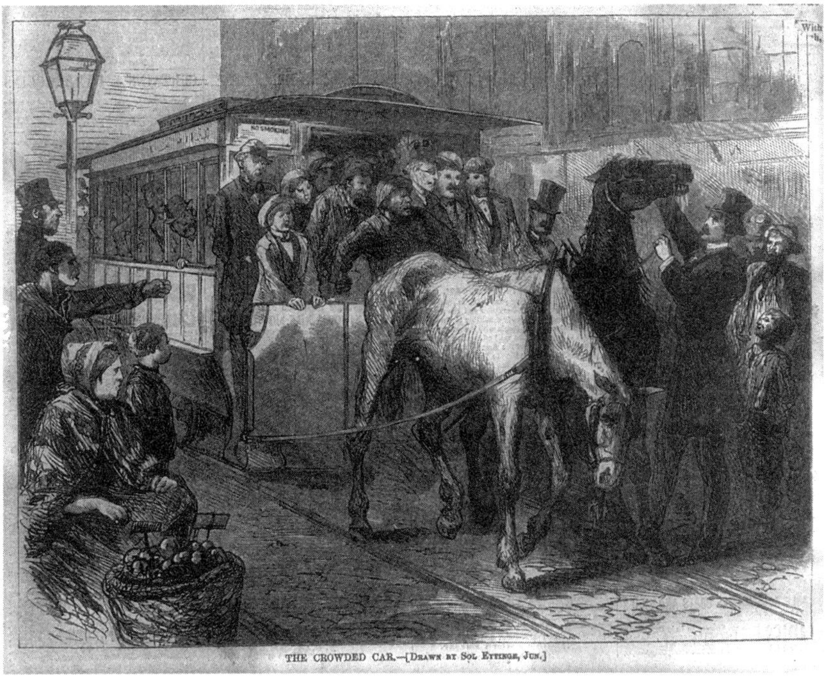

Just a few months before the Great Horse Flu struck, Sol Eytinge Jr. offered a remarkably perceptive representation of the concerns and conflicts that horse-drawn street railways triggered. Note the visible distress of the lighter-colored horse, its head drooped, its ribs exposed, and its spirit seemingly broken. Eytinge contrasts this pitiful creature with its darker partner, whose body is hidden from the viewer but who raises its head in response to the care shown by the well-dressed man whose dashing figure and mustachioed face both suggest that he was modeled after Henry Bergh of the American Society for the Prevention of Cruelty against Animals, who became a recognizable and controversial celebrity by 1872. As the humanitarian caresses the dark horse's muzzle, he and the horse lock eyes in a moment of palpable empathy across the species divide. Passengers lean out the windows and peer over the car balcony to take in this moment of communion. Meanwhile, onlookers bear witness to the horses' travails as well as the humanitarian's kindness. By contrast, those lining the sidewalk in the left foreground of the image, like those at the front of the car balcony, make no effort to hide their outrage. Presumably many of them were troubled by the animals' plight, but some of them seem even more angered by the wealthy man's intervention. Sol Eytinge Jr., "The Crowded Car," *Harper's Weekly*, September 21, 1872, 741, https://www.loc.gov/item/99614207/. Courtesy of the Library of Congress Prints and Photographs Division, Washington, DC.

Brooklyn City Railroad Company, told the *Herald* that "the public" was "literally killing our horses by overloading the cars," adding "that every man and woman who can walk to their homes at such a time as this is bound to do so. If things go on in this way," he warned, "there will be no horses left to perform the work . . . . All the horses want," Sullivan implored, "is rest. If they could get that, we should be all right in a very short time."[49]

Bergh, the ASPCA, and their journalistic allies bristled at Sullivan's allegations. Although the *Evening Post* agreed that "a horse afflicted in the least degree should have immediate rest," it averred that "the managers of the [street rail]roads hesitate to cease running their cars altogether to secure this object, and therefore compel the animals to work until they are completely prostrated." It was "all wrong" for creatures who were "exhibiting every symptom of illness" to remain on the job, given widespread agreement that "timely care" constituted "the one thing necessary to prevent fatal consequences."[50]

Bergh stepped up his anticruelty crusade by paying a public visit to the Third Avenue Railway's headquarters. Striding in unannounced with a *Herald* reporter in tow, the ASPCA founder overheard the company's officers "inveighing loudly against him." Once they realized that Bergh was in their midst, the managers shouted out in "surprise and anger." The railway president, intent on avoiding more bad press, then ushered Bergh into his office for a private conversation. An hour later, "when the door opened," the *Herald* writer recounted with palpable glee that Bergh was

> dictating to the President:—
>
> > MR. BERGH—It is agreed, then, that you shall not run sick horses on the road?
> >
> > THE PRESIDENT—Very well, but I beg of you to allow the cars to run today. Do not impede them, and tomorrow I shall not run a single sick horse on the road.

The streetcar executive then barked out a peal of orders: "Do not allow any emaciated horses to leave the stable," and "be careful that those which go out are the best that can be got." Bergh departed, watched by "a hundred scowling faces" peering down from the railway's headquarters, then wheeled around. "Look at that magnificent depot," he declared. "Think of the fine brown stone" mansions the managers who glared back at him inhabited, "all made by the toil of these poor animals. But they are not satisfied," Bergh snorted—not even "when the poor brutes are unable to put one foot before another."[51]

Bergh soon broadened his attacks on New York's largest employers of horseflesh through a public letter. How could it be, he asked in a missive republished as far away as San Francisco, that the horse, a creature who had distinguished itself throughout history as "the most generous and indispensable servant of mankind," seemed to be "held in lower estimate" in the United States than in other nations, "and more generally rated—particularly by large corporations—among their inanimate property"? Because, the ASPCA founder alleged, "the question of humanity" was "not an active principle" in corporate decision-making. "The disabled horse and the disabled car or stage," he asserted, "are placed in the same category!" The actions of transit companies, though, clearly demonstrated that they cared more for their rolling stock than for their animal property. "The careful housing, washing, oiling and repairing of the senseless vehicle," he objected, stood in "marked contrast to the inadequate consideration bestowed on the weary, maimed and emaciated creature, which, with dropping head and supplicating look, remains in the pelting storm or is domiciled in the damp, dark, foul smelling cellar below the street." Bergh concluded with a final dig: The street railways' exploitative stance toward their equine property, the humanitarian insisted, was "not only unprofitable" but also "something more—a crime," for "the horse, ever since his domestication, has been one of the greatest elements of human progress and happiness, and it is not exaggerating his importance to say that civilization would be almost impossible without him."[52]

Several competing transit companies soon joined the Third Avenue Railway in stabling all their horses. This move, though, was less a response to Bergh's pleading or the public's scorn, and more a result of the epizootic's amplification, which left New York's street railway corporations no real choice but to suspend operations. A few days later, several lines resumed service despite "Mr. Bergh's big crusade," including the Third Avenue line, which had reported more than a dozen equine fatalities during the previous few days. Three stagecoach companies then took the fight to the ASPCA; they "sued Bergh's society for interfering with their business," seeking an injunction plus $75,000 in damages.[53]

On the streets of New York, meanwhile, popular support for anticruelty policing began to waver. Newspaper coverage of the ASPCA's efforts to force numerous cars and stages out of service redirected frustration at flu-related transportation disruptions away from corporations and toward humanitarian activists. Uptown, for instance, a "very large party" of "sour-tempered and sore-headed" people found common ground by cursing Bergh and his fellow animal lovers for subjecting them to long, often fruitless waits for a spot on badly overloaded cars. The Bleecker Street Railway took advantage of this shifting sentiment by announcing on November 2 that it would resume operations "in open defiance of Mr. Bergh."[54]

The ASPCA's campaign against common horse workers also foundered. Small proprietors and their employees in the freighting sector "depend[ed]," as one journalist noted, "for their daily bread upon the earnings obtained by means of their carts or trucks and their horses." Equines "owned by the poor," the *Herald* added, usually "enjoyed less rest and attention" than those kept by wealthier New Yorkers. It was only "with the utmost reluctance that working men take their horses from the traces," the same journalist observed, "because of their inability to dispense with the services of their animals until the latter are no longer able to stagger under their burden." As in Montreal, common horse workers kept their animals on the job out of opportunism as well as desperation. One driver boasted, for instance, that he and his fellow hackmen could now clear twenty or even twenty-five dollars daily by compelling their animals to labor—rousing motivation indeed for men accustomed to earning fourteen dollars plus tips *weekly*.[55]

Humanitarian policing jeopardized efforts by working-class New Yorkers to get ahead as well as to get by. Little wonder, then, that some drivers responded to the ASPCA's interference with rage. In late October, Bergh and an associate approached Michael Feeny, a carter whom one paper described as "a tall, rough looking and muscular man, apparently quite poor," when they saw him "driving a sick horse troubled with the 'epizoot.'" After the anticruelty activists ordered Feeny to unhitch the animal and return it to its stable, Feeny snapped back at them in "the choicest language known to truckmen, hackmen and others of that ilk," a group of men whose skill at swearing might have made a sailor blush. Bergh used his police power to summon Feeny to court, but on arraignment at New York's notorious Tombs, the carter burst out of the dock and tried to batter his accusers.[56]

The ASPCA may have won this battle—the judge jailed Feeny so he could "repent of his ill-timed burst of temper"—but Bergh's broader crusade to rein in the continued use of flu-stricken animals by common horse workers soon flagged. Another *Herald* article, for instance, reproved a feckless ASPCA officer for pulling over "a poor carter" who was employing "a sorry-looking creature, frightfully afflicted with the prevalent malady" to draw a heavy load down Broadway. Bergh's deputy ordered the driver to halt and seek out a replacement for his ailing animal. Though well intentioned, the officer's orders left the sick horse to "stand with its burden" while his "unfortunate owner" desperately tried to find another horse to lease. When the carter finally returned, the animal he dragged behind him seemed even worse off than the one it replaced. Given the new horse's obvious ailments, the carter expressed disbelief that the officer "let me use him." Such arbitrary, ineffectual policing, the *Herald* opined, offered "a very fair example of such cases as Mr. Bergh's men provided for yesterday."[57]

Such criticism led the ASPCA to draw back, with ominous consequences for the horses humanitarian reformers were trying to protect. One reporter blamed the "great number of deaths" among New York's equines on "the enormous prices paid for cartage," which "tempt[ed] the owners to work sick horses." Street railways' constant push to squeeze additional profit out of flu-wracked animals, though, probably claimed even more lives.[58]

Similar dynamics played out in other cities, too. Local SPCAs in Chicago, Philadelphia, Boston, and beyond moved to forbid the driving of sick horses under penalty of arrest. Yet as in New York, all such campaigns faltered, often because of the limitations of state anticruelty statutes. Pennsylvania law, to cite a representative case, held street railway drivers and conductors—not their employers—criminally liable for abuse and neglect. The unpopularity of this provision, which struck many citizens as unfair, made indictments rare and convictions virtually impossible to secure, as an epizootic-related incident on the Girard Avenue Railway illustrates. At trial, eyewitnesses recounted how a horsecar had "filled outside and in" with eighty passengers. Its springs "bent way down" under the weight of mourners hoping to attend the funeral of Major General George Meade, hero of Gettysburg, the car started the journey to Fairmount Park. Soon, though, the horses charged with drawing this groaning load were "all in a foam" and "panting on their sides," with one of the team "bleeding at the nose." As a "steep grade" loomed before the "fagged out" beasts, "the passengers got out and pushed the car up." Frustrated at the delays occasioned by his exhausted, febrile horses, the driver proceeded to beat them "with a light whip." A watchful Pennsylvania Society for the Prevention of Cruelty to Animals agent then swooped in to arrest him. Despite compelling evidence of abuse, the judge dismissed all charges, perhaps because he reckoned that the driver was guilty of nothing more than trying to keep Philadelphians moving in the face of epizootic stoppages. As this and several similar cases demonstrated, state laws that insulated the nation's largest horse owners from direct responsibility for their horses' welfare ensured that humane policing gained little ground during the Great Horse Flu.[59]

The epizootic, as Thomas DeWitt Talmage had Charley Bucephalus argue in "A Horse's Letter," prompted Americans to reconsider how they thought about and related to equinekind. Intent on safeguarding their animals' lives and ability to labor, Northeasterners scrambled to understand and address influenza and its complications. Autopsies on the corpses of flu-stricken horses and donkeys underscored the dangers that pneumonia, dropsy, and other complications presented. Widespread claims that the outbreak was spilling over to afflict a variety of other host species, including people in a fast-growing number of communities, gave new life to old suspicions that influenza could afflict humans and horses in common. Americans doctored sickly animals by searching out cures in the news media, cooking up folk remedies, buying patent medicines, and hiring healers. Drawing on Canadian experience and extending consideration across species divides, most medical and veterinary experts urged the public to treat ill animals as they themselves wanted to be treated. This meant avoiding bleeding, blistering, and other so-called heroic therapies, which caused suffering and opened the door to complications, and choosing instead to rest sick equines while pampering them with supportive care. A combination of necessity, opportunism, and acquisitiveness nonetheless led many Americans to ignore this guidance. Recently established anticruelty organizations responded by trying to persuade or compel street railway corporations and common horse workers to give sick animals a break.

The kinder future that Charley Bucephalus and his comrades had glimpsed at the Great Horse Flu's peak soon slipped away. Media reports nonetheless show that for an all-too-transient moment, large numbers of people willingly prioritized the health of essential equine workers despite the costs and inconvenience this often entailed. In cities throughout the Northeast, newspapers praised local residents for keeping flu-stricken equines off the streets and in their stables. This precautionary approach became especially widespread in early November, after a flood of reports showed that animals who were forced back to work before fully recovering from influenza experienced sharply higher rates of dropsy, which killed perhaps half of the horses who contracted it.[60]

The MSPCA responded to popular concern for equine wellbeing with acclaim: "We have found our people—corporations and individuals—willing and anxious" to heed expert advice and "avoid working their horses." What no one could yet know, though, was that the public's embrace of the rest cure would soon combine with the epizootic's insidious effects to subject Boston to a disaster of monumental proportions.[61]

CHAPTER 4

THE GREAT HORSE FLU AND THE GREAT BOSTON FIRE

Ailing Animals, Aging Infrastructure, and Urban Disaster

The evening of Saturday, November 9, 1872, one Bostonian recalled, started off "unusually calm," with "a serene sky . . . bathed in the light" of a waxing moon. Yet by this time, the most destructive fire in Boston's long history was already roaring to life just a few blocks south of the city's heart. When the first company of firefighters ran up to the blaze in the basement of a hulking commercial warehouse at the corner of Kingston and Summer Streets just after 7:30 p.m., a veritable inferno confronted them.[1]

Later that night, the conflagration tore through one of the busiest, most densely built business districts in North America. Its flames grew "so great," recounted Louisa May Alcott, who had ascended to literary stardom soon after *Little Women* began rolling off a Boston printing press four years earlier, "that it created a whirlwind & an awful roar." A cleric claimed that newspapers could be read by the fire's light "at twenty miles' distance." Ship captains reported that the inferno was "visible by reflection three hundred and twenty-five miles at sea." A US signal officer posted north of Boston recalled "a flock of ducks" that "passed at a great height overhead," with "the fire reflected from their plumage" making "them appear as fire-balls passing rapidly through the air." Meanwhile, sixty miles inland, a locomotive engineer coming over a hill met the horrific sight of New England's largest city ablaze. When he pulled his train into Boston an hour later, the flames loomed "so high and so immense" that "many passengers jumped from the cars and left the train before it reached the station."[2]

As the fire leapt from building to building, one witness reported that "granite crumbled; brick and mortar fell away; and stout timbers glowed a moment, and then tumbled and crashed into the ash-heaps which seethed at the bottom of the fiery abyss." Cub reporter Sylvester Baxter remembered that architectural details dripped off buildings as when "molten wax or paraffine [*sic*] melts and runs down the side" of a candle. Marble and granite fell from the sky in pieces ranging from fine shards to massive boulders. "The red glare, the strange roar, the flying people, all made [the] night terrible," Louisa May Alcott shuddered, "& I kept thinking of the Last Days of Pompeii."[3]

John Stanhope Damrell, a brawny, snub-nosed North End native and chief engineer of the Boston Fire Department (BFD), recalled that as the conflagration advanced, collapsing buildings severed gas pipes buried beneath the city's streets. Soon "the whole atmosphere was thoroughly permeated with gas," which periodically coalesced into "dark, opaque masses" reaching "twenty-five feet in diameter." After a momentary shimmer, these gas pockets blew up in blinding, ear-shattering blasts that could be seen and heard several towns away.[4]

Containing the blaze required close to seventeen hours and more than 2,100 men from nearly a hundred firefighting companies—some coming from as far away as Biddeford, Maine, and New Haven, Connecticut. When the flames finally died down, the disaster's astounding extent and intensity came to light: Overnight, the Great Boston Fire had transformed sixty-five acres of downtown real estate containing what the *Boston Globe* rightly described as "nearly all our finest business streets and structures" into a "monotonous, dreary waste of fragmentary ruin."[5]

The scale and thoroughness of the annihilation defied comprehension. Many of Boston's "great thoroughfares of trade" and "principal business

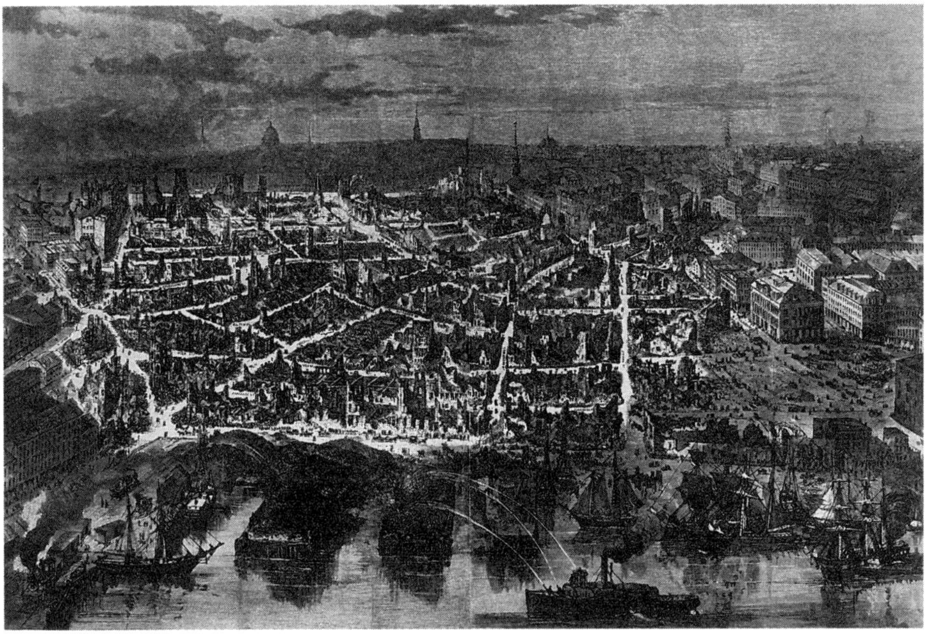

Combining photographic and cartographic techniques, this illustration depicts the former South End in ruins. Note the destruction throughout the foreground and the smoldering coal heaps at the bottom of the frame. "Boston After the Great Fire," reproduction of print from *Harper's Weekly*, December 14, 1872. Digital Commonwealth, https://ark.digitalcommonwealth.org/ark:/50959/xp68kr375.

squares," *Harper's Weekly* declared, had "vanished from the view, and not even a solitary lamp-post or curb-stone remains to tell their former location." Streets had been "so effectually obliterated" that "citizens clambering over the heaps of bricks and granite blocks" wandered about "utterly lost in places where before the fire they were most at home." For nearly a week after the flames died down, the haunting stretch of the city that instantly became known as the Burnt District gave off a "constant glow which in the night time lights up the field of ruin."[6]

Yet despite the conflagration's ferocity, it killed no more than nineteen people, most of them firefighters. Fortunate timing largely explained the fire's mercy, as it erupted an hour after quitting time in a stretch of the city where as many as twenty-five thousand men, women, and children labored but virtually no one lived. By 1872, the area obliterated by the Great Fire was inhabited by fewer than three hundred people, a startling reflection of the makeover the former South End had experienced in recent decades, with hundreds of stores and warehouses replacing upscale residences and scattered tenements that had once housed several thousand Bostonians.[7]

Property rather than people bore the disaster's brunt. Though nearly forgotten today, the Great Boston Fire of 1872 ranked as the second costliest urban fire in nineteenth-century North America. It was surpasssed only by the previous year's Great Chicago Fire, which killed several thousand people, destroyed roughly ninety thousand homes, and consumed property valued at nearly $200 million. Boston's Burnt District comprised some of the most valuable real estate anywhere on earth. The conflagration and subsequent gas explosions razed buildings valued at $15 to $20 million while destroying some $60 million worth of merchandise and possessions. Some of Boston's wealthiest families lost their fortunes; universities and other institutions that had invested their endowments in downtown real estate suffered major hits to their portfolios; and laboring folks, particularly "sewing women and clerks" employed in the buildings the blaze had reduced to rubble, faced the grim specter of unemployment as another unforgiving New England winter set in.[8]

Blame for the Great Fire soon fell on the Great Horse Flu. The *Chicago Tribune*, for instance, pointed out that "when the fire came, the lack of horses formed a serious obstacle in the way of the Fire Department." The relationship between these two concurrent but distinct disasters, though, was more complicated—and more instructive—than such simple cause-and-effect scenarios allow. Even though the novel influenza virus eventually struck every metropolis in the northern Americas, sickening most of the horses that human firefighters relied on to draw steam engines, no comparable conflagration ever erupted.[9]

This chapter traces a messier story of flu and fire, showing how the epizootic helped to subject Boston to a brutal one-two punch of calamity. The debility that influenza produced combined with the growing conviction that stricken horses could recover only if given adequate rest to lead Damrell and his lieutenants to stable the BFD's firehorses. By disrupting the circulation of goods through Boston, the outbreak also caused vast quantities of wool, cotton, leather, oil, and other combustible materials to accumulate throughout the former South End and other downtown districts. Once the fire started, the epizootic hampered efforts to keep coal-burning fire engines supplied with fuel and exacerbated property losses by hobbling efforts to rescue property from the flames. No less important, though, the Great Horse Flu made still other contributions to the Great Boston Fire by triggering submerged vulnerabilities stemming from the municipal government's failure to keep pace with the former South End's transformation from a fashionable residential quarter to a bustling hub for manufacturing, wholesaling, and retailing. The novel influenza virus played a key role in slowing firefighters' response to the conflagration, but the BFD's efforts to suppress and contain the blaze also fell short because of downtown Boston's aging water pipes, antiquated fire hydrants, and dearth of fire stations.

With compound disasters bearing unmistakable similarities to the Great Boston Fire growing alarmingly routine in recent years, excavating the connections between flu and fire points toward more robust and useful approaches for rethinking how infectious disease outbreaks interact with infrastructural inequalities to produce urban fires and other catastrophes. No less important, it shows how the Great Horse Flu's proliferating economic impact jeopardized the continuing growth on which Republican Reconstruction policies depended.[10]

Different from That of Any Other Horse in the World

The Great Horse Flu swiftly undermined the defenses that Bostonians had developed through long experience to safeguard persons and property against fire's menacing might. Chief Damrell of the Boston Fire Department later recalled how he and his subordinates reacted to news of the epizootic's ravages in Toronto with "seeming indifference, but as each succeeding bulletin announced its spread and that all horses of that vicinity were seriously affected," Damrell continued, "the alarm became general." The *Globe* expressed the logic behind this growing apprehension when it warned that "the well-being" of the BFD's force of roughly 130 horses had become "all-important to the safety of the city."[11]

Bostonians had struggled against fire ever since English Puritans founded the settlement in 1630 on lands they were wresting from Nipmuc, Massachusett, and Wampanoag peoples. As the Puritan cleric Cotton Mather famously growled in 1698, "Never was any town under the cope of heaven more liable to be laid in ASHES, either through the *carelessness* or the *wickedness* of them that *sleep* in it. That such a *combustible heap* of contiguous houses yet stands," Mather declared of a city that was still in its adolescence, "may be called a *standing miracle*," for "TEN TIMES has the *fire* made *notable* ruins among us."[12]

Between Mather's lifetime and the early 1870s, a succession of blazes great and small led Bostonians to develop elaborate but imperfect defenses. Town, colonial, and state governments authorized building codes; appointed bellmen and fire wards to keep watch over the city and sound alarms; empowered officers of the law to tear down buildings at risk of communicating flames to adjacent structures without compensating property owners; subdivided the city into fire districts; straightened several of the town's narrowest, most convoluted streets for easier firefighting; and incorporated volunteer firefighting companies.[13]

Devastating infernos nonetheless continued to afflict the city, with each disaster prompting new reforms. After a string of conflagrations in 1824 and 1825, Boston's newly incorporated city government established the municipally controlled and funded Boston Fire Department. In the decades that followed, the BFD continued to share firefighting duties with volunteer companies. Sprinting through Boston's streets pulling or carrying hand engines, hoses, ladders, and other apparatus, these notoriously unruly outfits engaged in running fights to beat competing outfits to fire scenes—and to claim whatever spoils they could by way of plunder and payment.[14]

Such continuities aside, the BFD's founding nonetheless marked a critical step in the long, halting process of modernizing, professionalizing, and centralizing firefighting efforts. From its inception, the department hitched its hopes to horses. City leaders responded to the fires of the mid-1820s, an early fire historian explained, by allowing the BFD's Engine Company 14 "to employ a horse to help carry that engine to and from fires." This "cream-colored" creature, whom firemen nicknamed "the 'charger,'" immediately proved its worth. Councilmen responded by authorizing every

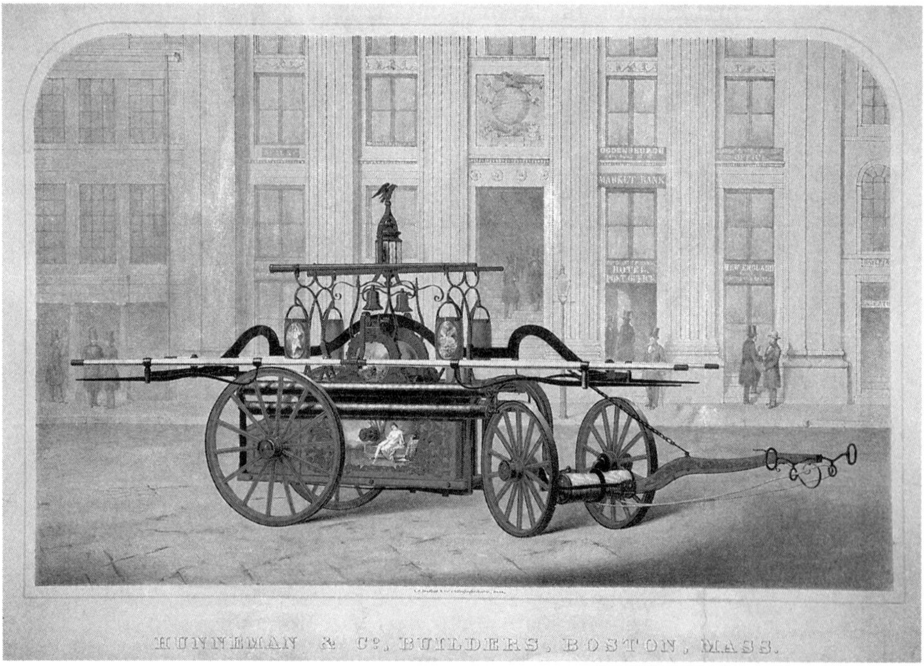

This print from the mid-1850s shows an ornate hand-powered fire engine on the streets of Boston. L. H. Bradford & Co., *Hunneman & Co. Builders, Boston, Mass.* (ca. 1855), pri-JLC_FIRE_001505, Jay T. Last Collection of Firefighting Prints and Ephemera, 1826–1907, Huntington Library, San Marino, CA.

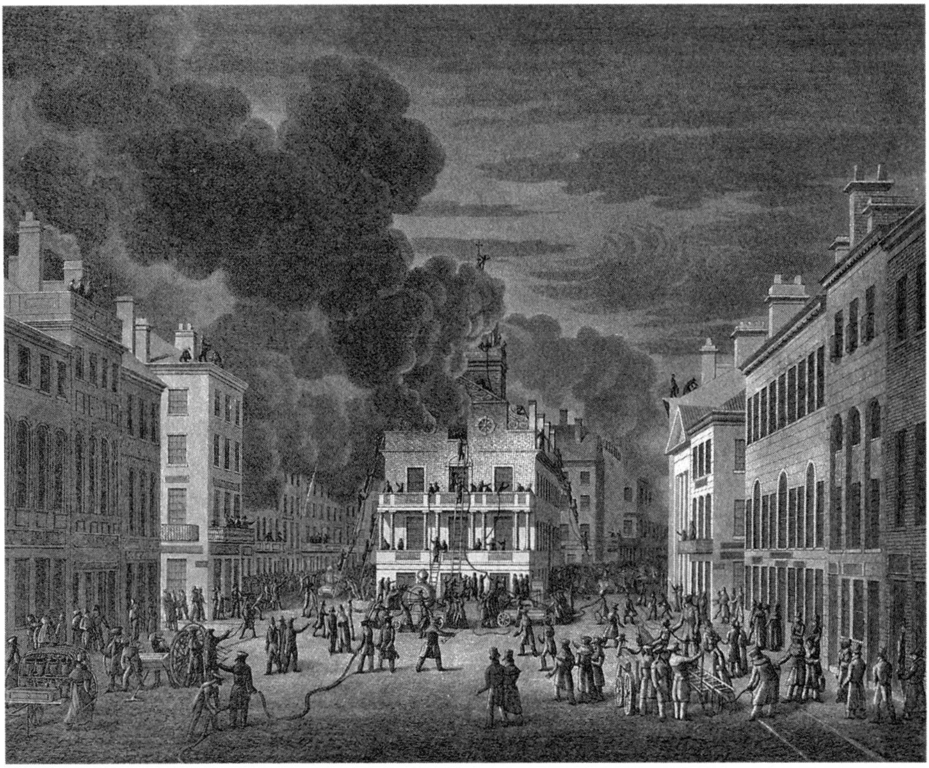

Note the use of hand-powered engines in this inset from a firefighter's certificate, which shows the 1832 Massachusetts State House fire. Thomas C. Amory, Boston Firefighter's Certificate, image dated 1833, certificate completed by Amasa Pray, 1846, pri-JLC_FIRE_001476, Jay T. Last Collection of Firefighting Prints and Ephemera, 1826–1907, Huntington Library, San Marino, CA.

engine company in the department to "employ a horse to assist in drawing the apparatus when the streets were in such a condition from rain, etc., that their progress was impeded."[15]

Firehorses became even more important after the BFD adapted steam-powered fire engines to the city's increasingly modern water infrastructure. It remained customary as late as the 1840s, fireman Charles Stearns recalled, "to have a couple of hundred brawny fellows on the line rushing to a fire" with "tubs"—small, hand-operated fire engines that were mounted on wagons, powered by teams of firefighters pumping in unison, and supplied with water transported by bucket brigades or suction pumps from public wells, cisterns, or Boston Harbor. Fire department leaders, though, were already turning decisively away from such old-fashioned methods. The

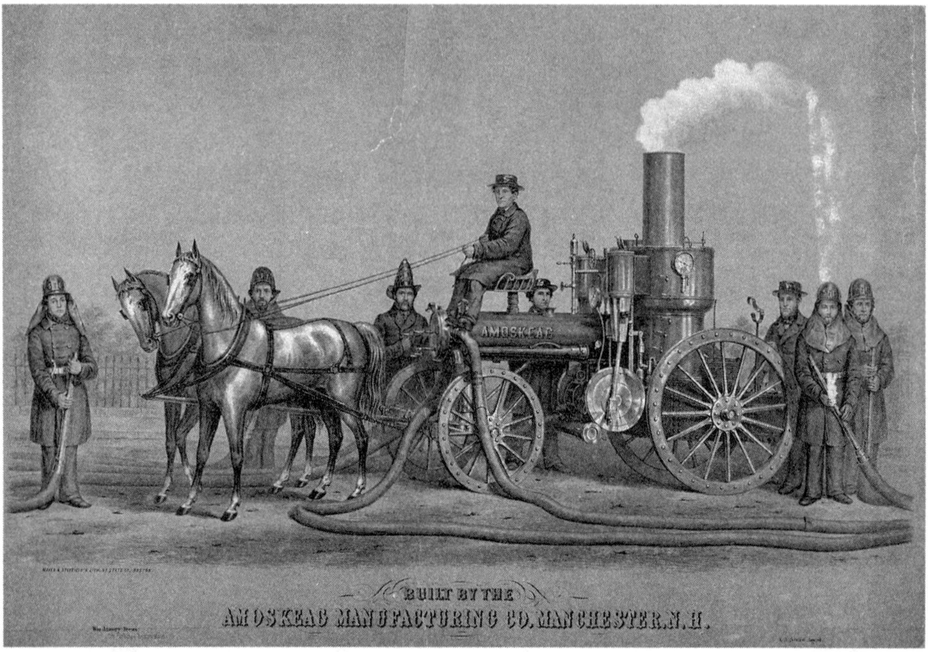

Coal-burning engines such as this model from New Hampshire's Amoskeag Manufacturing Company replaced Boston's hand-powered engines during the mid-1800s. Mayer & Stetfield, *Built by the Amoskeag Manufacturing Co., Manchester, NH* (ca. 1861), priJLC _FIRE_001497, Jay T. Last Collection of Firefighting Prints and Ephemera, 1826–1907, Huntington Library, San Marino, CA.

completion of an ambitious system of public waterworks in 1852 prompted the BFD's reorganization. It also enabled firefighters to couple engines and hoses to hydrants supplied by "over sixty miles of cast-iron pipes that workers had laid beneath every inhabited street in the city." These pipes led back, in turn, through several small reservoirs to the Cochituate Aqueduct and then to the lake of the same name, which impounded the Sudbury River twenty miles west of Boston. Meanwhile, a string of serious fires, including several within the future borders of the Burnt District, led municipal officials to experiment with new technologies for spraying what Bostonians habitually called "Cochituate water" onto budding blazes at much greater pressure and volume than hand engines could muster.[16]

In 1854, Boston's city council purchased a steam fire engine bearing the name of its builder, Cincinnati's fire chief. Weighing over four tons, the coal-burning *Miles Greenwood* was so heavy that even a teeming squad of burly firemen could pull it only a few blocks at a time. The engine nonetheless proved its worth in 1856, when it helped quench a massive blaze at the recently constructed Gerrish Market. This triumph seemed to offer clear proof, as the *Globe* would later recount, "that steam was superior to muscle in operating fire engines."[17]

Despite vocal opposition from volunteer companies, which rightly feared that such "steamers" would render them obsolete, the municipal government introduced a trio of momentous reforms between 1859 and 1860. In addition to dismantling volunteer firefighting outfits, which civic leaders successfully tarred as outdated, inefficient, and more committed to their own gain than protecting their fellow Bostonians, the city sold off all of the BFD's human-drawn, hand-powered engines and purchased a full team of firehorses for every engine house and hose company. Thereafter, Boston's efforts to keep fire at bay would depend on steam engines, municipal water supplies, an increasingly professionalized BFD, and—last but hardly least—a fleet of exceptional but vulnerable beasts.[18]

Firehorses, as the Massachusetts Society for the Prevention of Cruelty Against Animals (MSPCA) explained in its magazine, *Our Dumb Animals*, were carefully "selected for their size, strength and intelligence." Specific characteristics fitted individual animals for the distinct duties and demands of the BFD's three main divisions: engine, hook-and-ladder, and hose companies. "Old, partly broken down animals," including those who had aged out of more demanding duties, could draw hose carriages, which weighed a ton and a half at most. Engines and hook-and-ladder wagons, by contrast, required animals who possessed rarer qualities and were thus costlier as well as harder to procure. Hook-and-ladder wagons, which were heavier than hose carriages and had a higher center of gravity, could be pulled most easily by horses who were "higher at the rump than at the withers, and with long hind legs." "Short-legged and short-backed horses," meanwhile, proved "best for drawing engines," which rode lower but weighed even more (between three and a half and five tons as opposed to less than two tons).[19]

Firehorses performed "work . . . different from that of any other horse in the world." Their labors demanded "a peculiar combination" of innate qualities and learned behaviors. "Everybody knows," a contemporary observer intoned, "that a fire-engine horse is a large, strongly built, handsome animal, with a broad forehead and an intelligent eye." Every such horse, though, also had to learn "to take his place at the engine" when an alarm sounded, "all ready to be hitched up and started off." Each driver in the BFD took the lead in training the horses under his command, endeavoring to "convince his pupil, by gentle treatment, that no harm threatens him, and then to establish a connection in his mind" between the alarm signal and the subsequent "opening of the stall door." After mastering this sequence, horses learned to hasten from their stall and take their "station by the engine pole" so that firemen could lower quick-hitch harnesses over their heads before they could burst from station houses and gallop to fire scenes. Although some horses took just "three or four days" of training to perform the sequence of steps drivers expected them to perfect, others required two to three weeks of practice—and plenty of positive reinforcement.[20]

In addition to learning these procedures, though, firehorses also needed to evince a second, more elusive set of qualities. When confronted by the chaos and peril common to any fire scene, these animals had to check powerful evolutionary urges to fight, freeze, or flee. Firehorses, the *New York Evening Post* explained, had to be able to get "so close to a burning building that the heat almost singes their hair, and yet show no signs of fear . . . ; they must pay no heed to steam-whistles, excited crowds, men running hither and thither, the crackling of flames, nor the glare of a burning building." One firefighting magazine extolled firehorses' knack for standing calmly at blazes "for hours, exposed to all kinds of atmospheric conditions, blinded and half suffocated by the heavy smoke, sweltering in the fierce heat, or singed and blistered by the showers of sparks from the chimney of the steamer or the roof of the burning building, never moving nor showing any signs of discomfort beyond possibly an impatient tossing of the head or a fretful pawing of the pavement on which they stand." A horse called Grief—the BFD numbered its animals, but firemen insisted on giving them names—exemplified the courage a good firehorse had to possess. "He seemed to take a special delight in being in the midst of the sparks from the engine," a posthumous 1890 tribute noted, "and would shake his head and mane with every evidence of glee while the sparks fell upon him like snowflakes." Even when a collapsing building crushed the engine to which Grief was harnessed, this exemplary animal "stood immovable till led away from the rapidly approaching flames."[21]

Firehorses, then, were special creatures. Their unusual qualities—the body types that fitted them to draw different apparatus, the procedures they had mastered, and the composure they mustered in the face of hazards that made other horses cower—made them nearly impossible to replace. Imagine the concern, then, that gripped Chief Damrell, his subordinates, and other Bostonians as the novel flu virus raced through the BFD's station houses.

A Crippled Condition

The Great Horse Flu struck Boston nearly three weeks before an entire district of this city of 250,000 burned to the ground. Nowhere were the impacts of lost equine labors more apparent—or more pregnant with implications—than in the city's former South End, which the *Illustrated Christian Weekly* aptly described as "the seat of an extensive, flourishing, and opulent trade, chiefly in wool and woolens, dress goods, clothing, trimmings, and small wares, boots, shoes and leather, paper and twine, and drugs, paints and oils." With the epizootic making it "almost impossible," the *Globe* reported, "to move the goods" that the hundreds of firms comprising these industries had recently bought and sold, huge hoards of wool, leather, and other highly flammable substances piled up in the neighborhood's stores and warehouses.[22]

Meanwhile, medical and veterinary experts bickered about how best to remedy the equine scourge. On one crucial point, though, nearly all agreed: Any horse stricken by the epizootic needed ample rest. Many Bostonians nonetheless failed to heed this keystone therapy of flu care, as indicated by the *Evening Transcript*'s macabre mention on Halloween that rendering plants and other firms "in the business of utilizing animal remains" had grown "quite busy the last two days, with large orders ahead." Animals who "had to all outward appearance nearly recovered," it continued, had "fallen dead upon the streets in numerous instances" from "conjestion [*sic*] of the lungs, brought on by injudicious exposure to cold air."[23]

The dangers of making sick horses work and the accumulation of immense stocks of flammable goods in downtown Boston both weighed heavily on Chief Damrell. Just four days into the city's tussle with the epizootic, he addressed what he termed his department's "crippled condition" by ordering BFD drivers "to use every precaution to prevent any fatality" among firehorses. Damrell instructed his men to stable any animals displaying the epizootic's telltale symptoms of a "languid" demeanor accompanied by a "dry, hacking cough." Firemen tried to nurse flu-stricken horses back to health by placing steaming pots beneath their heads, bandaging their extremities, and prescribing a patent remedy touted by the municipal government's veterinary surgeon.[24]

Damrell's contingency planning did not stop there. He called a special meeting of the city council's Committee on Fire Department for Friday, October 25. There he commanded the BFD's drivers to hire horses when necessary and even "to seize, in case of fire, any horses they may find upon the street." The committee also authorized a delegation of three councilmen to buy replacement horses. Although this trio soon "visited all the sale stables in the city," the outbreak had nonetheless become so prevalent that these delegates proved "unable, either by purchase or hire, to secure any sound horses for use."[25]

The next day, with rain drenching eerily vacant streets and the condition of Boston's firehorses deteriorating alongside the weather, Damrell called an emergency joint meeting of the city council's Committee on Fire Department and the BFD's Board of Engineers. After this conclave finally adjourned at 10 p.m., Damrell's subordinates trudged to the chief's city hall offices and grabbed "drag ropes for each engine, hose, and hook and ladder company." With their horses sickly and stabled, these BFD officers had to heft these heavy hemp ropes on their backs to "the different engine-houses in the entire city," some of which were more than seven miles away. Damrell also directed his underlings "to obtain volunteers sufficient to double the number of men connected with the engine, hose, and hook and ladder companies." "Should the disease spread further" among the BFD's firehorses, the *Evening Transcript* explained, Damrell and his men planned to sound fire bells audible throughout the city as "a request to citizens to 'man the rope' as of yore." Councilmen pledged to pay "all good citizens" who answered the BFD's call a one-dollar premium (at least half a day's wages for most common laborers). Such precautions, the *Globe* reassured Bostonians, seemed enough "to ensure the city against any extensive conflagration." The *Evening Transcript* agreed, deeming "the Fire-Department arrangements . . . as complete as possible for emergencies."[26]

Within days, though, only a few firehorses remained sufficiently "fit to take from their stalls." Damrell, recalling that he felt "anxious about our suffering animals"—but "still greater" fear "for the welfare of our city should the department be called on"—summoned all his department's "officers and foremen" to meet over supper at Young's Hotel, where they "fully talked over" their predicament. After BFD leaders returned to their homes and stations, Damrell ordered that "in the event of a third alarm," firemen were to "seize and take possession of any horse they could lay hands on and make use of him." If the city council balked at paying "any bills caused by such action," the chief pledged to reimburse horse owners from his own pocket.[27]

But with the Great Horse Flu tightening its hold, where could Damrell's men scare up enough healthy animals to replace their ailing firehorses? And if disaster struck, what could Bostonians expect from creatures who were neither trained nor tested in the trials and tribulations of fire duty?

By Friday, November 1, perhaps 150 of Boston's horses had perished from the epizootic. Among the dead was the BFD's first flu-related fatality, from Engine 3. Sunny skies and warmer temperatures a few days later, though, led many to hope that the outbreak would soon relent. "Should the present weather continue a few days," the *Evening Transcript* ventured, "a general and quick recovery of the affected horses may be confidently predicted." When Tuesday, November 5—Election Day—dawned bright after a heavy frost that "nipped the foliage so effectually that the leaves were gently floating down . . . from the trees like a golden and crimson shower," the *Transcript* proclaimed Boston's streets "again lively with teams and vehicles." Oxen remained in widespread use, but horses returned in force.[28]

The epizootic's "decided decline" spurred misgivings alongside relief. A poem in the *Boston Advertiser* reflected of the horse that "we learn to esteem him in fearing to lose him." Yet this same piece of verse also concluded with a pointed reminder of the cruelties that seemed destined to resume once the epizootic relented: "He is better now—sponge off that lip— / Harness him up again. Get down the whip."[29]

As Bostonians wiped mucus from their horses' muzzles and armed themselves with quirts and lashes, humane reformers stepped up their policing, especially after heavy rains resumed. On Thursday, November 7, members of the MSPCA attempted to send "hundreds of teams—express, truck, market, milk, and private"—back to their stables, with "the owners generally acquiescing when made aware of the injury likely to result from a day's exposure to the moisture," given these animals' "present weak condition." The MSPCA also implored Boston's largest street railway, the Metropolitan, to suspend service, which it had only recently started up again. A public spat ensued. The corporation blamed the society's mollycoddling of Boston's horses for inconveniencing the public. The MSPCA, in turn, badmouthed the Metropolitan's decision "to continue their trips under these cruel and revolting circumstances."[30]

Fair temperatures and tranquil skies greeted Bostonians on November 9, the day of the Great Fire. City streets, according to the *Evening Transcript*, were "again lively, with teams, cars and omnibuses." Although most of Boston's equines were recovering from the epizootic, BFD veterinary surgeon T. S. Perry later painted a grim portrait of the condition of the department's firehorses on that fateful day. Nearly half, Perry testified before the five-member investigative commission that Mayor William Gaston appointed after the disaster "to investigate the cause of the recent fire and the efforts made for its suppression," were "ailing, and had been off their feed." The rest "were about recovering from the fever" but remained "prostrate and weak." Asked whether the BFD's recuperating equines "were fit to be used" when alarms began to toll on that lovely autumn evening, Perry answered that "it was only with extreme difficulty that they could be taken out of the stalls." Influenza had so sapped these firehorses' vitality that "almost all" of them "had . . . to be supported." Animals who could hardly stand or walk without assistance could scarcely be expected to tow steam engines and hose wagons at a gallop for more than a few blocks.[31]

When darkness fell on downtown Boston's stores, counting houses, and factories, the city's firefighting force remained almost entirely unhorsed. As had been the case since the epizootic's invasion, the safety of people and property continued to rest on the contingency plans Damrell and his associates had devised at the pair of emergency meetings the chief had called back in late October. Several fires had erupted since then, but in every instance, firemen and volunteers had heaved engines and other apparatus to the scene, then snuffed out the flames before they could ignite neighboring structures. After a BFD firemen died at a fire on North Street on November 6, Damrell ordered all of Boston's fire stations to be draped in black—a portent, perhaps, that trouble was poised to strike.[32]

Like a Living Furnace

Like the Great Horse Flu, the Great Boston Fire began with a single, unremarkable event that unfolded beyond the ken of human perception. That initial spark began its journey of destruction in the Klous Building, at the corner of Summer and Kingston Streets. Designed by architect John R. Hall in the Second Empire style that Boston's upper crust adored, it was named for its owner, Seman Klous, an entrepreneur and local real estate developer who had cofounded the *Boston Globe* just months before the structure had opened for business in 1866. Like most buildings erected since the 1850s in Boston's downtown, the seventy-two-foot-tall, granite-clad edifice was capped with a mansard roof that lent it a touch of faux Parisian elegance.[33]

Comprising four stories, a basement, and an attic, the Klous Building offered more than twenty thousand square feet of usable space. Its prime location at the heart of Boston's retailing and wholesaling districts enabled Klous to fetch premium rents from the building's three tenants. The ground floor accommodated a dry goods firm that kept its inventory in the basement; the second floor housed a purveyor of "gents' furnishing goods"; and the top two stories and attic were occupied by Alexander K. Young & Company, which produced "hoop-skirts and bustles" and employed 250.[34]

Together, the Klous Building's bulk, design, and dedication to manufacturing and commerce epitomized broader changes afoot in Boston's former South End. "Within the memory of middle-aged men," the retired Christian missionary Henry F. Bond proclaimed in an 1898 reminiscence, Summer Street had been widely "admired for its glory of trees and aristocratic residences." Bond recalled it as "a street of gardens and elm trees that branched over so as almost to meet across the way, with Edward Everett [a famous orator, politician, diplomat, and Harvard president] next door and excellent people on either side."[35]

Bond's paean dovetailed with early nineteenth-century travelers' gushing descriptions of the neighborhood. In 1838, for instance, a Philadelphian praised Summer Street as "decidedly the handsomest street in Boston. Town and Country seem here married to each other, and there is no jar between the husband and the wife. It is a harmonious union, and the source of many pleasures." At 27 Summer Street, which stood "village-fashion, back from the street, in an orchard and garden" behind "a bordering row of elms and Lombardy poplars," one biographer later noted, "Ruth Haskins Emerson gave birth to the famous philosopher and essayist Ralph Waldo Emerson in 1803 at her husband's parsonage." As the pursuits of Seman Klous's tenants indicated, though, the country lane where the charms of pastoral nature had first smitten a young Emerson had grown into an altogether different thoroughfare by the time the epizootic struck.[36]

No one has ever definitively determined the cause of the fire that began somewhere within the Klous Building around supper time on November 9, 1872. Nearly all who worked there had filtered out after ending their afternoon shifts. By roughly 6 p.m., when two partners in the ground-floor dry goods firm locked their doors to catch an evening train back to their suburban homes, the structure was devoid of human life.[37]

Policeman John Page noticed nothing amiss when his regular beat brought him to the corner of Summer and Kingston around 6:50 or 6:55. When Page circled back past the structure ten to twenty minutes later, though, his attention was immediately drawn to a "party of rough boys half way up Summer street, making some disturbance and noise." Page barked at the youths to disperse, but they responded with shouts of "Fire!" Page initially "supposed they were doing it to plague me." Glancing toward the Klous Building, though, the officer noticed flames dancing behind a basement window.[38]

Page beelined to the nearest alarm box—no. 52, a block away at the corner of Summer and Lincoln—to send a telegraphic signal that he hoped would summon firefighters. Introduced in 1852 and still used today in a few corners of Boston, the city's innovative fire telegraph system had captivated observers ever since its debut. Conceived by William F. Channing, a physician and son of famed Unitarian theologian William Ellery Channing, and realized by Moses G. Farmer, a "practical electrician" whom William F. Channing acclaimed as "one of the ablest and most ingenious telegraphic engineers in the country," Boston's fire alarm telegraph inspired both wonder and imitation. The system's "purpose," as Channing told an 1855 Smithsonian audience, was "to cover the surface of the municipal body as thickly . . . with telegraphic signalizing points as the surface of the human body is covered with nervous extremities or papillae, the whole being intelligently connected into a system by which the municipal body shall understand itself in every part, and shall have a common life and vital functions for its own essential purposes." To Channing, "the occurrence of a fire in a city" constituted "one of the exigencies in which rapid and intelligent co-operation is necessary between the members of the municipal body." Recognizing that "the extent of a conflagration depends, to a great extent, upon whether it is reached by the fire department within a short time or not," Channing warned that "the first ten minutes in directing the alarm is worth hours afterward."[39]

By 1872, the city's telegraphic fire alarm system comprised 164 boxes strategically placed throughout Boston. Once unlocked and activated by a special key entrusted to beat cops and other "key-holders," these alarms were supposed to communicate their unique number to the system's telegraphic nerve center, which was perched in a cupola atop Boston's city hall. At this "central and conspicuous position," the "literal net-work of wires" charged with defending what Channing called "the municipal body" converged.[40]

Two distinct arrays of overhead copper wires made up this "net-work." The first carried signals from alarm boxes throughout Boston to the city hall perch. The second fanned outward from the seat of municipal government, carrying pulses capable of tripping water-powered hammers to strike bells atop twenty-three churches, schools, and other public buildings distributed throughout the city. "When they were all making music together," John P. Kennard, the system's longtime superintendent later recalled, "the sound in the street was stirring if not startling in its effect." Additional wires in the outbound network sounded gongs located in every fire station as well as in the homes of Chief Damrell and other members of the BFD's top brass.[41]

The number of times each bell or gong tolled indicated the alarm's box of origin; if necessary, the same bells and gongs could later signal second, third, fourth, and fifth alarms to summon firefighters from increasingly distant locations. It was the responsibility of a lone human operator to mediate between these two electromechanical systems, translating inbound signals from the boxes dotted throughout the city into alarms that identified a blaze's location and severity.[42]

By 1872, the integration of telegraphic innovation, fire department professionalization, and horse-powered firefighting neared its zenith. In Boston's newer engine houses, the *North American Review* explained, "the electric current which gives the alarm unhitches the horses from their stalls at the same time, and those which have been trained instantly take their places at the pole, without any word of command." Thanks to this intricate choreography between humans, horses, and technological systems, it took just "fourteen to twenty seconds," a local journalist noted, "from the time the bell strikes for men and horses to be already to go, and the horses are as eager for a start as the men." "Often, perhaps commonly," another observer declared, firehorses galloped onto Boston's streets with apparatus in tow even before their station's gong had "finished telling the number of the box" whence the alarm originated.[43]

This is what was supposed to happen—but did not—after Officer Page opened Box 52 at the corner of Summer and Lincoln Streets and pulled its slide around 7:08 p.m. Page later testified that he heard the box "ticking." This sound led him to assume—incorrectly, as it turned out—that the alarm had dispatched an electrical signal to city hall that should, in turn, have sent firefighters racing toward the Klous Building. Not until Page returned to the box and again activated it at 7:24 would telegraph operator Charles Stearns sound the first of the eight alarms that would echo that evening throughout Boston and beyond. After the Great Fire had incinerated much of the former South End, the mayor's blue-ribbon commission decried this approximately quarter-hour delay as "disastrous and strange": "disastrous" for obvious reasons, "strange" because no one could explain why Boston's vaunted fire telegraph alarm system had left the city in the lurch.[44]

Even before alarm bells and firehouse gongs finally began to ring, news of the blaze at the Klous Building was already spreading throughout downtown and even across the river to Charlestown. James Powers, for instance, remembered that he was rounding a corner more than a mile away from the former South End when, "as sudden as a flash of lighting, . . . the sky was illuminated, and immediately there was a hurrah in the street from children, boys and girls. They sang out 'Fire,' and all, of course, ran in that direction." By the time the first alarm tolled at 7:24, several Boston firefighters also heard cries of "fire," saw the blaze, or both, and firemen from Hose 2 and Engine 7 were already dashing to the Klous Building.[45]

Few people inhabited the blocks nearest the fire scene. Yet in the minutes that yawned between Page's failed attempt to activate Box 52 and the sounding of the first alarm, residents of a Kingston Street boardinghouse had front-row seats to the blaze's fearsome metamorphosis. When Olin Paine noticed "light . . . reflected" in his third-story window, he looked across the street and saw the Klous Building's basement glowing "like a living furnace." Moments later, the sound of the building's glass "cracking" interrupted William Halsall, his wife, and their companions as they prepared for an evening at the theater. When the group looked out Halsall's second-story "chamber window," they witnessed the fire erupt "up the elevator . . . very rapidly, the same as a blast would." "The instant it went into the elevator," a neighbor of Paine's and Halsall's testified, the blaze "ran up as though there had been a train of powder laid there." The flames took less than a minute to climb from the building's basement to its roof. On their ascent, they ignited all four stories of the structure and its attic. "If [the building] had been saturated with something inflammable," declared Halsall, a sign painter who knew plenty about volatile substances, "it couldn't have burned quicker."[46]

Disastrous and Strange

Chief John Damrell reached the Klous Building about ten minutes later, around 7:32. Damrell later told investigators that when the gong in his house struck, he hastened to dress—though "not as fully" as usual, for he knew Box 52 "to be, as we term it, a very bad box" due to its location in Boston's most fire-prone section. Just a few months earlier, Damrell had taken a visitor to the alarm operator's room atop city hall. His guest praised the beauty of the business blocks stretching southward from the cupola. Damrell admitted that the edifices comprising this bustling commercial district were "pretty to look at, but" hastened to point out that they were "dangerous firetraps in their construction . . . . Some day," he gloomily predicted, "we will have a fire that will sweep them all out of existence."[47]

After Damrell hustled the half mile from his Beacon Hill home to the corner of Kingston and Summer Streets, this nightmare was fast becoming reality: The Klous Building, the chief later remembered, was "on fire from the basement to the top, presenting, as it were, one vast furnace." In "twenty-five years" of firefighting, Damrell claimed that he "never saw such a sight as was presented that night." Already the blaze was giving off such heat that the building's stone facade was exploding. With twenty-pound pieces of stone "flying in every direction," firefighters found it "impossible to get within fifty or seventy-five feet." L. E. Shaw, a twenty-year BFD veteran who rolled up to the Klous Building with Engine 7 soon after Officer Page sounded a second alarm at 7:29, corroborated Damrell's recollections, describing the blaze as already having reached "a very far advanced state from what we usually find" on arrival.[48]

Shaw reached the Klous Building as part of the first of two waves of firemen. In all, the early arrivals included six engine, six hose, two ladder, and two chemical extinguisher companies; all began their journeys at central Boston firehouses. A third alarm at 7:45, followed by subsequent alarms at 8:00, 8:06, 8:07, and 8:24, summoned the rest of Boston's firefighting forces—more than two dozen additional companies in all. Starting with the arrival of an East Cambridge steamer at 8:12, firefighters from other municipalities also entered the fray. By the next day, nearly sixty companies from other parts of Massachusetts as well as Rhode Island, New Hampshire, Maine, and Connecticut rallied to Boston's defense.[49]

The Great Horse Flu occasioned only minor delays for the first wave of firefighters, who originated in downtown stations within two miles of the Klous Building. Over short distances, crews of human pullers managed to draw steamers and other apparatus as fast as firehorses could—and sometimes faster. Nathan Brown, foreman of Hose 2, the first company to spray water onto the Klous Building, reckoned that "our hose-carriage . . . arrived at the scene of the fire even sooner than we should if we had a horse." Brown claimed it had taken mere moments to recruit dozens of "hangers-on" to pull his company's two-wheeled spool of hose to Summer and Kingston. A hook-and-ladder company reinforced Hose 2 between 7:30 and 7:35 and immediately began "attempting to break in the doors" of the Klous Building. Steam engines, the BFD's heaviest and most important category of apparatus, arrived soon after. Daniel Marden estimated that it took "inside of two minutes" for around one hundred volunteers to pull Engine 7 to the scene. Joseph Pierce, Engine 4's acting foreman, likewise claimed that he and his comrades covered the ground between their station and the fire at "what I should call a good trot," taking no more than three minutes longer to reach the scene than it would have taken had their horses not been down with the flu.[50]

The second wave of fire companies, by contrast, faced longer journeys—and hence suffered graver delays. As informed observers had feared since the epizootic reached Boston three weeks earlier, humans could not match the strength, stamina, and speed of firehorses over distance. George Upton, former head of Nantucket's fire department, was among the crowd of several thousand onlookers drawn to the fiery spectacle as the first firemen pulled up to the Klous Building. By the time Upton arrived, he later recalled, "the fire was getting the entire control." Upton was horrified to find just a lone steamer (presumably Engine 7) pumping water onto the blaze. "Where in heaven's name," Upton remembered asking his fellow gawkers, were the BFD's "other engines"?[51]

The answer to Upton's question, it turns out, had as much to do with municipal miserliness as it did with the Great Horse Flu, and brings us to one of several underlying vulnerabilities that magnified the epizootic's contributions to the conflagration: The central city had far fewer fire stations than its prominence and valuation merited because elected officials and bureaucrats had failed to keep up with the unintended consequences of Boston's astounding economic growth.

By 1872, the city's fire stations were concentrated in newer neighborhoods, as well as in Roxbury and Dorchester, two formerly independent towns annexed by Boston in 1868 and 1870, respectively. "The old portion of the city" on the Shawmut Peninsula hosted just six of Boston's twenty-one engine companies—precisely as many as the middle-class bedroom community of Dorchester, even though the central city's assessed value dwarfed Dorchester's by $514 million to $31 million. Damrell later reminded the mayor's investigating commission that in the years preceding the disaster, he had "constantly" warned his fellow citizens as well as the municipal government "that this entire district, comprising nearly all the wealth of Boston" and accounting for some "eight-tenths of all the fires" that broke out each year, "ha[d] been entirely destitute of steam engines."[52]

Hammered by ferocious criticism in the disaster's wake, Damrell defended himself by excoriating the local government for failing to keep up with the times. All six of Boston's downtown engine houses occupied locations chosen decades earlier, when one- to three-story buildings covered the Shawmut Peninsula and hand-powered, human-drawn engines represented the vanguard of firefighting technology. Financial considerations, especially skyrocketing property values, led city councilmen to table Damrell's requests for more station houses. City hall's stinginess compelled the BFD to fight fires in some of the continent's busiest manufacturing and commercial neighborhoods with one hand tied behind its back.

When Lawrence Curtis, a clerk who worked in the former South End, reached the fire around 7:40, the blaze was still "confined." Suddenly, though, "parts of the building fell in" and "large sheets of flame flew out and across the street." With an ever-increasing crowd looking on aghast, a flagpole attached to a structure opposite the Klous Building caught fire. Flames immediately raced down the flagpole, then inched along "wooden cornices" high above the street. According to Curtis, "it burned very slowly, apparently attracting little notice from the department, who were pumping vigorously into the solid flames, that nothing could control." When one of his companions complained that "the firemen did not seem to be doing much," Curtis responded with a touch of sympathy, "If I was a fireman I should not know what to do; because it seemed as if nothing could possibly be done."[53]

As Curtis's despair suggests, the first wave of firefighters proved no match for the blaze exploding outward from the Klous Building. More engines would certainly have made a difference. Yet from the earliest stages of the Great Boston Fire, firefighters faced other problems, too.

"The water did not seem to make any impression," one eyewitness recounted of the BFD's opening salvos against the blaze. At least one company of firemen tried to take the fight to the fire by entering the Klous Building and running a line of hose up its stairs, only for searing heat and fast-moving flames to force a hasty retreat. After this failed attempt to combat the blaze directly, firefighters kept to the streets rather than rushing into burning structures. Everyone involved with the BFD knew that few buildings in the former South End had fire escapes, so ordering axmen and hosemen into the district's towering structures might well have doomed entire fire companies to injury or even death.[54]

And yet in firefighting as in warfare, sticking to the low ground made for an uphill struggle. J. M. Crafts, who reached the fire scene at 7:45, observed how the BFD's hoses "were playing quite uselessly on the fronts" of the buildings facing Summer Street because of the "lack of power in the stream; it couldn't be carried high enough," for "the fire was above the point that the water reached."[55]

The water shortages that plagued firefighters throughout the night resulted from the same governmental tightfistedness that had left the former South End woefully undersupplied with fire stations. Over the previous decades, the neighborhood had grown into perhaps the densest, most highly capitalized, and most combustible stretch of the city. Yet as flames started surging outward from the Klous Building, firefighters had no choice but to rely on a quarter-century-old water supply system that, as Damrell later bemoaned, had been "placed there when that territory" was overwhelmingly residential. This system, the chief complained, had "never been changed, while the buildings have been changing constantly," with "high stores hav[ing] taken the place of the dwellings" throughout the former South End.[56]

The area's water supply led from the six- and eight-inch pipes that ran below most of the neighborhood's thoroughfares to a twelve-inch main under Bedford and Broad Streets; this, in turn, led back to a twenty-four-inch main beneath Washington Street. The Great Fire revealed these pipes to be undersized and clogged with years of accumulated rust and sediment. Corrosion had narrowed the usable diameter of the six-inch pipes below Summer Street and most of the district's other roads to an estimated four and a half inches, reducing their carrying capacity by almost half. The usable diameter of the four-inch lines that branched outward from these pipes to feed most of the area's fire hydrants, meanwhile, had constricted by an inch or even an inch and a half, enabling them to carry just 39 percent as much water as when they were installed.[57]

The former South End's hydrants were as outdated and inadequate as the pipes that supplied them. For years Chief Damrell had begged municipal officeholders to replace Boston's old fireplugs with a newer model, the

Lowry hydrant. Unlike the city's existing hydrants, which provided just one coupling where firefighters could attach hoses, the Lowry furnished six. Rather than drawing water from four-inch feeder lines, moreover, these newer hydrants connected directly to water mains. These features enabled Lowry hydrants to feed several engines and hoses simultaneously without losing water pressure. This permitted firefighters, in turn, to mass many more engines at a fire scene than the old hydrants, which were spaced a few hundred feet apart, could supply.[58]

After Damrell witnessed an impressive performance of the Lowry hydrants' supremacy a few years before the Great Fire, the chief repeatedly lobbied the Boston Water Board and municipal officials "for larger mains, for more hydrants, and for the more efficient hydrant" throughout Central Boston. Yet these pleas, like those to locate additional fire stations in the former South End, failed to persuade municipal leaders to make costly investments to protect downtown. The city's government *did* install hundreds of Lowry hydrants in the late 1860s and early 1870s—but they placed nearly all of them in East Boston, Dorchester, and Roxbury, bedroom communities where these hydrants' superiority over the old model was pretty much overkill. According to Damrell, these decisions left the former South End's water supply system so deficient that it kindled grave concerns among "every one who had anything to do with the Fire Department."[59]

The Burnt District was created, in short, not just by the Great Horse Flu but also by the reluctance of pennywise but pound-foolish officeholders and elected officials to foot the bill for additional fire stations, wider pipes, and updated hydrants to accommodate the former South End's transmutation from a neighborhood of elegant residences to a bustling hive of commerce. Systematically neglecting the yawning mismatch between the labyrinth of commercial buildings that towered atop Emerson's childhood stomping grounds, on the one hand, and the BFD's capacity to respond to alarms in the district and drown small blazes before they erupted into colossal conflagrations, on the other, Boston's government was quite literally playing with fire.[60]

The Cost of These Minutes

As flames pushed outward from the Klous Building between 7:40 and 7:45 p.m., they coursed along two main routes. One flame-front dashed southeastward down Summer Street toward Boston Harbor. Brigadier General William Burt, Boston's postmaster and judge advocate general for Massachusetts throughout the Civil War, later recounted that after the fire "took in the corner" of Summer and Bedford Streets, "the wind carried [it] almost in an angle from the old Church Green block," a site left vacant by the 1868 demolition of New South Church. The blaze subsequently "beat up to the windward faster in the course of an hour," Burt testified, "than at any fire I ever saw."[61]

Meanwhile, another tongue of flames hurtled northward up Kingston Street. After navigating a jog in Boston's mazelike street system, it pressed up Otis Street. Onlookers recognized that "as soon as it crossed" that roadway "and spread down towards Winthrop square," an open area that would give full vent to the blaze, there was no way to stop the conflagration from mushrooming into "a very serious fire."[62]

As this pair of flame-fronts pushed outward from the Klous Building, the second wave of firefighters began straggling onto the scene. The fourth alarm at 8 p.m. called in the BFD's remaining outfits from outlying parts of Boston. Three engine companies judged their firehorses sufficiently healthy to do their jobs. Every other company in the second wave hastily rounded up volunteers, took hold of the drag ropes that BFD officers had lugged back from city hall two weeks earlier, and heaved their apparatus as fast as their muscles would permit over distances ranging from two to seven miles.[63]

These gangs of human pullers performed surprisingly well. Damrell claimed that a team of firemen and volunteers from Engine House 19 in the Mattapan neighborhood had kept up "neck and tie" with a four-horse team from a nearby station for most of their nearly seven-mile journey into the former South End. Even this exceptional crew, though, flagged on the home stretch, reaching the vicinity of Box 52 some four minutes after their horse-powered neighbors. Most companies in the second wave, though, experienced even longer epizootic-driven delays.[64]

Firefighters from adjoining municipalities also hastened into Boston to assist the BFD. The alarms that pealed through the night air from the city's churches and public buildings were audible in Charlestown, Cambridge, and other towns; flames and smoke from the blaze soon became visible from miles away, too. Although many out-of-town companies had already responded to these sights and sounds by rushing toward the former South End, Chief Damrell started dispatching desperate telegraphic pleas for backup by 8:30.[65]

As the firefight intensified, Damrell called in reinforcements from increasingly distant municipalities. Since the Great Horse Flu continued to grip most of New England, the fire companies that rallied to Boston's aid mostly relied on manpower to draw engines and other apparatus to nearby train depots, where waiting crowds hefted them onto train cars. The moment the locomotives hauling these reinforcements pulled into downtown depots, crowds of citizens swarmed in to lift steamers onto Boston's streets so that volunteers could pull them toward the conflagration.[66]

After sitting through weeks of testimony on the Great Boston Fire, the mayor's investigating commission acknowledged in the preface to its 688-page report on the disaster that "the difference of speed between horse-power and hand-power is less than the general public suppose," yet the commissioners also lambasted the Great Horse Flu for causing delays ranging "from three to five minutes for the nearest" companies to the Klous Building "to forty minutes for the most distant" BFD engine companies. "No one," they somberly noted, "can tell what was the cost of these minutes to our city."[67]

The true magnitude of that toll first became apparent as the fire's northern salient roared from Otis Street into Winthrop Square. Damrell later lamented how he had "got the Boston and Charlestown departments massed" at this critical juncture in hopes of blocking the fire's path, only for the water to give out. "If we had a sufficient supply," Damrell asserted, he had "no doubt" he and his forces "could have kept [the] fire there." Even under the best of circumstances, though, downtown Boston's pipes and

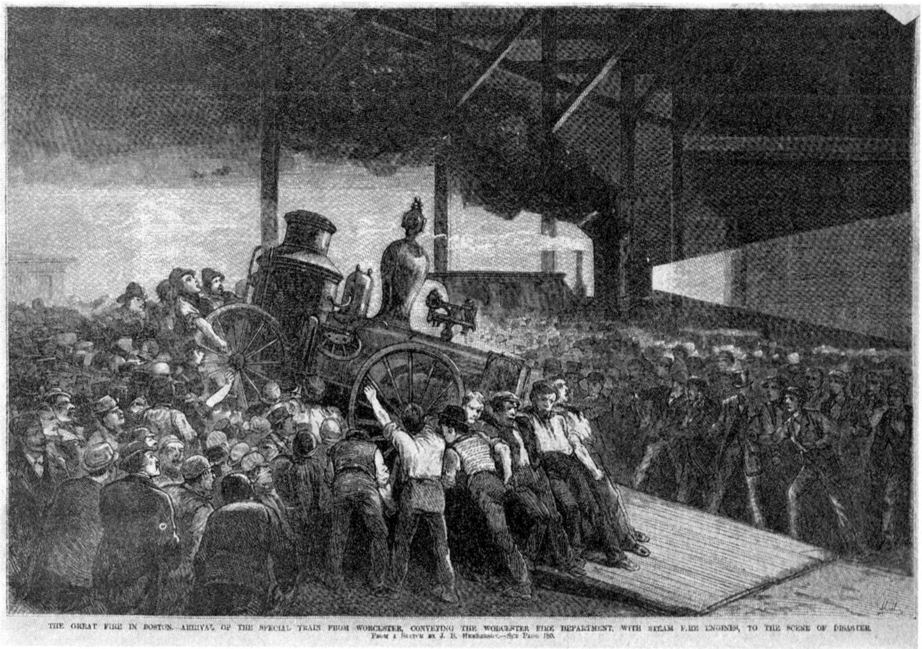

Crowds gathered at Boston's railroad depots to help firefighters from other towns and cities to unload their fire engines. With Boston's horses ailing, people then powered these machines to the fire scene. J. B. Henderson, "The Great Fire in Boston.—Arrival of the Special Train from Worcester . . . ," *Frank Leslie's Illustrated Newspaper*, November 23, 1872, 179. Digital Commonwealth, https://ark.digitalcommonwealth.org/ark:/50959/xp68kr439.

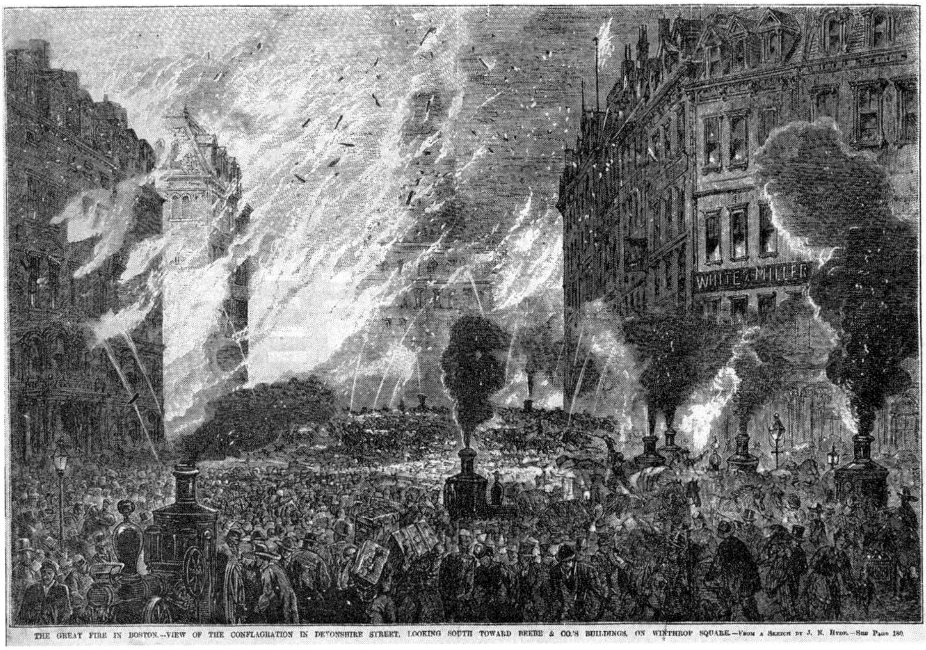

The foreground of this scene comprises a jumble of fire crews, panicked Bostonians removing their possessions from harm's way, and gawkers. Especially telling is the evident mismatch between the paltry streams of water firemen were attempting to spray into buildings where the fire was coursing and the imposing height of the structures that enclosed Winthrop Square. The Boston Fire Department and the fire companies that had raced to its assistance on November 9, 1872, proved unable to hold off the conflagration at this crucial juncture. John H. Hyde, "The Great Fire in Boston.—View of the Conflagration in Devonshire Street, Looking South Toward Beebe & Co.'s Buildings on Winthrop Square," *Frank Leslie's Illustrated Newspaper*, November 23, 1872, 178. Digital Commonwealth, https://ark.digitalcommonwealth.org/ark:/50959/xp68kr41r.

hydrants could have supplied only about forty-two simultaneous streams of water—far less than Damrell and his comrades needed to extinguish so big and ferocious a blaze. Rather than risking his firefighters' lives, the chief thus ordered them to stand down and retreat before the fast-advancing flames.[68]

Alderman and longtime BFD member William Woolley summed up the dire consequences of Boston's failure to upgrade its water system. If the city council and Water Board had heeded Damrell's pleas for thicker pipes, newer hydrants, and more engine houses throughout central Boston, Wooley averred, "the fire would not have extended over one-twentieth part of the territory" that lay in ruins by Sunday, November 10.[69]

The forceful gusts generated by the inferno added to the dangers and difficulties firemen faced. "There was such a draft of wind," Charlestown Fire Chief William Delano recounted, "that it was almost impossible to get a stream up on the narrow streets." The height of the buildings bordering Winthrop Square further hampered the firefight. An engraving in *Frank Leslie's Illustrated Newspaper* vividly depicted this mismatch by showing more than a dozen engines pumping piddling streams of water that rarely reached even the third story on buildings that soared one hundred feet or more above street level.[70]

Gorgeous Tinder Boxes

The same illustration captured another key factor in the fire's rapid thrust from the Klous Building outward through Winthrop Square and Church Green: the mansard roofs that crowned at least three-quarters of the former South End's buildings. High above the reach of firefighters' hoses, the dodgy construction of these fashionable and cost-conscious features hastened the conflagration's growth.

Named after a pair of French architects who collaborated on the Palais de Versailles and other baroque chefs d'oeuvres, mansards became a defining feature of Second Empire architecture, which enjoyed widespread popularity throughout the Atlantic world starting in the 1850s. Although mansards jibed with nineteenth-century Bostonians' enchantment with all things French, these roofs' attractions had as much to do with money as with style. Architects favored mansards, one magazine explained, because they combined "beauty of effect" with "economy in height and room." Other roofing designs, another journalist noted, saddled landlords with "an attic story, an unattractive, inconveniently shaped and poorly lighted place only suitable for a rubbish room." Mansards, by contrast, pitched steeply upward from a building's perimeter to enclose attics that proved "equal to and quite as desirable" as main-floor rooms.[71]

Despite the extra revenue the style promised, Americans nonetheless sought to squeeze additional savings from mansards by building them almost entirely from wood. In contrast to European builders, who preferred to fashion such roofs from fire-retardant iron, slate, or copper, American architects almost always restricted these costly materials to cornices, trim, and other superficial features—or dispensed with them altogether. Given that downtown Boston's buildings loomed 80 or even 120 feet above street level, after all, it took a trained eye to distinguish wood expertly finished to look like metal or stone from the real thing.[72]

Just a few years before the Great Boston Fire, the dangers of wooden mansards garnered widespread attention when fire consumed Chicago's Drake Block, leading one newspaper to excoriate this building's ornate roof as a "gorgeous tinder box." This 1870 disaster heightened concerns regarding the safety of wooden mansards, but no one seriously considered removing them from the Klous Building or the hundreds of other structures they crowned throughout downtown Boston. The city's weak building codes, moreover, did nothing to prevent hundreds more from going up in the years following the Drake Block's destruction. David Chamberlin, who became Boston's first building inspector in 1871, invariably instructed builders to construct mansards from "non-combustible material—galvanized iron and copper." Yet he was also the first to admit that municipal ordinances gave him "no power" to enforce the city's haphazard building codes.[73]

Beginning with the blaze's initial spread from the Klous Building to neighboring structures, the Great Fire often leapt from one wood-framed roof to the next. George Gardner, a businessman who joined the crowds of rubberneckers who packed into the former South End throughout the firefight, later described how a mansard consisting of "thirty to forty feet . . . of wood-work" went up like "a great bonfire in the air." Physician Henry Bigelow, meanwhile, recounted how such roofs fueled the conflagration's expansion far above the reach of firefighters' streams. "When one store was pretty well burned," Bigelow later testified, "the upright roof of the next one (for they were most all of them French [i.e., mansard] roofs) began to smoke at a dozen or so small points between the slates. After a while, a few little tongues of fire appeared here and there," Bigelow continued. "Then came the flame, perhaps not larger than your finger or your wrist. Presently somewhere a place as big as your head was burned through, and then the whole roof was on fire." When the mayor's investigating committee asked David Chamberlain why the fire had become "so uncontrollable," the inspector offered a five-word summation: "*Mansard roofs on high buildings*."[74]

Although firefighters from outlying BFD stations as well as other communities periodically reinforced Damrell and his men, the Great Fire continued to engulf widening swaths of the former South End. A *Globe* retrospective later recalled how the inferno "assumed such terrible proportions that all the buildings" on several of the former South End's streets "were swept out of existence, and any attempt to resist the march of the fire through those streets would have meant loss of apparatus and the death of men." By 10 p.m., Postmaster Burt later remembered, the fire had erupted "beyond our control." In the hours that followed, the survival of the former South End—and, at times, even Boston itself—teetered in the balance.[75]

Like Oil Factories

Several subtler consequences of the Great Horse Flu further complicated the firefight while making the Great Fire even more destructive than it might otherwise have been. Consider, first, the matter of fuel. In the brave new era of steam, it took fire to fight fire. But with nearly all of Boston's firehorses sick or convalescing, and most other equines throughout New England still too unwell to labor safely, the forty-five engine companies who spearheaded the struggle against the inferno had trouble keeping their boilers burning.

Fuel shortages frequently forced firemen to retreat. Each BFD steamer should have started off with roughly five hundred pounds of coal—enough to continue pumping water from hydrant to hose for roughly one hour. The typical procedure was for drivers to unhitch their horses from the engine once a second alarm sounded, then drive them to the nearest station house or fuel cache so drivers could hitch their team to a wagon preloaded with two

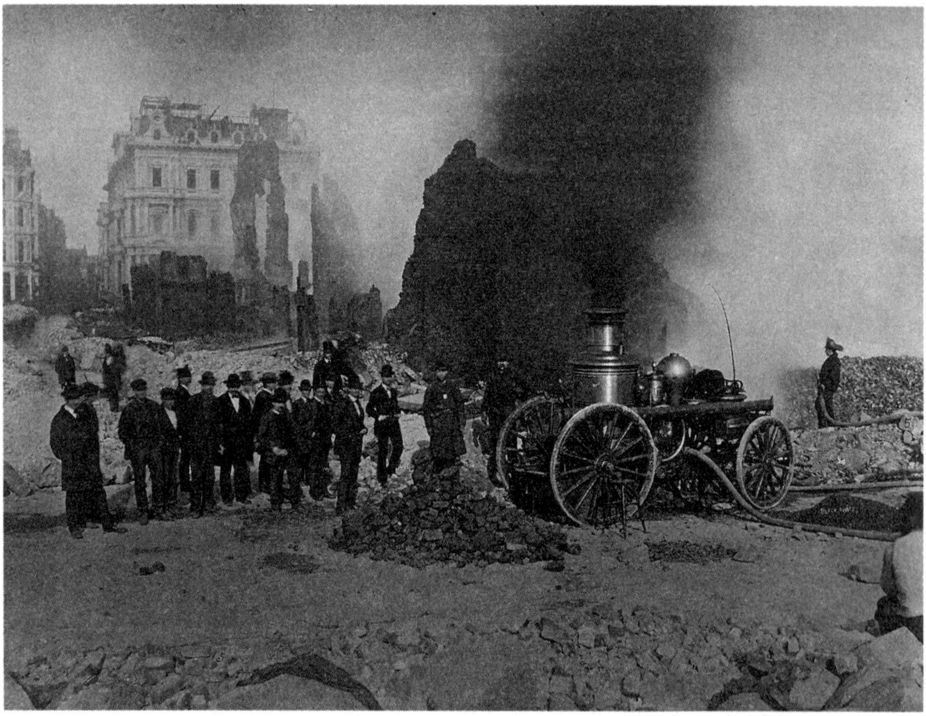

This photograph shows a steam engine pumping water onto the smoldering ruins of the former South End. Note the large pile of coal in front of the engine. James Wallace Black, *Federal St. (Post Office . . . Fire Engine)*, photograph (ca. 1872). Digital Commonwealth, https://www.digitalcommonwealth.org/search/commonwealth:2801pj69f.

to two and a half tons of English cannel coal. Returning to the fire scene, they would next "dump some two hundred or three hundred weight of coal alongside" any engine that blew "three sharp whistles" to signal that it was low on fuel, then repeat these rounds until firefighters had doused the blaze.[76]

The Great Horse Flu bedeviled this routine. After the first wave of engines burned through their payloads, one witness recounted, they became "very clamorous for coal." Growing desperate, firemen scared up whatever fuel they could find. They harvested wooden boxes and pallets from the district's stores and warehouses, raided logs from residents' woodpiles, and even pried boards off fences and outbuildings. Engine 4's John Regan later granted that "there was a want of coal" throughout the firefight's early phases, then added that engines nonetheless "had plenty of fuel" from scavenged wood. Later in the night, a man-powered wagon began delivering coal to steamers, enabling several engines that had been out of service for twenty-five minutes or more to resume pumping. Before long, though, the armada of engines arrayed against the conflagration outstripped fuel supplies. Postmaster Burt recalled that he "counted around me some thirty-two steam fire engines, actually running. No previous forethought," he argued, "could have supplied so many with coal or fuel."[77]

Chief Damrell tried to meet the need by ordering his drivers to press into fuel supply service the few BFD horses who had drawn their apparatus to the former South End. Animals donated by the post office and several public-spirited citizens soon joined horses from Hook and Ladder 5 and Engines 6, 7, and 17 in pulling wagons loaded with coal between stations, fuel caches, and the fire scene. By midday on Sunday, November 10, the engines arrayed against the conflagration had burned through more than a hundred tons of coal.[78]

Earlier in the night, a city councilman handed Chief Damrell the reins to his horse, then declared, "Your horses are sick; I have a good horse; use him if you kill him." This councilman's steed apparently managed to survive working all night to supply steamers with coal. His comrades in Engine 17's team, though, proved less fortunate. Still suffering from lingering flu symptoms, they had pulled their company's engine four miles from Dorchester to the former South End, then pulled countless loads of coal to feed fuel-starved steamers. These feats proved too much for these animals to survive, and Damrell attributed their demise to "the effects of their use" in combatting the Great Fire.[79]

In addition to exacerbating the BFD's fuel supply problems, the epizootic also made it harder for Bostonians to prevent their property from going up in smoke. With so many horses still suffering from influenza and its complications, bulkier items proved especially difficult to move from harm's way. Making matters worse, the police barred vehicular traffic within the fire zone to discourage looting and protect fire hoses from being crushed or punctured. Nor was it clear where people could take their belongings for safekeeping. Most streets in the former South End were notoriously narrow, and firemen needed all the space they could get to reposition engines, ladders, and hoses as fast-changing circumstances demanded. Many residents and business owners thus resigned themselves to losing anything they could not haul away under their own steam—or that of boys who, as Louisa May Alcott recounted to her sister, "were hired at high prices to become beasts of burden for awhile." Several storekeepers even began inviting bystanders to help themselves to merchandise that was otherwise doomed to certain destruction.[80]

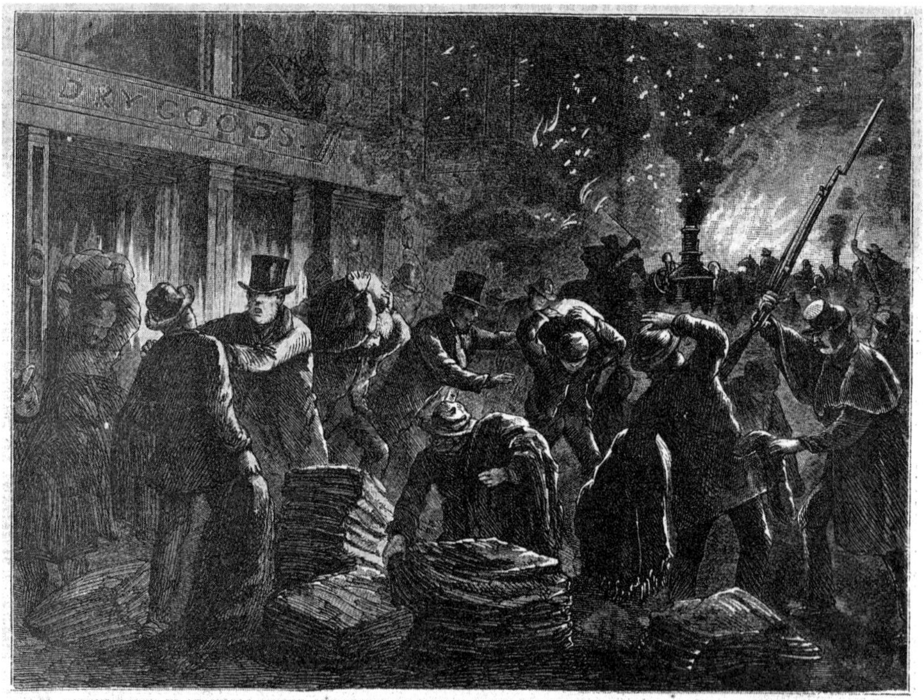

BOSTON—SCENE IN CHAUNCEY STREET—MERCHANTS DEFENDING THEIR GOODS AGAINST THIEVES AND ROUGHS.—[See Page 934.]

The Great Horse Flu made it difficult for merchants in the former South End to protect their property and inventory against the flames. Thieves and looters descended, while policemen and troops tried to keep the peace. "Boston—Scene in Chauncey Street," *Harper's Weekly*, November 30, 1872, 932. Digital Commonwealth, https://www.digitalcommonwealth.org/search/commonwealth:q811kn125.

Finally, early in the morning of November 10, policemen allowed horse-drawn vehicles back into parts of the former South End. They also opened the gates of Boston Common, a few blocks west of the Great Fire's western edge, "to allow people to cart their goods there," with Fort Hill serving the same purpose for those located nearer the waterfront. As Sunday dawned, piled-up possessions, makeshift shanties, and canvas tents were already offering shelter from the firestorm for hundreds of displaced residents and more than a thousand burned-out businesses.[81]

While the epizootic hindered efforts to fight the Great Fire, the outbreak made perhaps its most consequential contribution to the disaster well before the first spark in the Klous Building had even come to life. Three weeks of flu-fueled transportation disruptions caused vast inventories of combustible raw materials and finished products to build up in stores, factories, and warehouses throughout the former South End. This accumulation of goods, in turn, fed the conflagration's growth and aggravated its economic impact.

Because "the horse distemper" had "prevented the delivery of wool," Boston's stock of that highly flammable fiber "was probably at its very largest" in recorded history. The *New York Times* described how "the wool-houses" lining Federal Street exploded "like oil factories." The Great Fire, the *Times* explained, "could never have attacked at a more dangerous time; crammed from cellar to garret, hundreds of thousands of dollars' worth were on hand that might have been delivered to customers had it not been for the horse disease." Much the same story unfolded along Pearl and High Streets, "reputed the most extensive shoe and leather market in the world," where a quarter million cattle hides carried to Boston from throughout the world went up in flames.[82]

Even as the "sickly smell of smouldering leather and wool" hung thick in the air, unprecedented stocks of other goods fanned the fire's advance. "The paper-houses came next," the *Times* alleged, burning out "the majority of the large city dealers." Cotton merchants, clothiers, newspaper and magazine publishers, and other businesses also suffered outsized losses because the novel influenza virus had gummed up Boston's commerce.[83]

Across the Waste

As midnight approached, the conflagration that had begun with a mysterious spark somewhere in the Klous Building's basement stood poised to obliterate the former South End. With firefighters seemingly powerless to stop the blaze's expansion, many observers now feared that the Great Fire might push onward to South Boston, jump Washington Street to spill into

Boston Common, and perhaps even incinerate the State Street corridor, the city's political and financial core. A cadre of influential politicians and leading citizens thus took it upon themselves to pressure Mayor Gaston and Chief Damrell into authorizing the use of explosives to create fire breaks. At an emergency meeting held in Gaston's city hall chambers around 1 a.m., they beseeched Damrell to consent to their gunpowder scheme.[84]

A year before, Damrell had ventured to a burned-out Chicago to question General Philip Sheridan, who had played an instrumental role in combatting that city's Great Fire. When Damrell asked Sheridan about the "glowing accounts of your success in staying the conflagration in Chicago"—newspaper accounts had alleged that "only through the medium of gunpowder was any part of the city saved"—Sheridan retorted that this tactic had instead proven "a signal failure." Boston's top firefighter, like virtually every other expert to investigate the matter, decided that the potential risks of blasting down buildings to deprive the fire of fresh fuel outweighed the benefits. Yet with flames tearing through his own city and several of Boston's biggest power brokers turning the screws, Damrell caved and permitted Postmaster Burt and other private citizens to mine and detonate more than a dozen structures. These efforts to create firebreaks failed, just as Damrell and other skeptics anticipated they would. Most explosions failed to demolish their intended target. Instead of containing the inferno, these blasts accelerated its growth while also forcing firemen to retreat to safer positions.[85]

Where gunpowder failed, conventional tactics succeeded. Firefighters waged a series of crucial stands throughout the night and early morning. Many such efforts met with defeat, but success at several key junctures blocked the blaze from expanding beyond the former South End. Firemen used a tugboat hastily outfitted with "a fire pump," to cite just one instance, to save the Hartford and Erie Railroad bridge and stop the flames from coursing down the former South End's wharves and into South Boston. Chief Damrell and the vast army of firefighters who had valiantly answered Boston's call received less credit than they deserved for these victories. Meanwhile, within the former South End itself, platoons of private citizens risked life and limb to save Hovey's Store, Boston's new post office, and a few other structures by manning bucket brigades, protecting wooden windows and roofs with wet blankets, and deploying a host of other time-honored but increasingly passé techniques.[86]

As dawn finally broke on Sunday, November 10, nearly two thousand firefighters continued to battle the Great Boston Fire. Every inbound train brought additional reinforcements. That morning, Emily Marshall Eliot, a fifteen-year-old from a prominent Boston family, joined the crowds flocking to the Burnt District "to look at the sad state of things." "Trinity Church was burnt down last night," she lamented in her journal: "Where shall we go to church?" The fire, Eliot noted, was "still raging & raging. God help us."[87]

Later that afternoon, firefighters finally got the upper hand. On Sunday night, though, smoldering fires began on several occasions to blow up into larger blazes punctuated by numerous explosions of gas that had leaked from the Burnt District's shattered pipes. For weeks to come, the rubble continued to smoke.[88]

In late November, a reporter offered a pen portrait of the former South End's ruins. "Looking across the waste," they could discern "nothing but a solitary tall chimney, here and there a tottering corner or side wall, and heaps on heaps of chipped blocks of granite, disjointed bricks, and twisted iron-work. The streets are all obliterated by the *débris*," they continued, "the landmarks are all gone, the eye wanders from side to side in perplexity, and the air is filled with smoke and gloom."[89]

Even as the Great Fire smoldered, Bostonians tallied their losses. "The calamity," one souvenir history bemoaned, "swept out of existence millions of property, impoverished hundreds of business men, and broke all but two of the local insurance companies of the city," the investors in which ranged from wealthy Brahmins to folks of humbler means. Against total fire-related losses approaching $80 million, property owners and tenants held just $55 million of insurance. American and British insurers took months to make good on the claims against them; more than a dozen firms dissolved without making their policyholders whole. Among the biggest losers were Harvard College, Boston University, and Simmons College, each of which suffered losses of $200,000 on real estate holdings in the burn zone.[90]

Labor, however, arguably suffered even more than capital. In obliterating what one observer rightly described as "the accumulation of honest toil of days and nights, weeks, months and years," the Great Boston Fire forced at least twenty thousand clerks, factory operatives, and other workers into joblessness. In the following weeks and months, most of these laboring people could only keep food on the table and roofs over their heads by drawing on the donations that flooded into Boston from across the United States and well beyond. Alas, elite Bostonians quickly established control over these relief funds and doled out short-term aid with Yankee stinginess. The only consolation for the unemployed was the fact that the conflagration, like most such catastrophes, generated plenty of work—not just to clear the wreckage but also to rebuild the former South End. As they had before the Great Fire, laborers toiled alongside Boston's recovering horse population in "carting away all of value that may remain of the millions of dollars' worth of property which was engulfed in the fiery maelstrom." Teams hauled innumerable cart- and wagonloads of rubble from the Burnt District to the waterfront, where the remnants of the former South End served as landfill for another encroachment of the Shawmut Peninsula into Boston Harbor. Although the *Evening Transcript* boasted on Wednesday, November 20, that the "horse distemper has nearly disappeared in this vicinity," the epizootic's ongoing effects made horses hard to procure well into December.[91]

Meanwhile, other Americans joined New Englanders in counting their lucky stars that the flames had largely spared what *Harper's* called "the historic relics of which Boston is so proud." "Nothing," the *Hartford Courant* agreed, "could have replaced the Old South Church with its memories of the past two centuries, or Faneuil Hall, the 'cradle of liberty,' which has stood the trials of one hundred and thirty years." The list of human casualties from the firestorm also proved reassuringly short, though not short enough to save the Abbott family of Charlestown from wrenching loss. As the brothers Lewis and Albert Abbott helped make a courageous stand to prevent the blaze from jumping across Washington Street, a collapsing building trapped them. Albert's comrades managed to pull him from the rubble, but his injuries were so severe that he lingered for weeks "at the point of death at the City Hospital." Each day, a third Abbott brother, Nathan, returned to the ruins to search for Lewis's remains. More than two weeks after the Great Fire, Nathan, already mourning Lewis's passing, suffered a brutal double blow: His mother died from "a fever, brought on by the excitement caused by the misfortunes which befell her children," and Albert Abbott passed into the great beyond later that day.[92]

Wherever the epizootic reached, the novel influenza virus and its complications hit fire departments and firehorses hard. In all but a few instances, though, the use of human volunteers and other contingency plans staved off disaster. The most notable exception was a blaze that struck Lexington, Kentucky, a little over a week after the Great Boston Fire. After the Great Horse Flu had "disabled all the horses of the fire department," a blaze broke out in a planing mill. Because steam engines "drawn by citizens" were "considerably delayed in reaching" the scene, "a strong northwest wind" turned this small fire into a veritable inferno that razed nineteen structures, most of them "tenements," wire service reports maintained, "principally occupied by negroes."[93]

There were many reasons the Massachusetts capital proved the only place to experience a district-destroying conflagration during an epizootic that paralyzed fire departments in every stretch of the northern Americas for weeks on end. Several wildcards played a role, including the after-hours timing and basement location of the initial Klous Building blaze as well as the unexplained failure of the city's telegraphic alarm system to sound when Officer Page first attempted to activate Box 52. Ultimately, though, the Great Boston Fire revealed the Great Horse Flu's capacity to expose and exacerbate the long-standing infrastructural problems that Chief Damrell and other informed observers had long urged city leaders to remedy: inadequate water supplies, antiquated hydrants, and, perhaps most of all, insufficient fire stations to safeguard the city's rapidly commercializing downtown against catastrophe.[94]

On the Great Fire's one-year anniversary, the *Evening Transcript* marveled that "within twelve months," the "mass of smoking, jagged, and unsightly ruins" that had blanketed sixty-five acres of Boston had been replaced by "fine and symmetrical structures, far exceeding in general attractiveness and beauty those covering any other metropolitan locality of the same dimensions in the United States." As they reconstructed the former South End, Bostonians also tried to remedy at least some of the vulnerabilities that had contributed to the district's destruction. In addition to widening seventeen Burnt District thoroughfares, extending four others, and carving Post Office Square from Water Street, the municipal government also replaced central Boston's undersized and corroded pipes with new eight- and twelve-inch conduits while swapping out 83 of the area's out-of-date hydrants for 113 Lowry hydrants spaced no more than 260 feet apart—close enough together for fleets of fire engines to quench incipient blazes before they could grow too menacing.[95]

As one local paper philosophized, "Occurrences calamitous in their first effects sometimes result in important material good." Yet many of the problems that vexed firefighters in November 1872 endured. City leaders, fearing that growing municipal debt and rising taxes would lead even more wealthy and middle-class Bostonians to decamp for fast-growing horsecar suburbs beyond city limits, flinched at the expense of stationing additional fire companies in the former South End, with the exception of a new engine house on municipally owned land atop Fort Hill, on the Burnt District's southeastern fringe. At least the mansard roofs that had done so much to hasten the Great Fire's progress soon fell out of fashion; many builders also incorporated stronger fireproofing measures, although proposed improvements to Boston's building codes foundered in the face of concerted lobbying by deep-pocketed construction interests. As for the BFD, a sweeping new ordinance passed in the wake of a late May 1873 fire that destroyed four acres of buildings valued at $1 to $2 million placed the department under an independent commission instead of the city council; provided for more rigorous building inspections; tightened regulations on "the manufacture, storage and sale" of volatile substances; and made all firemen permanent municipal employees (a status enjoyed by only 90 of the 475 Boston firefighters who squared off against the Great Fire).[96]

As for the Great Horse Flu, it was already galloping through the Upper South and Great Lakes by the time the Great Fire broke out. The damage the epizootic soon wreaked on these overwhelmingly rural regions added to the growing economic toll levied by the scourge's Northeastern disruptions as well as the former South End's destruction, with dire consequences for the newly reelected Grant administration as well as the ruling Republican Party's efforts to rebuild a war-torn nation.

CHAPTER 5

A MOST UNWELCOME GHOST

Unsettling Rural Economies in the South and Midwest

As Bostonians licked their wounds and tallied their losses, the Great Horse Flu replicated now-familiar disruptions as it hurtled deep into the South and Midwest and even crossed the Florida Straits to Cuba. As a newspaperman journeyed from Cincinnati to New Orleans, he complained that he "could not outrun" the scourge, which "was, it seemed to me, omnipresent." Mere days after striking St. Paul in late November, Minnesota's capital resembled "a vast Equine Hospital" because "all her horses are invalids." More than a thousand miles to the southeast, a Louisiana paper quipped in early December that it was "no longer 'news' to tell of the appearance of Epizootic in any particular locality. It has become a Southern 'institution.'"[1]

"Nothing is thought of or talked of but . . . the prevailing epizootic," observed a visitor to the South's biggest and most powerful city, "and no wonder. Only consider how New Orleans straggles for miles along the bank of the river, and sprawls backwards into the swamps, utterly regardless of the ground she covers; remember that not a car is running throughout the length and breadth thereof, . . . and you will be able to form some idea of the extent of the calamity which has befallen us." Fording the Mississippi River in mid-December, the Great Horse Flu brought turmoil to St. Louis: "It is very curious to watch the various substitutes for the missing horses," a visitor from Kansas exclaimed. "Freight wagons, milk carts and buggies drawn by oxen—here and there a light vehicle propelled by three or four men—now a couple of dogs trot by coaxed to their novel task by their little owners, and again a poor coughing horse, blanketed to his very feet, with his neck enveloped in red flannel, and looking as if he would like to know what it is all about."[2]

"No horse," declared the *Columbia (SC) Phoenix* in early December 1872, "can escape the epizooty." "This remarkable epidemic," the *Hagerstown (MD) Herald and Torch Light* declared, "has extended itself over almost our entire country, as we hear of its prevalence in every district and neighborhood." After remarking that "the inconvenience resulting from it is very great," the Maryland journal took heart in "the consolation, if it be a consolation, of knowing that other people and other communities, from one of this vast country to the other, are suffering from the same general cause. The disease," the *Herald and Torch Light* continued with palpable amazement, "has spread in every direction, North, South, East and West, and seems to disregard all the laws and conditions of climate, prevailing as extensively in a mild as in a severe temperature." The horse plague, as another American editor presciently declared, seemed "destined to sweep the entire country"—and indeed it would.[3]

As the outbreak convulsed the South and Midwest, it revealed that people in these regions were no less reliant on equines than their counterparts in eastern Canada and the northeastern United States—and just as defenseless against the Great Horse Flu's ravages. Equines proved indispensable from cotton plantations to coal mines, logging camps to wheat farms, rustic crossroads settlements to sophisticated cities. Singly or in teams, they powered plows, mine cars, hoists, and other implements and machines. Horses, mules, and donkeys also drew passengers and freight in drays, carts, carriages, wagons, and other conveyances, especially over short and medium distances. The epizootic adeptly exploited this dependency to hobble equine-driven capitalism throughout the South and Midwest. The resulting downturns added to the disruptions and losses the Great Horse Flu and the Great Boston Fire had already inflicted, threatening the continued growth on which Republican control over Reconstruction was premised.

Four years of bitter disunion and ruinous warfare had killed more than eight hundred thousand people—more than 2 percent of the US population—while maiming hundreds of thousands more. It also destroyed more than a third of the Confederacy's horses and over 40 percent of its livestock while mangling vast swaths of the South, leveling many of the secessionist republic's towns and cities, and dismantling chattel slavery, which had generated enormous wealth by appropriating African American labor and turning enslaved persons into commodities in their own right. In all these ways, the war, as W. E. B. Du Bois perceptively argued in his landmark work *Black Reconstruction in America 1860–1880* (1935), "brought anarchy" to the American economy.[4]

Reclaiming order from this chaos proved no easy feat. By 1872, Americans had enjoyed seven years of relative prosperity, yet the South's recovery remained both partial and precarious. Populations of horses, mules, and other livestock had not yet returned to prewar levels, while total agricultural production in the South remained nearly 25 percent lower than before secession. Although Americans disagreed vocally and incessantly about economic affairs, nearly everyone grasped that a rising tide lifts all ships—that reconciling their abundant differences would be much easier, and thus much likelier, if the heady growth of the postwar period continued. "The Republican government that protected civil rights," as one historian points out, pursued policies that "were bound up with a vision of harmonious interests" in which "economic progress would create a fluid social order open to upward mobility . . . . As long as the economy performed well, voters overlooked" Republican shortcomings. But "when economic circumstances soured, things changed quickly."[5]

The Great Horse Flu did not singlehandedly stem the growth on which Republican rule and Reconstruction's destiny depended. As the novel virus flooded the South and Midwest, though, it exacted a steep and mounting toll. This phase of the epizootic brought additional downturns in production and exchange, inflicted further losses in wealth and productive capital by killing off huge numbers of equines and subjecting many more to long-term debility, and impeded the flows of money and credit that sustained the national banking system by binding Northeastern financial centers to the South and Midwest. Even in combination, none of these dynamics sufficed to turn the tide of postwar growth—yet all portended troubled waters ahead.

Near to the Standstill Point

The Great Horse Flu sowed disorder throughout the Southern and Midwestern countryside. Massachusetts fish dealers struggled to get the day's catch to market before it spoiled, railroad construction in several places faltered, and many of the factories and mills that dotted rural America faced slowdowns or suspended production. The epizootic's rural ravages generated less drama and attracted less attention than the urban turmoil the novel influenza variant had unbridled on its path from Toronto and Montreal through New York, Boston, and beyond. Yet because countryfolk often leaned at least as heavily as city dwellers on equines and the labors they performed, the scourge's proliferation upset all manner of pursuits. Three key sectors—lumbering, mining, and agriculture—suffered especially serious and costly downturns.[6]

As a Wisconsin newspaper noted in late November, the outbreak's arrival at a juncture when "lumbermen [were] making extensive preparations for the coming winter campaign among the pines" caused "serious inconvenience" to the logging industry. Each year as the first blushes of autumn began to color the North Woods, lumber firms began buying or leasing horses (and sometimes mules) from farming regions to the south. Equines not only provisioned remote logging camps by hauling food, tools, and other necessities, but also dragged logs to sawmills, rivers, and railroads. No wonder, then, that another Wisconsin journalist encountered "great consternation among lumbermen" when horses who had "been taken down sick on the road" filled barns between Oshkosh and the pineries to its north.[7]

From Maine and Pennsylvania in the east to Minnesota in the west, horses and mules soon became so ill that they could no longer haul in supplies or drag off felled timber, delaying the logging season's start by several weeks. The *Bangor Whig* griped that "lumbering is going on under great difficulties" because most horses in Maine's logging camps had "been much weakened by the epizootic, which affected them just before going into the woods, and many of them had the disease again." A Minnesota correspondent calculated that similar "difficulties" threatened to slash production in that state's pineries by roughly 50 percent, adding that this was "true of all the northwestern lumbering districts."[8]

People in many parts of the South and Midwest used wood not just for lumber but also to keep their home-fires burning. By making it harder to transport fuel cut from woodlands in the countryside to towns and cities, the epizootic's expansion sent cordwood prices skyward. As the outbreak infiltrated Tennessee's forests, for instance, Nashvillians soon had to fork over "nearly double" the usual price of four to five dollars per cord. As the Great Horse Flu dragged on, costs climbed even higher, eventually topping out at fifteen dollars per cord. As an Indianapolis paper noted, soaring fuel prices translated into "untold suffering upon the poor and needy, who could by no possibility be prepared for such a state of things," since people in most of the American interior continued to rely on wood to heat their homes and cook their food.[9]

The Great Horse Flu also hobbled the extraction and transportation of coal, which was fast becoming the preeminent household and industrial fuel throughout much of the eastern United States. By mid-November, newspapers described influenza as "becoming general through the coal regions" of Pennsylvania. The trouble started on the region's canals, where flu-stricken equines struggled to draw boats loaded with coal from Pennsylvania's collieries to urban consumers. Before long, the virus extended its reach from canal ponies to mine mules. People initially hoped that these hardy hybrids—humans bred mules by placing estrous mares in pens with male donkeys—might prove "too tough and stubborn to catch the horse disease," but it soon became evident that mules were just as powerless as horses to stave off infection. At a colliery near Wilkes-Barre, the first creature to fall ill was "one of the toughest old mules ever known," an animal who reportedly had not "seen daylight for eight years." A wire service report noted that many miners believed "that a stroke of lightning wouldn't hurt him; but the epizootic fetched the old sinner to his knees." Outside La Salle, Illinois, the epizootic began preying on mules who "live four hundred feet below the surface of the ground, and haven't been within whinnying distance of a horse for a year, and have had no opportunity of catching it from above, except through the medium of the air." In nearby Braidwood, sick mules' "hacking coughs" likewise "echoed through the mines, and there was no work done."[10]

With equines at dozens of other collieries also too weak to continue hauling coal out of the earth and into the region's fast-growing energy markets, miners faced layoffs of days or weeks without pay. Coal prices soared as supplies dwindled. Dealers in Wheeling, West Virginia, for instance, "more than doubled the price of fuel and are reaping a golden harvest from the disease that has disabled so many of the horses."[11]

The Great Horse Flu's impacts on agriculture, the foundation on which most of the Midwestern and Southern economy rested, caused especially widespread distress. The timing of the scourge's invasion of these regions—after the harvest but before preparations for the next growing season began—softened the outbreak's impact. It also helped that some crops—potatoes and corn, for instance—could remain on the stalk or under the soil for weeks or months after maturing without much risk of spoilage. Many countryfolk, moreover, continued to keep oxen, whom they could readily harness up when their horses and mules became too sick to work. Yet despite all these mitigating factors, the epizootic nonetheless caused serious headaches for those who made their living by husbanding stock and cultivating crops.[12]

Markets for horses and mules suffered for obvious reasons. Each year, as the weather cooled, people in the Deep South sought to renew or expand their force of equine workers by purchasing horses and mules raised in Kentucky,

Tennessee, and Missouri. Upper South breeders timed their annual Southern sales trips to start off "before winter, when it might be necessary to purchase expensive feed." In late 1872, though, more and more stock fell sick with the epizootic as drovers whipped them along country byways leading to Georgia, Alabama, and other markets. Quarantines imposed by local and state governments intent on keeping the scourge at bay and the reluctance of stable-keepers and landowners throughout the Deep South to accommodate ailing equines added to these sellers' woes. "The excitement over the disease is so great," a Kentucky horse dealer reported from Walker County, Georgia, in early December, "that it is with extreme difficulty that a trader can get quarters for his stock." Those drovers fortunate enough to make it to their destinations found prospective buyers unwilling to purchase any creature suspected of harboring influenza. Some sellers responded by taking out newspaper ads declaring that their stock had already recovered from the epizootic—and could thus be presumed immune to the novel influenza virus—but demand nonetheless languished. In early December, for instance, a Tennesseean reported from Selma, Alabama, where he had ventured overland with "sixty head of mules and horses" who "all" showed clear signs of flu, that he "could not sell the best horse in Alabama for $25 now"—a telling statement, since the average value of an American horse at the time was $73.[13]

The epizootic had even weightier consequences for those who grew, traded, or otherwise depended on the South's three most important cash crops: tobacco, sugar, and cotton (the rice-growing regions along the Atlantic and Gulf coasts suffered less in comparison, probably because of their easy access to water transportation). Farmers and planters in the border states and the defeated Confederacy, like growers throughout North America, employed horses, mules, and the occasional donkey to work their land as well as to transport their harvests to steamboat landings, railroad depots, and urban markets. The epizootic unsettled these everyday routines, with costly consequences that reverberated throughout the American economy.

The outbreak struck tobacco-growing regions beginning in early November. A Richmond, Virginia, newspaper exclaimed that with the scourge settling in, the cost "to haul a hogshead of tobacco from the depots to the warehouse" shot up from fifty cents to "*five dollars per hogshead*"—a 1,000 percent increase. Another journal reported that "panic . . . prevails among the country people" outside Petersburg. When "five wagons loaded with tobacco came near," the same account continued, they stopped dead in their tracks "outside" Petersburg's limits "when their drivers heard of the horse disease."[14]

Less tobacco reaching towns and cities and higher costs for moving the fall harvest spelled trouble, but the epizootic proved even more disruptive in Louisiana's cane-growing parishes. The scourge, the *Times-Picayune* observed from New Orleans, struck "the sugar plantations at a critical period of sugar making." The many planters who had still "not finished" the time-sensitive process of cutting down cane, grinding it up in mills, and boiling down the dense liquid thus produced before temperatures dipped below freezing and ruined the entire year's harvest worried that the horse plague would cause "a vexatious delay" that many feared would "result in the loss of a part of the crop." No statistics document how much sugarcane went bad before it could be processed, but given the outbreak's intensity and timing, many planters' balance sheets probably dripped with red ink.[15]

The Great Horse Flu struck King Cotton with even more force than the South's sugar- and tobacco-producing regions. Cotton played a paramount role in the US economy. Accounting for more than 60 percent of total national exports by value in 1870, its significance rippled outward from Southern farms and plantations to commodities exchanges, textile mills, and financial centers in the North and Europe. Substantively and symbolically, cotton had bound the antebellum United States together. And even though the Cotton Kingdom's westward expansion did much to stretch long-standing sectional fissures beyond their breaking point, efforts to reunify and rebuild the nation following the Civil War relied more on this fluffy fiber than on any other crop.[16]

The Great Horse Flu invaded the Cotton Kingdom at an especially perilous juncture. As one Georgian later recalled, "The people were led by the high price of cotton just after the war into a craze of cotton-raising . . . . They usually went into it upon borrowed money, and if it so happened that cotton declined greatly in price, or some other disaster happened to the planter, he was unable to meet his obligations." Despite this commitment, cotton production still had not recovered from the disruptions of the Civil War and emancipation. The annual harvest for 1871–72 languished at just under 3 million bales, a far cry from the 5.3 million bales picked in 1860. The Great Boston Fire, moreover, had "burned up twenty-five millions of dollars worth of cotton goods"—an "amount . . . fully equal to two months' productions of all the cotton mills in the United States." Cotton's tribulations extended from New England to the Deep South. The *Atlanta Constitution* asserted that "one-half of the cotton was entirely killed" in October 1872. "The damp cloudy weather" that followed then "mildewed" a quarter of the standing crop, "turn[ing] it blue" and sharply reducing its value. With the Great Horse Flu bearing down on Memphis and poised to "affect all manner of business," the *Public Ledger* complained that "at this particular season, when money is tight and business not what was expected, and cotton so low [in price], the epizootic is a most unwelcome ghost of a visitor."[17]

Seven years after the Confederacy's defeat and approaching Radical Reconstruction's apogee, many freedpeople remained wary of field work. "There is much cotton in northern Mecklenburg and southern Iredell [Counties] standing," a typical objection published in the *Charlotte Observer* read, "which needs picking badly. The farmers complain of a scarcity of laborers." A wage increase surely could have helped, but sickness among both humans and horses added to planters' distress. After smallpox struck North Carolina, Harnett County's cotton harvest was "entirely suspended." The few bales that field hands managed to pick, the *Raleigh News* hastened to add, "cannot be sent to the market on account of the Epizooty." Some growers tried to get ahead of the curve by shipping out as much of the crop as freighters could haul in advance of the Great Horse Flu's arrival or hastily importing oxen from "nearby plantations."[18]

Despite these precautions and workarounds, the epizootic nonetheless threatened the cotton trade with ruin. As the *Memphis Avalanche* reasoned, "When cotton can't be moved it can't be sold, and that as a matter of course would produce temporary extreme financial stringency." During ordinary times, horses and mules pulled immense quantities of fiber between fields, railway depots, levees, cotton presses, warehouses, and wharves. While on assignment for the *New York Times* in western Louisiana before the Civil War, Frederick Law Olmsted encountered "numerous cotton waggons [*sic*] . . . drawn by three of four pairs of mules or oxen." Each vehicle carried five four-hundred-pound bales, "and the cotton," Olmsted exclaimed, "comes in this tedious way, over execrable roads distances of 100 and even 150 miles" from the fields where it was picked to the nearest riverboat landings. Olmsted surmised that "the profit remaining, after paying the charges of transportation and commission . . . must be exceedingly small in ordinary years." Given these fine margins, even relatively minor, short-lived hikes in the expense of freighting could easily turn profit into loss.[19]

The Great Horse Flu made it more difficult and expensive to haul cotton in the city as well as the country. After "the great demon of the day, the epizootic," hit Memphis, the *Appeal* grumbled that "business in cotton, as well as in other articles, came near to the standstill point." Horses and mules even powered the hoists used in Southern ports to lift cumbersome bales into ship's holds. With Savannah's horses convalescing, a local tinkerer introduced a steam traction engine to help stevedores load cotton onto Baltimore-bound vessels. "On level ground," a journalist claimed, the contraption "worked well enough, but when she came to up-hill work it stalled" and "had to be pushed up by hand," leading many merchants to fork over the flu-inflated rate of one dollar per bale that local draymen could fetch if they were willing to risk their horses' health.[20]

In late November, with the epizootic bearing down on New Orleans, business leaders in the South's commercial epicenter took extraordinary steps to ensure that the cotton harvest could continue flowing through their city en route to Northeastern and European markets and mills. With the flu's invasion just days away, "joint committees from the Cotton Exchange, the Cotton Press Association," and several major railroads held an "important meeting" at which they joined forces to build an emergency spur to connect the city's two largest rail lines. When completed on November 30, this new track enabled railcars to carry cotton atop New Orleans's street railways, which, as one newspaper noted, had been "abandoned for passenger travel by reason of the prevailing epidemic." Thanks to "these arrangements," the *Times-Picayune* predicted "no delay in moving cotton, horse disease or no horse disease." Before long, the Jackson Railroad had hauled "fifteen hundred bales from their cars" on tracks recently vacated by horses, mules, and the streetcars these equines ordinarily powered. This improvisation protected "the up-town cotton presses against any serious embarrassment." A few miles down the Mississippi, meanwhile, the Harbor Towboat Company agreed to ferry cotton "to and from the steamboat landing and railroad depots and to ships, without intermission or delay." Collectively, these contingencies succeeded, as one newspaper crowed, in lowering the "expense of receiving and delivering freight." The *Times-Picayune* nonetheless painted a bleak portrait of New Orleans at the epizootic's height: "Cotton languishes on the Levee," it griped in early December, "sugar sweetens under the sheds, and the horses and mules sicken in the stables." This bad situation soon deteriorated even further when the epizootic expanded to the city's cotton presses, which could do "but a meagre business" without horses and mules to draw bales within their confines.[21]

People in major cotton shipping points drew on Northeastern precedents by resorting to other prime movers, especially oxen and manpower. As the outbreak peaked in Memphis, "a large number" of draymen, carters, and wagoners continued to work animals who "were evidently very bad" with influenza; "the drivers and owners excus[ed] themselves" for risking their equines' well-being, one journalist explained, "on the ground that the work would have to be done." Already, though, "about one thousand handcarts were in active operation," and "wagons hauled by relays of stout colored men" raked in "big prices for transporting cotton." Yet as had been the case in Canada and the Northeast, such substitutes fell far short of satisfying demand. "Cotton bales lie on the wharves in mountains," the *Boston Globe*'s

New Orleans correspondent bemoaned on December 6, "but it is impossible to ship them, even with regular teams of men harnessed."[22]

"Truly," the *Times-Picayune* editorialized, "our horses have never before been properly appreciated." "I dare say if we could know what the beasts are thinking that are shut up so closely in the stables," the *Globe*'s Crescent City correspondent speculated, "we should find them enjoying our dismay. If one could interpret the wheezes and coughs and stampings that issue so mysteriously from the closed windows and doors," the same author speculated in an expression of interspecies sympathy that would have heartened Henry Bergh and Charley Bucephalus, "they would read very much after this fashion: 'Oh yes, they are always beating and abusing us, let us see how they will get along without us for awhile.' . . . There is no doubt," the correspondent quipped in conclusion, "that we are, in national parlance, 'in a regular fix,' and that it is beastly."[23]

For weeks to come, "unprecedently low" water levels and harsh winter weather aggravated the impacts of that "beastly" fix, further hampering cotton shipments throughout the Lower Mississippi Valley. The epizootic soon grew "to such an extent in the country" surrounding Memphis that "interior railway stations" outside that Mississippi River port were described as "crammed with cotton." With equines throughout the Cotton Belt too unwell to work, "ginning and baling cotton" was "entirely suspended" in large stretches of the countryside. On an early December tour that took him "through a considerable portion of the cotton-raising district of the South," an Englishman remarked that several of the biggest traders had "telegraphed planters to hold back" shipments "owing to horse disease." A Nashville paper reported that demand—and, with it, prices—had plunged because potential purchasers were "afraid to buy, fearing their inability to move cotton to the depots and landings." By mid-December, cotton receipts in Memphis had declined 50 percent, while those in many "interior towns" stood at "only 75 per cent. of last year." Even several weeks later, entire fleets of railcars continued to sit idle on sidings, stuffed to their roofs with cotton. The *Republican* described all "the railroads centering" in New Orleans as "pushed to the utmost extent of their transportation power," making it "difficult to prevent an accumulation of freights." Already more than a thousand bales choked the city's railway depots.[24]

Cotton shipments began picking up again in many parts of the South after the New Year. Even so, a Nashville newspaper later reported that beginning in February 1873, cotton prices had suffered a "calamitous fall to extreme low figures . . . due to the epizootic and excessive cold weather . . . . This unlooked for turn of affairs," the *Union and American* griped in September

1873, "threw the markets not only of this country, but also of Europe, into a chronic state of dullness from which there has been no healthy recovery." The *Atlanta Herald* characterized the "business year" that concluded that same month as "one of general disasters and gloom." The epizootic had combined with other misfortunes to bring about "crushing speculative losses in cotton, by which it was estimated that $13,000,000 in hard cash was swept out of Georgia and put in the hands of New York speculators," leading to many foreclosures and bankruptcies while draining the South of currency.[25]

As cotton's travails illustrate, and as loggers in the North Woods, miners in the Appalachian and Midwestern coalfields, and stock-raisers and farmers throughout the continent all discovered, the novel influenza virus exerted forceful curbs on extraction, cultivation, production, processing, and commerce—all of which added up to big trouble for the US economy.

Tighter Than Number Six Shoes on Number Nine Feet

Not just in the South but throughout rural America, the Great Horse Flu threatened equine-powered exchange between rural areas and the villages, towns, and cities that purchased their produce and supplied a growing proportion of their wants and needs. In sapping these commercial relationships, the epizootic strained the networks of association that Americans entrusted to reunify the nation by rebuilding the market relationships, political cohesion, and sense of shared purpose that secession and war had rent asunder.

Even before the epizootic reached them, country folk like the tobacco farmers who stopped short of Petersburg began steering clear of flu-stricken towns in hopes of protecting their horses and mules from influenza. "Very few horses were to be seen on our streets," the *Plymouth (IN) Weekly Republican* complained, "not because the horses were all sick, but mainly for the reason that owners of horses in the country were afraid to drive them to town." Having "heard terrible stories of the existence of the horse epidemic in Plymouth," one farmer told the *Republican* that he "left his horses at home and walked eight miles to town."[26]

Farmers' efforts to avoid exposing their equines to influenza meant potential ruin for townspeople, whose livelihoods often depended directly or indirectly on trade with the surrounding countryside. Trade in many small towns quickly dried up. "Frightful reports" of "the fatal effects of the epizootic," fretted a newspaper in Sedalia, Missouri, "have the tendency to prevent farmers at a distance from coming to the city, and also materially diminishes the usual supply of produce brought to market." Midsize and larger commercial hubs experienced even more dramatic downturns. "Business, in a retail way," lamented the *Nashville Tennessean*, "has experienced a decline on account of the exaggerated reports carried into the country to the effect that the epizootic was raging" in Tennessee's capital, "thus preventing the country people from visiting our city."[27]

Townspeople's irritation sharpened after farmers began cashing in on the produce boom the epizootic incited. "Every article brought to the markets from the country," bemoaned the *Richmond (VA) Dispatch*, "is higher by a good deal than heretofore, and scarce at that." At "the present rates of increase," the *Nashville Union and American* postulated, anyone "who owns a market garden near the city and includes a hand-cart among his earthly possessions, will soon become a blooded aristocrat, provided the horse disease hangs on long enough." Soon, the same journalist predicted, "the scenes of the old Confederate days will be revived, and we will see housekeepers on the way to market, carrying their money in a market basket and returning with their purchases in their pocketbooks." A Pennsylvania correspondent explained that the outbreak "compelled" those seeking to take their crops to market "to trudge weary miles on foot, sometimes pushing along a well filled wheel-barrow or 'go-cart.'" Rural folk who went to the trouble of bringing produce to town under their own steam discovered they could reap "war prices." Such invocations of "old Confederate days" and wartime inflation show that in contorting urban markets, the epizootic recalled the tensions the Civil War had aggravated between city dwellers and country folk in the Union and the Confederacy alike.[28]

Urbanites responded to high produce prices and dwindling stocks by trying to convince rural people that they could maintain or resume their trips to town without threatening their animals' health. Editors, cognizant of the advertising revenue their newspapers earned from local businesses, often spearheaded such efforts. The *Atlanta Constitution*, for instance, reasoned that "the farmer's horse in the mountains of North Georgia is as liable to be attacked as the city horse that draws a dray—if not indeed more liable, because of the colder temperature of the atmosphere in the mountains than here." Another article in the same paper trumpeted the "settled" fact "that the disease is not contagious, but atmospheric," then drew a predictable lesson: "Our country friends need entertain no alarm" in visiting the city. A Wisconsin paper expressed much the same anticontagionist logic; because the outbreak was "of atmospheric origin," it argued, "the idea entertained by many of our farmers . . . that their horses will not take the epizootic unless brought into actual contact with the disease is erroneous. They can neither retard or assist its spread," this editor insisted, for "the air is infected and as long as their horses continue to breathe they are liable to the infection. Hence the absurdity of neglecting business and running away from localities where the disease prevails is apparent."[29]

As the Great Horse Flu wore on, evidence regarding its spread reinforced such pleas. The press dismissed quarantines as ineffective. The "preventing measure" enacted by South Carolina's governor, the *Charleston Courier* noted in a typical jibe, "really did no good"—a conclusion applicable to every other effort to establish a cordon sanitaire against the equine scourge.[30]

As the outbreak continued scything south and west, editors turned the breadth and uniformity of its expansion into additional ammunition against farmers whose caution threatened trade with stagnation. With reports that the epizootic was increasingly hitting towns and their hinterlands simultaneously, newspapers stepped up their campaign to convince rural people to harness their horses and drive to town. Editors soon claimed victory. "Many farmers," Ohio's *Highland News* approvingly noted just before Christmas, "express indifference as to having their horses come in contact with the diseased stock." "The country people, who were wont to attend our market," the *Nashville Republican Banner* declared with palpable relief, "no longer regard it as an obstacle in their coming into the city."[31]

As these accounts indicate, the disruptions the Great Horse Flu brought to urban-rural exchange networks eventually abated—but not before they exposed deeper problems. Throughout late 1872 and early 1873, the press grumbled that epizootic slowdowns and spiking prices were exacerbating the nation's tight money supply, with potentially ominous consequences. To "stop the exchange of commodities," expounded the *Chicago Inter Ocean*, was "to stop the circulation of the money which represents them and their movements." Each autumn, currency streamed from Northeastern financial centers to cities, towns, and rural neighborhoods in the South, the Midwest, and beyond. The ability of specie to move during this "particularly critical" season of "enormous capital flows," however, depended in no small part on reciprocating streams of cotton, tobacco, sugar, lumber, coal, wheat, and other goods, virtually all of which required horses or mules for at least some portion of their journeys. By making it difficult or impossible for equines to continue hauling the countryside's produce to urban markets, the epizootic deprived rural producers and small-town merchants of the funds they needed to settle debts with creditors in bigger towns and cities.[32]

The Great Horse Flu consequently led the US money supply to grow "tighter," as one correspondent griped from New Orleans, "than number six shoes on number nine feet." In Memphis, as in the Crescent City, the core problem, as the *Avalanche* explained, was that "cotton, no less than the general trade of the city, seems to be, like the horses, suffering from the epizootic." Bankers and cotton factors, "fearful of the spread of the horse disease to an extent that would seriously embarrass business," had tightened credit and "ceased remitting money to the country." A Pittsburgh paper bemoaned that "the slowness of country merchants"—not just in the South but throughout rural America—to make good on the obligations they had encumbered over the preceding year was inducing mayhem "in all departments of trade." This state of affairs made it "extremely difficult," in turn, "to make collections, and so long as this continues, business will, as a matter of course, be considerably contracted, as there is no object in expanding when there is no prospect of getting returns."[33]

The short-term economic upheavals the Great Horse Flu unloosed in the Midwest and South, in short, soon mutated into enduring checks on growth. Little wonder, then, that after a financial panic metastasized into a full-blown depression in late 1873, some observers insisted that the epizootic was at least partially at fault.

A Strange Fatality

The Great Horse Flu's advance caused immediate drop-offs in production and trade that often dragged on for weeks. Compounding the outbreak's negative economic effects, the novel influenza virus and the complications that followed in its wake also wiped out significant amounts of wealth. At an estimated mortality of rate of 1 to 2 percent in rural areas and 2 to 4 percent in towns and cities, between 97,100 and 194,300 horses and mules perished from the epizootic in the eastern half of the United States, with about 45 percent of those deaths occurring south of Virginia and west of Indiana. Together, the total value of the animals killed in the East by the Great Horse Flu and its complications would have reached $7.1 million to $14.2 million—roughly 0.1–0.2 percent of total US annual production and a loss equivalent to tens of billions of dollars in present-day terms. As the epizootic rolled south and west, moreover, it became increasingly clear that two types of equines—donkeys and newborn horses—succumbed at disproportionately higher rates. By zeroing out the investment farmers had sunk into these animals in hopes of cashing in on their labor power and reproductive capacity, the Great Horse Flu caused losses that compounded for years to come.[34]

Tennessee stock farmer George T. Allman was among the first to notice that the Great Horse Flu struck donkeys dead with startling efficiency. Although influenza had "prevailed in a mild form" among his horses, Allman noted in December 1872 that his "jack stock" (his male donkeys) had "suffered immensely." Three of Allman's asses had already perished, and two seemed on the verge of death. "The disease attacked them in a very singular way," Allman told *Turf, Field and Farm*: "They became stupid, refused to eat, and then thumped as badly as a horse with the heaves, death ensuing in less than forty-eight hours" (thumping is a serious condition in which an equine's diaphragm spasms, often in time with its heartbeat, making sounds resembling human hiccups). Donkeys died with shocking frequency in other places, too. "A strange fatality has fallen upon the jacks throughout the country," bemoaned the *Andrew County Republican* of Savannah, Missouri; "in nearly every instance where they took the epizootic it proved fatal." The *Louisville Courier-Journal* went so far as to claim that "three-fourths" of Kentucky's jacks had died from the epizootic, along with a smaller but still high proportion of jennets (female donkeys). The US Department of Agriculture alleged that overall mortality for donkeys during the epizootic ranged from twenty to "50 and 67 percent of animals attacked." Recent studies confirm that influenza almost always kills donkeys at a faster clip than horses or mules, though there is no consensus regarding why this is so.[35]

Newborn horses also began dying off in droves once the late winter foaling season began. Several observers attributed these fatalities to influenza's transmission from mares to their young. "There is no doubt," the *Buffalo Commercial* asserted, "that many brood mares which suffered from the epizootic last autumn and which were supposed to have entirely recovered still retain some of its effects lurking in their systems." A *Missouri Republican* correspondent offered a more sweeping take: "There are lingering traces of the epizooty in the land, and many of the spring colts are dead and dying, as the result, in several localities." The *Sioux City Journal* detailed the outbreak's fatal impact in western Iowa. "A most singular and fatal epidemic is raging among the spring colts in this part of the State," it gravely pronounced. "Over sixty" succumbed in just a single township "within a few days. As soon as the colt is foaled," the *Journal* continued, "it develops rapidly all the symptoms of epizootic. In fact, when foaled, many of them are running at the nose, and are so weak that they are unable to take nourishment, and hence die within a few hours." Even newborn horses who seemed "well and strong enough at first" would soon "begin to cough, flow at the eyes, run at the nose," and manifest other "symptoms of horse distemper in epidemic form. All efforts to relieve them," the Sioux City paper lamented, "seem to prove abortive, and the only way is to let them die." Drawing on this and other wire service accounts, a Pennsylvania journal arrived at a startling conclusion: "The epizootic turns out to be a hereditary disease in Iowa."[36]

Genetics, though, had little to do with these foals' demise. Instead, newborn horses probably faced heavy mortality because of common American husbandry practices. Many farmers took pains to separate foals, whose immune systems afforded little to no protection against pathogens, from their mothers. This routine deprived newborn horses of the antibodies that their mothers would ordinarily have provided through their colostrum.

Wyoming rancher John Wanless, for instance, noticed that on his spread, "all the colts that had been taken from their dams" had fallen sick with the epizootic, while "those that were left at large" and continued to nurse from their mothers "were not afflicted." Wanless's observations square with what we now know about the differences between humans, who enter the world armed with antibodies their mothers pass along to them through the placenta, and equines, who, as one scientist explains, are "born immunologically naïve."[37]

The epizootic caused long-term troubles for rural households not simply by destroying valuable animals who were capable of doing work and begetting offspring but also by saddling some equines with lasting, occasionally fatal debilities. Although most flu-stricken equines eventually waged full recoveries, a significant subset had difficulty fighting off the virus. Singling out protracted cases of epizootic in the historical record—long flu—is difficult. The novel influenza variant undoubtedly continued to circulate for weeks or months after its initial arrival in any given place, making it hard to draw clear distinctions between lingering infections and new cases. Numerous observers, though, remarked that some equines suffered persistent symptoms from influenza and its complications that made it nearly impossible for them to labor either as much or as well as they had before falling ill. "The most marked feature of the disease," as veterinarian James Law told the Ithaca Farmers' Club, "was its weakening influence. The weakness lasts even after the animal is comparatively well," Law reported, "and he is in a very unfit condition to go into work." A month after the outbreak reached Wheeling, West Virginia, a local paper acknowledged that the epizootic "leaves the animals very weak," with "hardly strength enough left to digest their food properly."[38]

Lethargy and other flu symptoms caused ongoing ordeals. In April 1873, five months after the outbreak's peak in West Chester, Pennsylvania, a local newspaper lamented that "many horses" still had "not fully recovered from the effects of the Epizootic last fall." That same month, "many of the farmers through the country" outside Decatur, Illinois, were reportedly "complaining that their horses have never fully recovered from the epizootic and that in damp weather the animal[s] are very weak and unable to do as much work as before." A year after the outbreak reached the Chesapeake, numerous animals employed by the Baltimore and Yorktown Turnpike Road Company still could not complete a full day's work. Horses who "go out apparently well in the morning before night have to be taken out of harness," the company groused, "and carefully attended for ailments which are regarded as the effects of the epizootic." Long flu took such a toll on equine productivity that a New York editor bemoaned that "sometimes, the horse is ruined by it."[39]

Long after the outbreak moved on, newspapers continued to carry stories on epizootic fatalities. Six weeks after Chicago's tussle with the Great Horse Flu began, for instance, the *Evening Mail* remarked that "although all traces of the epizootic have disappeared from our streets," the horse plague's "effects . . . are still shown in an unusual mortality among horses." Over the preceding week, 127 horses had perished, "nearly all" from "dropsy or pneumonia"—a fraction of the weekly death toll of around 400 at the epizootic's peak but more than two and a half times above pre-outbreak mortality rates. Deep into 1873, newspapers continued to link the deaths of individual horses to the epizootic. That February, a Columbia, Tennessee, man reported that he had "lost one of his best horses . . . . He thinks it died from the effects of the epizooty," a local paper related, "as it had never appeared well since it had it." Two months later, outside Harrisburg, Pennsylvania, local farmer William Wolf "lost two horses" from influenza; that Wolf had been "offered four hundred dollars" for one of these animals just the day before it first got sick hints at the financial losses that fatal cases of long flu inflicted.[40]

The epizootic, in short, caused widespread rural disruption and jeopardized the exchange networks and monetary flows that maintained ties of common interest between cities and their hinterlands, as well as between the Northeast, Midwest, and South. The Great Horse Flu also destroyed tens of thousands of costly creatures while sapping the strength of many more for weeks or even months. In all these ways, the epizootic hobbled the US economy, with dire collective and cumulative consequences. These developments proved less dramatic and more diffuse than the Great Boston Fire, but they ultimately proved even more damaging. Together, flu and fire undermined the continued growth on which Reconstruction's destiny depended, although the magnitude of these conjoined disasters would not become fully apparent until one of New York's preeminent banking houses collapsed in September 1873, sparking years of depression and ending the postwar boom on which efforts to reunify and reconstruct the United States relied.

Pineapples, Polar Bears, and the Star of Empire

The new names that Americans continually coined for the Great Horse Flu as it galloped through the Southern and Midwestern countryside spoke to the epizootic's shape-shifting capacity. Cornell's James Law was among several contemporary observers who perceived the malady as remarkably malleable. After "giving some of the numerous names applied to the disease" before a packed house at the Ithaca Farmer's Club in mid-November, Law proclaimed the epizootic "*extremely Protean in its nature*," with "scarcely any two cases being exactly the same and having different symptoms at different stages." Law's description echoed an early November report by the veterinary editor for the *Prairie Farmer*, who declared that influenza was "*essentially a protean malady*."[41]

Like Proteus, an "old sea deity" who assumed a succession of guises to elude capture by a Spartan king, the epizootic continually assumed new forms. The novel influenza virus often stuck around for months after the outbreak's leading front decamped, but claims that some equines caught a second case of epizootic suggest that new variants sometimes sickened animals who had already fought off one or more cases of the flu. In March—more than four months after the outbreak hit central North Carolina—a Charlotte paper alleged that "a number of farmers . . . report that the epizootic has returned and attacked their stock with increased virulence." The previous month, a wire service item claimed that "the epizootic has broken out a second time at Lawrenceville, Georgia." The simplest explanation for these claims is that equines who contracted multiple cases of flu probably encountered different strains, since the antibodies these creatures' immune systems had acquired in fighting off an initial infection should have protected them against any strain that had already infected them.[42]

Widespread reports claimed that the Great Horse Flu mellowed as it expanded from the city to the country, and from the heavily urbanized Northeast to the less densely populated South and Midwest. "In the country," claimed the *Sunbury (PA) Gazette*, "the epizootic cases have been much milder in their symptoms than in the cities, and have rarely been fatal." "In all the South," a Tennessee journal declared, "it is in a much milder form than in the North." A Davenport, Iowa, newspaper posited that the Great Horse Flu "seems to have spent its force the further it goes West, and it appears to have reached our city in a subdued form," while a Missourian likewise boasted that it was "consoling to know that the malady is not nearly so serious and stubborn in the west as it proved to be in the east."[43]

Human expectations may have stoked suspicions that the Great Horse Flu was losing vigor. The epizootic's first few days in any new locale, after all, must have seemed underwhelming to those who had consumed the catastrophizing reports that wire services had circulated throughout the outbreak's Northeastern peak. Several other factors also contributed, including more favorable climates; better conditions and care for equines in rural neighborhoods and smaller settlements; "the success which has attended the more rational mode of treatment adopted by veterinary doctors" when compared to the perils posed by heroic therapies; and the supposed ruggedness evinced by what one Missouri journalist termed "the stout and hearty stock of the western prairies." Common assertions that the Great Horse Flu's virulence—its capacity to cause serious illness or death—slackened even as the scourge continued to infect 90 percent or more of equines nonetheless

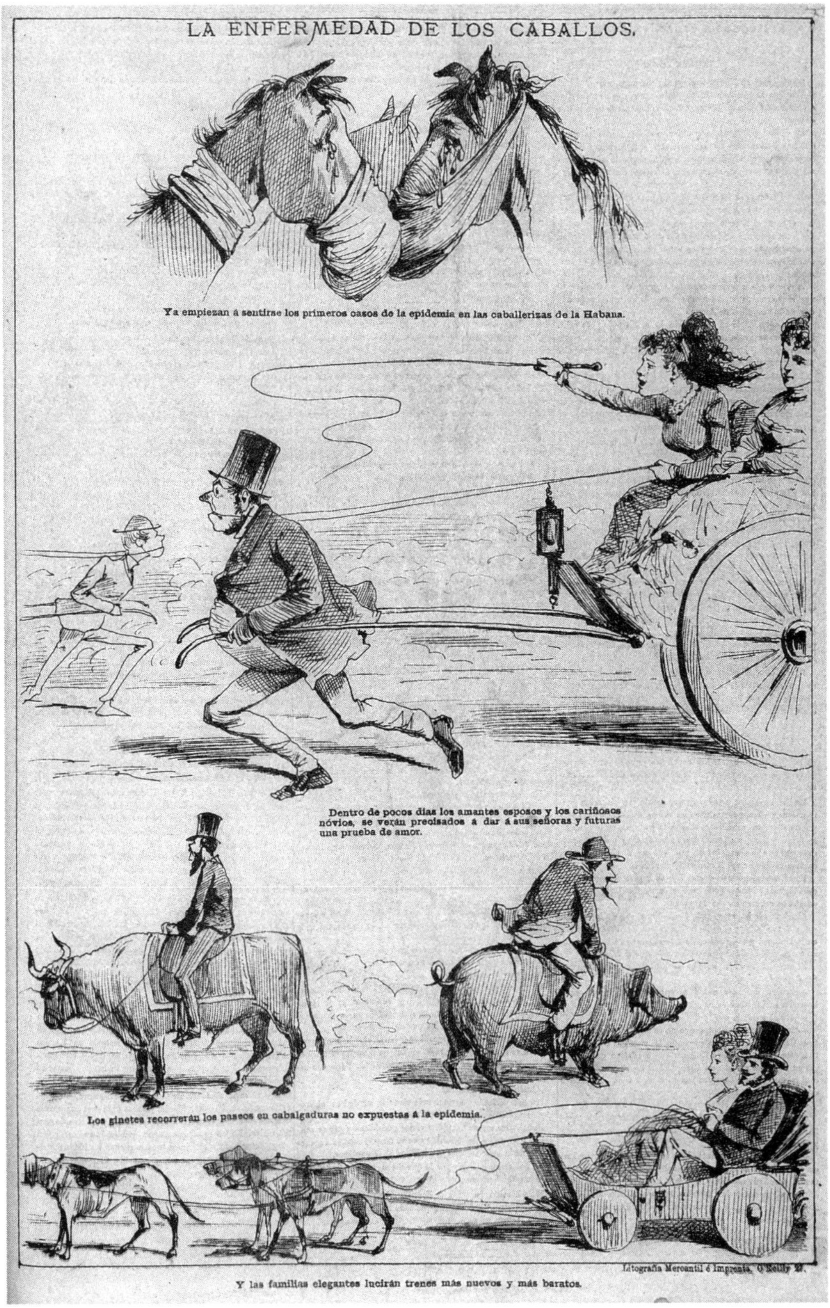

From the top, these Spanish captions translate to "The first cases of the epidemic have already begun in the stables of Havana," "In a few days, loving husbands and loving fiancés will be pleased to give their wives and future brides a token of their love," "The riders will travel the promenades on mounts not exposed to the epidemic," "And the elegant families will be sporting newer, cheaper teams." Víctor Patricio de Landaluze, "La enfermedad de los caballos," *Juan Palomo*, December 15, 1872, 21. Courtesy of University of Miami Libraries, Cuban Heritage Collection.

suggest that the virus may also have evolved to produce milder variants as the outbreak pushed south and west.[44]

As the Great Horse Flu shifted shape, it also gained ground. "The first cases of the epidemic in the stables of Havana are already beginning to be felt," a Cuban magazine proclaimed in mid-December. "All the horses walk down the street coughing," another article in the same publication stated, leading their owners to clothe the beasts in "mantles that make them look like the kings who come out in the operas." Soon telegrams and letters described the surge of death the epizootic visited upon the island colony. Horses imported from the United States allegedly suffered from a "lighter" version of the disease than their "creole" or Cuban-born counterparts, while mules were "attacked even more severely." With "very few veterinary surgeons in Havana, and only one or two of them" possessing "any knowledge of the disease," the *Chicago Tribune* declared just after Christmas, the death toll was "becoming very great." In late December, wire services reported that "a malignant type" of the epizootic was infecting oxen in Cárdenas and Cienfuegos. "In many cases," one account observed, "death follows almost immediately upon the animal being attacked." By mid-January, the *Panama Star and Herald* called the outbreak "general and severe" in Cuba, adding that "traffic in the streets of Havana by horses has stopped almost completely." So many cavalry mounts had been struck down by influenza that the colonial government, which had been battling rebels seeking independence from Spanish colonial rule and the abolition of slavery, imported horses purchased in Mexico.[45]

Dispatches on the Great Horse Flu's Cuban ravages hit American newspapers alongside reports that the outbreak was recrossing the international border to invade Manitoba. The epizootic, one journal declared, was a "universal traveler" that was "not restrained by distance nor place." No matter "whether it is a climate for pine apples [*sic*] or white bears," it continued, "it is all the same to the epizooty."[46]

As 1872 turned to 1873, though, it became evident that the Great Horse Flu was destined to write its next chapters not in the subtropics or the subarctic but, rather, in the settler heartlands beyond the Missouri River. "'Westward the star of empire takes its way,'" one editor prophesied, "and the epizootic has followed the well-beaten way of civilization so rapidly that it will soon overtake the star."[47]

CHAPTER 6

VIRAL LIES AND INFLUENZA'S PROGRESS

Indian Country, the Great West, and Partisan Plagues

On March 1, 1873, with the Great Horse Flu fast approaching the eastern flank of the Sierra Nevadas, Joseph Walkup, a newspaper editor and prominent citizen of Auburn, California, published a pair of arresting stories in that town's *Placer Herald*. The first perpetuated and elaborated on old falsehoods by attributing the Great Horse Flu to ponies plundered by American troops after they massacred a smallpox-stricken Piikani village in Montana Territory in January 1870 (the Piikani are known to most English speakers as Piegans). The second item, which appeared just below the first, marked the arrival at Walkup's office of *American Progress*, an engraving designed by tourism impresario George Crofutt and created by John Gast, a Berlin-born, New York–based painter and lithographer. This twelve-by-sixteen-inch color print would soon adorn the walls of tens of thousands of homes and businesses, becoming one of the most iconic representations of US expansionism ever produced—what cultural historian David Scobey aptly calls "a handy meme for 'Manifest Destiny' or 'the frontier thesis.'"[1]

Together, these two short articles printed in a single column in the same issue of a small-town newspaper in California's Gold Country speak to the undeniably human dramas of dispossession, violence, and migration that marked the winning—and losing—of the West in the Civil War's wake. When analyzed together, though, Walkup's articles also hint at the vital roles that equines, influenza, and other nonhuman entities played in settler colonialism. Using these adjoining stories as its point of departure, this chapter explores the Great Horse Flu's thrust from the Great Plains to the Far West. In the process, it examines what we can learn about the transformation of Native American homelands into integral parts of the United States and Canada by tracing the epizootic's westward migration, the meanings that various participants and observers made of the outbreak's growth, and the viral lies about conquest, disease, and politics that Walkup and other strident opponents of the Grant administration and the Republican Party cooked up to account for influenza's expansion.

A Beautiful Picture

The first of the two curious stories to appear in the *Placer Herald* praised "a beautiful chromo"—a chromolithographic engraving made from as many as thirty separate stone or metal plates, each of which applied an additional color or tint. The *New York World* praised this recently perfected technique for mass-producing "wonders of modern imitative art" that were "true to a hair, and finer, if necessary, than the naked eye can discover."[2]

Walkup's article featured a succinct but illuminating discussion of the print he had just received by mail. Walkup's fellow editor, George Crofutt, had commissioned John Gast, a twenty-nine-year-old Prussian-born artist, to make a painting to serve as source art for an engraving. Crofutt, an "old-time Coloradan" and author of several popular travel guides to the transcontinental railroad, edited a New York–based magazine, *Crofutt's Western World*, that endeavored to sell tourists, settlers, and investors on the bounty and beauty of recently conquered Indigenous homelands. The editor, who decided to title Gast's work *American Progress* even before brush met canvas, provided Gast with detailed instructions for the print, which the artist dutifully carried out.[3]

Throughout late 1872, Crofutt's magazine hawked Gast's engraving as "a present" available to anyone willing to pay the *Western World*'s $1.50 subscription fee. Yet production problems kept delaying the chromo's debut. Finally, on February 15, 1873, the first batch of ten thousand prints arrived at Crofutt's Lower Manhattan office. The editor and his small staff devoted the next three days solely to "the work of mailing them." At least one of the prints Crofutt and his crew dispatched during this flurry of activity subsequently traveled 2,800 miles, to Auburn, California, landing in late February on the desk of Joseph Walkup.[4]

Walkup, a bushy-bearded, big-bodied fifty-three-year-old, had been born and reared in Miami County, Ohio. His parents had ventured westward from Virginia in 1812 to farm. While Walkup was still a young man, he relocated to New Orleans, where he applied his carpentry skills to building ships and steamboats. He joined the California gold rush in spring 1849 and, after sailing through the Golden Gate, ventured up the North Fork of the American River from Sacramento to the mineral-rich foothills above.[5]

There Walkup joined other invaders in prosecuting what many local settlers forthrightly described as a "war of extermination" against the area's Nisenan inhabitants. In spring 1850, residents of the newly established town of Auburn celebrated the killings of at least twenty-five Nisenan men, women, and children by exhibiting "several scalps" as trophies. As Auburn solidified its commercial dominance over upstream goldfields violently wrested from the Nisenans and other Indigenous peoples, Walkup distinguished himself as a merchant, rancher, mining investor, and farmer.[6]

Parlaying economic success into political power, Walkup served two terms in the state senate, one term as California's lieutenant governor, and a stint as warden of San Quentin. Hailed as a "strong partisan" of the Democratic persuasion, Walkup gained renown as a vocal critic of Abraham Lincoln and the Union war effort. After becoming proprietor and editor of the *Placer Herald* in 1868, Walkup used the paper to inveigh against the Republican Party, the Grant administration, the Central Pacific Railway, and Chinese immigration.[7]

Walkup had no way to reproduce *American Progress* in his newspaper, so he painted a word-picture of the image instead. He began by describing the "central figure" in Gast's composition—"a female with a book" (Walkup did not mention that Gast had labeled the tome "Common School") who hovers above the plains "unwinding a telegraph wire that spans the continent." As this goddess-like eminence glides westward, her head emblazoned with what Walkup recognized as "the star of empire," the West's indigenous occupants—"the buffalo, the savages, the bear, deer and other wild animals"—turn tail. Into the vacuum left by this seemingly bloodless exodus pour "the emigrant train, the prospectors, the pony express, and in the rear," Walkup continued, "is the overland stages, followed by the husbandman and the railroad train."[8]

Walkup's seventeen-line item drew liberally from descriptions of Gast's print that Crofutt started circulating even before *American Progress* began rolling off the press. A half-page advertisement in *Western World*'s February 1873 issue probably scripted how Walkup and others made sense of Gast's mythic tableau. This ad began by framing the conquest and transformation of the continent's western reaches as a drama of world-historical significance. "This rich and wonderful country—the progress of which at the present

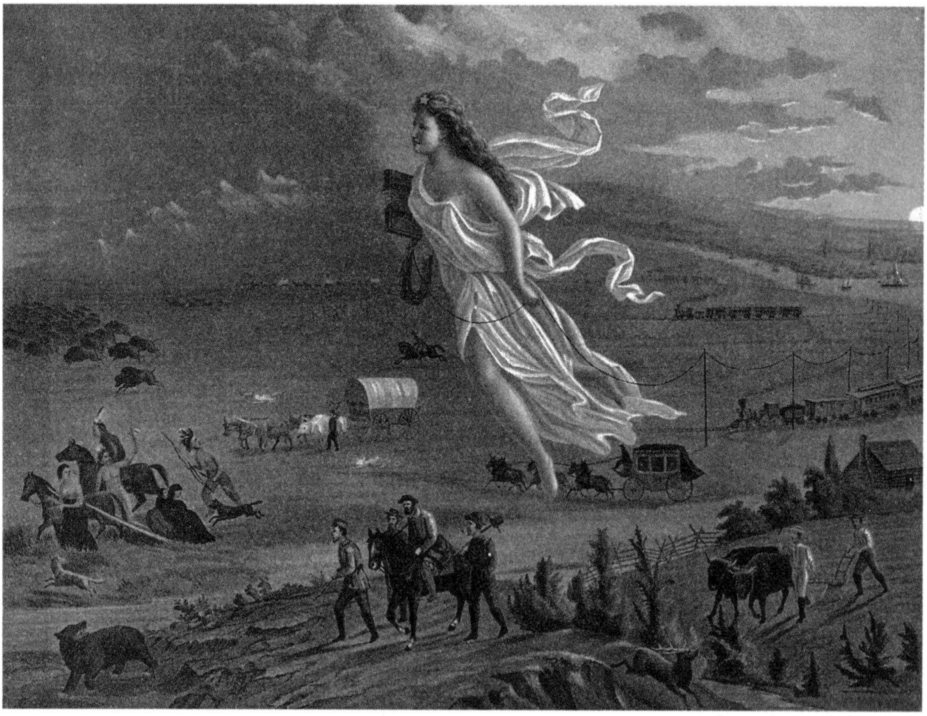

John Gast made this painting according to detailed instructions from George Crofutt, the author of several popular mining and travel guides as well as *Crofutt's Western World*. Gast then turned the painting into the chromolithograph that reached the desk of Joseph Walkup, a former lieutenant governor of California and newspaper editor. Walkup lauded the engraving as a "beautiful picture" and described it in detail next to a second story that circulated a viral lie blaming General Philip Sheridan—and, by implication, the Grant administration—for instigating the Great Horse Flu by massacring a Piikani camp in Montana Territory in 1870 and stealing the village's ponies. John Gast and George Crofutt, *American Progress* (1872–73). Courtesy of the Library of Congress Prints and Photographs Division, Washington, DC.

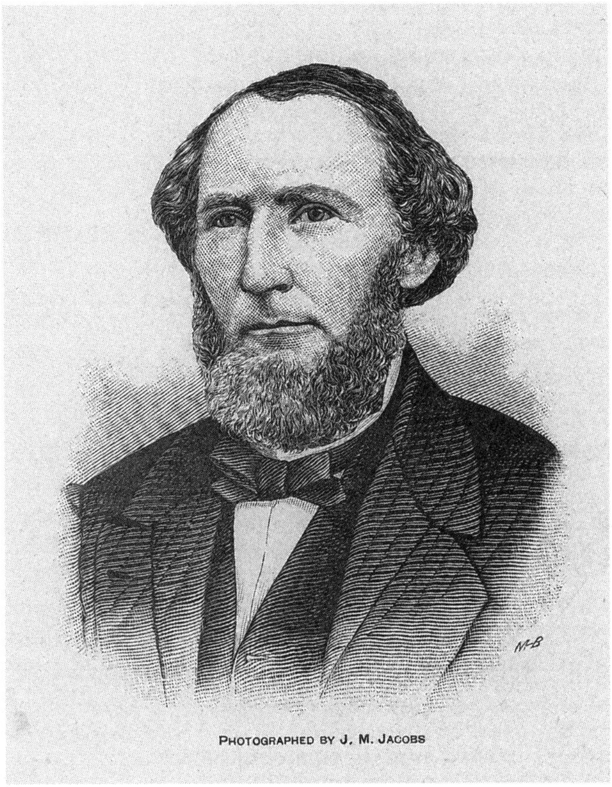

This portrait of Joseph Walkup was published after his 1873 death. "Joseph Walkup," in [Myron Angel], *History of Placer County, California, with Illustrations and Biographical Sketches of Its Promiment Men and Pioneers* (Oakland: Thompson & West, 1882), between 176 and 177. Courtesy of Western Historical Collections, Denver Public Library.

time, is the wonder of the old world," Crofutt averred, "was, until recently, inhabited exclusively by the lurking savage and wild beasts of prey." Recent years, though, had witnessed the radical transformation of "the 'Far West,'" which Crofutt prophesied was "destined at an early day, to be the vast granary, as it is now the great treasure chamber[,] of our country." The point of *American Progress*, this advertisement explained, was to celebrate "how this change has been wrought, and by whom."[9]

Crofutt cast *American Progress* as an unapologetic salute to the conquest of Indigenous peoples and wild nature. "The general tone of the picture on the left," where Gast showed Indian peoples and wild creatures warily retreating, "declares darkness, waste and confusion, while from the right, life, activity, light, flash their influences upon the scenes depicted." As the ethereal female figure whom Crofutt named "Progress" extends her reign across the image's foreground, Indigenous Westerners avert "their despairing faces," for "the 'Star,'" as Crofutt proclaimed, "is *too much for them*."[10]

Crofutt's "Description" concluded with a breathless paean to *American Progress*'s broader import:

> What American man, woman or child, does not feel a heart-throb of exultation as they think of the glorious achievements of PROGRESS since the landing of the Pilgrim Fathers, on stanch [*sic*] old Plymouth Rock! What home, from the miner's humble cabin to the stately marble mansion of the capitalist, should be without this GREAT National picture, which illustrates in the most artistic manner all the gigantic results of American Brains and Hands! Who would not have such a beautiful token to remind them of our country's grandeur and enterprise, which have caused the mighty wilderness to blossom like the rose!!!

Joseph Walkup evidently concurred with Crofutt's plaudits, for he titled his little article on Gast's engraving "A Beautiful Picture."[11]

Westward the Star of Influenza

As the first copies of this iconic embodiment of US frontier ideology rattled west, they retraced routes recently traveled by the Great Horse Flu. "The epizootic," a Kansas newspaper declared in late November, "follows Greeley's advice and 'goes west.'" Several other observers, as we have seen, also linked the unbridled expansion of the novel influenza virus to that of the American nation.[12]

Our best guess is that the copy of *American Progress* which Crofutt had dispatched to Walkup overtook the equine scourge somewhere in Nevada. By that time, the epizootic's growth was assuming a clear and fascinating pattern that mapped onto Gast's lithograph in unexpected ways. The epizootic spread most swiftly along equine-powered thoroughfares connecting major settlement corridors, more slowly astride the recently completed transcontinental railroad, and slowest of all in Indigenous homelands. Counterintuitively, the grinding consequences of conquest and colonialism—especially the decimation of Indigenous populations, the destruction of Native American horse herds, and the demobilization of First Nations—delayed the virus's advance through Indian Country while masking the epizootic's impacts on tribal nations.

Two main east–west routes provided especially ideal conditions for the scourge's transmission. The first brought the novel influenza virus to Nevada's Comstock Lode from eastern Nebraska via Colorado's Front Range, Utah's Mormon settlements, and mining camps in eastern and central Nevada. Meanwhile, the second and more southerly path of diffusion led from central Texas toward southern California, with one branch unfurling into northern Mexico. As it pushed toward the Pacific along these corridors, the Great Horse Flu also spun off tendrils to the north, south, and sometimes even the east until it eventually permeated the Interior West.

Settlers began reading about the epizootic's progress months before the scourge itself arrived. As the flu bore down, though, its capacity to infect entire populations of equines within mere days inspired wonder alongside worry. Salt Lake's *Herald-Republican*, for instance, pronounced in early January that "the horse disease . . . has broken out *almost simultaneously* along the eastern slope of the Rocky Mountains for many hundreds of miles." Nearly a month later, Nevada's *Virginia City Enterprise* published a "frightful account" provided by a "well-known surveyor" who reported that "many wagons loaded with merchandise" could be found "standing in the deserts" of eastern Nevada and western Utah because "so many" of the area's horses and mules had "died of the disease . . . that not enough were left to draw the vehicles." The Great Horse Flu, the *Enterprise* declared, had "spread over a thousand miles of ground with the swiftness of a flash of lightning. It was everywhere at once."[13]

Neither railroads nor waterways—long the main conduits along which epidemics spread from European, American, Canadian, and creole traders and settlers to Indigenous peoples—played much role in carrying the epizootic westward. By the winter of 1872–73, only one transcontinental railway, the Union Pacific–Central Pacific (UP-CP), was in operation. From roughly the 97th meridian to the crest of the Sierras, the only other functioning railways were the Kansas Pacific and Denver Pacific (allied lines that linked Kansas City, Denver, and Cheyenne), as well as several short lines scattered across Colorado, Utah, Nevada, Oregon, and Washington. When horses, mules, and asses in Denver, Georgetown, and other Colorado settlements began in late December 1872 to hack with a dry cough, equines in Cheyenne—the largest town on the UP's line between Omaha and Ogden, Utah—remained unaffected. It took the malady a few additional weeks to hit Wyoming's capital, reportedly arriving not by train but instead via a team of horses who had contracted the epizootic on a visit to Colorado. No less revealingly, the malady struck Salt Lake City by January 11, 1873, yet took until late February or even early March to reach Evanston, Wyoming, eighty miles east of Salt Lake along the UP.[14]

During these same weeks, the Great Horse Flu was racing beyond the railroads' reach to suffuse southern Colorado and northern New Mexico. It took the disease less than three weeks to leap from Denver to Santa Fe, around four hundred miles away, only the first hundred miles of which were served by rail. By early February, the epizootic halted mail service between Santa Fe and the two closest railway termini (Pueblo and Kit Carson, Colorado); officials at one New Mexico stage company lamented that "every one of their mules and horses" was "badly infected with the disease." As had been the case in the South and Midwest, the outbreak levied an especially heavy toll on the territory's asses. In early February, the *New Mexican* lamented that in northern New Mexico, the epizootic was proving "very fatal, especially among the burros." Donkeys, a federal official reported, were "dying off in great numbers," with "the wood roads leading" into Santa Fe from the mountains above "dotted with defunct burros—victims of the epizootic and ill usage." These deaths presumably dealt an especially hard blow to Hispanos who relied on burros to transport produce, firewood, and other necessities on the territory's twisting trails and primitive roads.[15]

A San Francisco newspaper perceptively summarized the single most important driver of the Great Horse Flu's growth: "The horse complaint traveled across the continent," the *Evening Bulletin* pointed out, "because there was a chain of animals" to communicate the virus, as well as "continuous settlements for its transmission." The epizootic, the *Evening Bulletin* asserted, thus held vital "lessons" for public health officials and ordinary Westerners alike. "The barriers which heretofore have kept pestilence away from us," it cautioned, "have been thrown down, and . . . for the future we shall have to take our chance with the other communities of the world when general sickness falls upon humanity." What held true for humankind evidently applied to horsekind, too.[16]

These insights point the way, in turn, to a counterintuitive but compelling reinterpretation of *American Progress* as an unintended study in viral transmission and pathogenic colonization. The rapidity and relentlessness with which the Great Horse Flu sickened equines throughout the Interior West demonstrates how the very same processes touted by George Crofutt, John Gast, and Joseph Walkup as hallmarks of "American progress"—transportation improvements, Indigenous displacement, and quickening integration into national and global economies—combined to imperil settlers and their equines.

To reread this iconic image in epidemiological terms, begin in the picture's brightly lit upper-right corner, where New York looms as the seedbed for the epizootic's Western adventures. The railways connecting the Empire City to the main subject of *American Progress*—the frontier scenes in the image's foreground—haul passengers, freight, and livestock over the prairies before petering out on the Great Plains. Neither these railroads nor the telegraph wires unspooled by the angelic, toga-clad female luminary who flutters above the center of the scene seem capable of conducting the horse disease beyond the midcontinental interior.

This is where the equines who canter, gallop, and pace across Gast's print come into play. In this reinterpretation, the sprinting horse of the Pony Express, the trusty burro hefting prospectors' supplies in the image's central foreground, the trio of teams pulling emigrant wagons across the mountains' base, the stage horses who trot just in front of the female figure, and the rest of the equines who far outnumber humans in *American Progress* materialize not simply as vital agents of American conquest but also as viral agents for the Great Horse Flu's advance.

The Great Horse Flu in Indian Country

Take a closer look, though, and other equines beckon. Gast's print portrays several small groupings and larger herds of Native American ponies. Carrying their people—and their people's lodges and possessions—toward the blank space beyond the canvas's western margin, these animals seem destined to share their owners' destiny of dispossession, dislocation, and disappearance. The separation Gast depicted between Indigenous horses and settlers' stock raises an intriguing question: What became of the Great Horse Flu in Indian Country?

Despite the rumors that Joseph Walkup broadcast through the *Placer Herald*, the evidence clearly shows that the epizootic reached Indian Country *after* it infected the main corridors of US settlement. The outbreak also seems to have caused less concern in Indigenous communities than it occasioned among westering Americans. These findings might seem surprising. Infectious diseases introduced from Eurasia and Africa had long histories of devastating Native American societies; imported pathogens including brucellosis and canine distemper exacted heavy tolls on bison, dogs, and other Indigenous creatures; and many of the West's First Nations undoubtedly ranked among the most equine-dependent cultures anywhere on earth.[17]

Little evidence documents the Great Horse Flu's impact on Indigenous Westerners. In January 1873, newspapers claimed that the virus had reached Lakotas and other Northern Plains nations. After striking Manitoba's Red River Valley later that month, though, the epizootic seemed to stall. The horse plague presumably percolated throughout Indian Country by the time the outbreak died down in late summer 1873, but that year's annual report of the US commissioner of Indian affairs hardly mentioned it. This omission seems especially odd, since the same document contained the most thorough census yet tabulated of human and equine populations in the West's tribal communities. The outbreak's differential impact on the US Army and

Indigenous resistance fighters also suggests that the flu struck the former more severely than the latter. In March and April 1873, American forces in Arizona as well as the California-Oregon border region contended with sick horses and mules, but the extensive news coverage on these wars of conquest made no mention of illness among the horses and mules kept by Modocs, Yavapais, and Dilzhę'é Apaches.[18]

If the Great Horse Flu indeed decelerated on reaching Indian Country, it probably did so because the West's Indigenous Nations presented the novel influenza virus with distinctive—and distinctly challenging—epidemiological conditions. As veterinary surgeons, physicians, and other experts noted, the epizootic spread fastest where equines were densely concentrated, exposed to large numbers of kindred kinds, and housed indoors. In early 1873, for instance, a Colorado rancher kept fifteen of his horses in a stable while leaving seventy others "running out" on the range; "all" of the animals he kept indoors contracted the flu, while "none" of the others "show[ed] any signs of the epizooty." While settlers often confined their equines in stables, barns, and corrals, Native Americans mostly allowed their animals to run free. Indigenous-held horses and their kin usually spent even the harshest winter nights spread out beneath open Western skies, a practice that probably fettered the Great Horse Flu's growth.[19]

Second and more significantly, nearly every Indigenous Nation in the West had suffered devastating population losses in the decades leading up to the epizootic's emergence. Scholars have shown how a perfect storm of assaults—including the loss of key resources (especially land), disruptions to Indigenous foodways, purposeful efforts to make Indigenous peoples dependent on Euro-American trade goods, sexual violence against Native American women and children, and forced dislocations from tribal homelands to reservations and residential boarding schools—traumatized Native communities while blazing transmission routes for infectious diseases. The consequent decimation of Native populations in most parts of the Interior West reduced Indigenous demand for equines while making it much harder for tribal nations to maintain existing herds. Estimates place the population of Native Americans in present-day California, for instance, at 150,000 in 1846; by the early 1870s, no more than 30,000 Indigenous Californians survived, a loss of 80 percent. Even Native polities who had thrived as late as the 1840s, most notably the Lakotas and Comanches, began in the 1850s to mourn the deaths of large numbers of kinfolk. Demographic declines probably intensified during the Civil War, when Union armies stepped up assaults on several Indigenous Nations and long-standing fissures within many Native communities, especially the Five Civilized Tribes in Indian Territory, erupted in violence. Between 1861 and 1865, to cite an especially dramatic case, the Cherokee Nation's population dropped from 21,000 to 14,000 because of scorched-earth conflicts that nineteenth-century ethnographer James Mooney rightly decried as leaving "their whole country in ashes."[20]

Prior to the 1860s, nations such as the Yavapais and Dilzhę́'és whose homelands lay distant from colonial epicenters may have suffered rarely if at all from introduced diseases. Thereafter, though, members of virtually all of the West's Native nations experienced repeated epidemics as well as violent settler incursions that targeted not just human victims but also the plants, animals, water sources, sacred places, and storied lands that had sustained Indigenous peoples since time immemorial. One authoritative study reckons that in 1800, 600,000 Native Americans populated the area within the present-day boundaries of the United States; the early 1870s, though, saw this figure plummeting toward an all-time nadir of approximately 240,000 in 1890. Canada's First Nations declined apace, with the Confederation's Indigenous and métis population of roughly 125,000 in 1867 creeping toward a historic low of 113,724 in 1921.[21]

We know only a little about how these Indigenous holocausts affected Native horse-holding. As Native peoples grappled with human tragedies of imponderable proportions, though, it is difficult to imagine how they could have sustained their herds at preexisting levels. Horses, mules, and burros can be needy beasts, after all, so the disasters that befell First Nations communities probably made it harder for survivors to muster the time, energy, and expertise their equines demanded.[22]

The precise mechanisms by which cratering Native populations translated into smaller herds remain unclear. Several well-documented practices, though, probably contributed. Indigenous peoples commonly slaughtered horses and mules as part of their mourning and mortuary rituals. Traveling up the Missouri River in 1862, for instance, ethnographer Lewis Henry Morgan recorded the story of Blackbird, a venerable Omaha leader who "directed his followers," Morgan claimed, "to lash his body after death upon his best horse, and take [them] down to a high bluff on the river, and bury both horse and man together . . . . The horse was buried alive," Morgan's Omaha informants told him, "with Black Bird upon his back and a large mound raised over both." Comanches, Yavapais, Apaches, and members of many other tribal communities also ate equines, often as a prized foodstuff but also as a hedge against starvation amid sharp declines in bison and other game. Moreover, Indigenous peoples sometimes sold off entire herds of horses, mules, and donkeys to outsiders. Supplying equines to fur trappers, ranchers, miners, and even Louisiana's cotton and sugar planters enabled Natives to turn surplus equines into trade goods. In addition, intertribal warfare claimed the lives of large numbers of horses and mules throughout the middle and late 1800s, as widespread depictions of wounded and dying equines in ledger drawings and winter counts made by Indigenous memory-keepers indicate. Still another factor was the targeting of Indigenous equines by the US Army. Soldiers had always tried to seize or slaughter the horses and mules on whom the West's Native peoples literally mounted their resistance to settler colonial invasions. Starting in the 1850s, though, US officers introduced a new tactic: After assaulting Indigenous villages and running off their equines, Army leaders ordered troops to slaughter the horses and mules they took so that Indigenous foes could not reclaim them.[23]

One final dynamic hindered the Great Horse Flu's progress in Indian Country: Both the United States and Canada did their utmost to demobilize Indigenous Nations. Despite some important disparities, North America's two most expansive settler states pursued similar Indian policies. Both Canada and the United States sought to concentrate Indigenous peoples and limit their movements with the ultimate goals of neutralizing Native independence, gobbling up Indigenous lands, and assimilating Native individuals and nations into the dominant society as subject and subordinated peoples.[24]

This shared rationale explains close similarities between the treaties that delegates from Ottawa and Washington forged—sometimes quite literally—with tribal nations in the 1860s and early 1870s. Compacts signed on either side of the US-Canadian border took aim at Indigenous mobility by creating reservations and reserves, then promising rations and annuities to those who remained within these circumscribed domains. Many treaties also divvied up communally held tribal lands into privately owned allotments, shunted nomadic hunters toward sedentary agricultural lifeways, and ripped Native children away from their families and sent them to distant boarding schools.[25]

Colonial attempts to crack down on conflict between Indigenous Nations placed additional obstacles in the Great Horse Flu's path through Indian Country. Treaties often contained clauses in which Native signatories pledged to remain at peace with neighboring peoples. Some Indigenous leaders, meanwhile, vied to align themselves with settler governments by taking the initiative and promising not to take up arms against their foes. Turning from legal agreements to everyday practices, the bureaucrats who helmed US reservations and Canadian reserves often tried to stop Native peoples from going out on horse raids. Indian agents deprived suspected offenders of annuities and rations, prosecuted them in US and Canadian courts, and repeatedly called in the military to wage retributory warfare against entire First Nations after settlers accused tribal members—often baselessly—of stealing horses or other livestock. Similar dynamics were also at play in the US-Mexican borderlands, where the US Army, Mexican *federalistas*, and local militias composed of Mexican and American settlers all sought to check raiding by Comanches, Kiowas, Kickapoos, Yavapais, Chiricahua and Western Apaches (including Dilzhę́'és), and many others. By the early 1870s, raiding almost certainly became rarer, less lucrative, and less extensive than in previous decades, when Native war parties often ventured hundreds of miles to seek out other peoples' horse-wealth, frequently returning with hundreds of equines in tow.[26]

Sweeping ecological changes reinforced colonial efforts to restrict Indigenous mobility. Longer-distance travel was becoming especially unrewarding for Native buffalo hunters. Although one federal official still counted "plenty" of shaggy bovines grazing along New Mexico's Cimarron River in the winter of 1872–73, bison numbers were already free-falling across most of the Great Plains. "In former times," the agent for the Mandans, Hidatsas, and Arikaras noted in his annual report for 1873, "the buffalo roamed over the country, but they have receded and are now some two or three hundred miles away." Although bison were holding on in parts of Canada, many Plains Cree nonetheless faced hunger by the early 1870s, one trader lamented, because of "the visible diminution of the buffalo, their sole support." Sweet Grass, "the Chief of the Country," consequently implored dominion officials to "make provision for us against years of starvation." Members of many other Indigenous horse nations responded to the demise of the West's once-prolific buffalo herds by shortening or canceling their hunts. With Indigenous peoples and their equines staying closer to home for more of the time, the novel influenza virus had less opportunity to reach new hosts.[27]

The Great Horse Flu's progress through Indian Country, in short, was constrained not simply by Indigenous husbandry practices but also by many of the same dynamics of conquest and colonization that Crofutt, Gast, and Walkup commended in *American Progress*.

Chickens Coming Home to Roost

In most instances, the epizootic rippled into Indigenous American communities after striking nearby US settlements. Walkup, though, told a very different story about the outbreak's origins in the short article he wrote and placed immediately below his description of *American Progress*. Rather than tracing the Great Horse Flu's movements by analyzing the heaps of epidemiological information carried over wire services and mail routes since the outbreak first began, Walkup seized on and amplified trumped-up rumors blaming the scourge on an 1870 atrocity.

"The horse epizootic," the editor intoned, "is traced to General Sheridan. It may be remembered," Walkup continued, "that Phil Sheridan killed a lot of sick squaws and papooses of the Piegan Indians, on the plains, some years ago." Walkup was undoubtedly referring to the bloodbath known as the Marias or Baker Massacre, which took place beside Kiaayoai'tahtaa (Bear River, which Meriwether Lewis renamed the Marias in 1805 after his cousin Maria Wood). In this vicious January 23, 1870, atrocity, US troops overran a peaceful village of Piikanis—a nation that Americans usually referred to as Piegans and one of four constituent nations of the Niitsítapi or Blackfoot Confederacy—led by Issokui-omachkan (Heavy Runner). Major Eugene Baker and his troops cut a swath through the village, killing nearly two hundred people, as part of a larger campaign authorized by Lieutenant General Philip Sheridan, commander of the US Army's Department of the Missouri. Walkup alleged that after Baker and his men murdered sleeping villagers, they "stole all their robes and ponies."[28]

Walkup's curious account of the Great Horse Flu's origins hinged on the claim that these plundered goods bore hidden pathogenic burdens. Piikani robes, he explained, "contained the virus of the small-pox." Once these robes "got into the Eastern market," Walkup alleged, they served to "spread the small-pox, which killed its thousands of victims." As for the stolen "ponies," Walkup asserted that they "were afflicted with a terrible distemper, but finally partially recovered." After these plundered horses kicked the malady, Walkup asserted, they "were driven into Canada and sold, and from them the epizootic broke out, crossed over into the United States, and has well nigh swept all over the country." The Californian concluded his article with a parting moral: The Great Horse Flu, he declared, "is chickens coming home to roost with a vengeance"—cosmic payback for Baker's acquisitiveness and Sheridan's brutality.

Walkup erected this alternative origin story for the epizootic atop a foundation of partisan grievance. Though an Ohioan by birth, Walkup imbibed his Virginia-born father's enduring allegiance to his boyhood home. The time Walkup spent building ships in New Orleans during the 1840s reinforced his Southern sympathies and proslavery politics. After venturing to California, Walkup remained a staunch Democrat, representing his party as lieutenant governor (1858–60). Myron Angel's 1881 *History of Placer County, California* summed up the ideology of a man who "had grown to manhood and to maturity in the West and South, impressed with the sacredness of the Constitution and the constitutionality and patriarchal origin of the institution of slavery; devoted to the principle of the independence of the States in all domestic matters and that this was essential to maintaining the liberties of the people from encroachment by the overwhelming votes of great

States or the centralization of power in a distant and unappreciative central government." Walkup, Angel continued, ardently believed that "the Democratic party was the embodiment of these principles." Lincoln and the Republicans, by contrast, "threatened to overthrow and obliterate every tenet of [Walkup's] sacred dogmas. With many democrats of like education and belief," the former state senator and lieutenant governor thus "maintained that coercion was unconstitutional and was unnecessary to preserve the Union." After eleven Southern states seceded from the United States, Walkup kept up an implacable barrage against the Union war effort. In 1864, for instance, he chaired a meeting of local Democrats, shepherding a resolution to passage that compelled the party's nominees for local offices to urge federal leaders to negotiate "a speedy and honorable peace" with the Confederacy while doing all they could to undermine "the policy of the present National Administration," which Walkup condemned as "subversive of the Constitution, the Laws, and the Union of our Fathers."[29]

Walkup's misgivings extended from the White House to the US Army's top brass. The Californian reserved special scorn for Philip Sheridan. Sheridan, who had waged war against several Indigenous Nations on the Pacific Coast as a young military officer in the late 1850s, rose to Union fame—and Confederate infamy—by executing Ulysses S. Grant's August 26, 1864, order to reduce Virginia's Shenandoah Valley, birthplace of Walkup's father, to a "barren waste." (Sheridan's old West Point pal George Crook, a central figure in the next chapter, commanded a corps of Sheridan's army as a brevet brigadier general.) In his memoirs, Sheridan remarked that Grant had "concluded that it was time to bring the war home to a people engaged in raising crops from a prolific soil to feed the country's enemies," adding that the Union commander had "endorsed the programme in all its parts, for the stores of meat and grain that the valley provided, and the men it furnished for [Robert E.] Lee's depleted regiments, were the strongest auxiliaries he possessed in the whole insurgent section." Months after making it significantly tougher for the rebels to glean food for themselves and fodder for their horses from the Shenandoah's farmsteads, Sheridan's cavalry helped to corner Lee's Army of Northern Virginia. After obliging Confederate forces to evacuate Petersburg, Sheridan and his men then captured nearly a fifth of Lee's hard-pressed army at Sayler's Creek on April 6, 1865. Three days later, Lee, his retreat blocked by Sheridan's cavalry, laid down his sword to Grant at Appomattox Courthouse.[30]

After Walkup took over the *Placer Herald* in the late 1860s, he constantly disparaged Sheridan for his role in the US Army's occupation of the defeated Confederacy. The editor criticized Sheridan, for example, for releasing several African American prisoners from a Louisiana jail after these parolees were accused of sexually assaulting white women. After Sheridan assumed command of the Army's Department of the Missouri, which was prosecuting warfare against several Indigenous Nations, Walkup reported with palpable glee that a grand jury was considering indicting the general for a fatal shooting blamed on a member of the vigilance committee Sheridan had led after Chicago officials declared martial law in response to the Great Fire of 1871.[31]

The Marias Massacre afforded Walkup plenty of ammunition against the general he loved to hate. Walkup's *Placer Herald* joined Democratic papers throughout the United States in lampooning "Piegan Phil" as a butcher and fiend. Although Walkup occasionally sympathized with the travails of the West's Indigenous peoples, he remained deeply reactionary on matters of race, insisting that the Democrats were "the only party that will protect the white men and women of this country." Walkup's manifest racism helps us better understand his ultimate goal in linking Sheridan and the Great Horse Flu: to stoke readers' outrage with President Ulysses S. Grant, the Republican Party, and GOP policies ranging from railroad land grants to African American civil rights.[32]

Walkup's partisanship combined with his combativeness to shape the style and purpose of his article purporting to trace the epizootic to the Marias Massacre's aftermath. The Auburn editor, as his counterpart at another gold-country paper aptly quipped, "wielded a battle-ax rather than a rapier." For Walkup as for virtually everyone else in Reconstruction America, politics represented the continuation of war by other means.[33]

Contagious Rumors

Walkup's staggering claim that Baker's attack on Piikanis led by Heavy Runner begot the Great Horse Flu riffed on an older refrain of grisly falsehoods that conflated two distinct smallpox epidemics. The first broke out in 1869 and decimated the Piikanis and their Indigenous neighbors on the Northern Plains. The second, meanwhile, reached North America's Atlantic coast in 1871. Walkup followed other Democratic newspapermen in mischaracterizing the latter outbreak as a continuation of the first. In these editors' telling, the Marias Massacre marked a pivotal epidemiological event. Scourges that had been ravaging Piikani communities and herds, these partisans contended, jumped to settlers and their equines as a direct consequence of Sheridan's ruthless campaign—a scenario that flies in the face of the evidence.

The earliest version of this story seems to have appeared in the *Cincinnati Enquirer* in November 1871, more than twenty months after Baker's forces rampaged through the village beside Kiaayoai'tahtaa. "Prominent gentlemen here," the *Enquirer* averred with equal measures of earnestness and vagueness, "attribute the spread of the small-pox in Philadelphia and other cities to the sale of buffalo robes there, taken from the Blackfeet and Piegan camps, where the disease prevailed two years ago." Two months later, the *Fayetteville (TN) Observer* moralized on the rumors the *Enquirer* had instigated. "The massacre of the sick men, women, and children, even the babies, of the Piegan tribe of Indians," it hissed, "which Sheridan, the Virginia barn-burner, was the only man to applaud, has wrought retributive justice to the white man, if we are to believe the story that the buffalo robes on that disgraceful occasion were the means of disseminating the small-pox in New York and elsewhere."[34]

A few weeks after this article appeared, Walkup related in the *Placer Herald* that smallpox "has been raging in a virulent form in the eastern cities, and as far west as Chicago, and lately at Omaha and Salt Lake, and has now reached this coast and county." This epidemic, Walkup alleged, "is believed to have started in Philadelphia, from buffalo robes and other camp equipage captured from the Peigan [*sic*] Indians at the time of the Phil Sheridan massacre."[35]

The straight lines that Walkup and other Democratic editors drew between the smallpox outbreak and the slaying of nearly two hundred Piikanis rested on half-truths and outright lies. Many perpetrators, survivors, and bystanders of the US attack on Issokui-omachkan and his people maintained that US troops had immediately set fire to all the Piikani property they had pilfered. One of Baker's subordinates, for instance, later testified that the commander "wouldn't let us take anything," least of all "anything that belonged to [the Piikani], for they had the smallpox among them."[36]

Other witnesses, though, insisted that soldiers had seized and kept hundreds or even thousands of bison robes. Documents from the massacre's aftermath lend credence to such allegations. Secretary of War William Belknap received so many reports of a suspicious spike in the number of robes and furs brought into Montana trading posts that he issued orders to quarantine any goods believed to have been stolen from Heavy Runner's village. An Indian Office functionary near Fort Benton (a fur-trading post that had long served as the epicenter of tensions between Piikanis and American invaders), though, defied these orders by permitting the sale of one lot of robes widely believed to have been stolen from the massacred Piikanis. He justified this exception by alleging that the consignment in question had "not spread or caused any contagion or disease among persons handling or using them." This pretext meant that at least some of the Piikani belongings that perpetrators of the Marias Massacre had purloined probably would, in fact, reach what Walkup called "the Eastern market."[37]

Yet even if this consignment of robes indeed carried smallpox virions from Indigenous peoples on the Plains to US settlers on the Eastern Seaboard—and there is no reason to think that it did—attempts by Walkup and other Democratic partisans to pin the variola epidemic on Sheridan's forces still fail to hold water. The first localized eruptions of smallpox in the Northeast, after all, did not break out until more than a year after the January 1870 annihilation of the village along Kiaayoai'tahtaa by Baker and his troops. In the interim, western Europe experienced its worst smallpox outbreak in nearly a century. Researchers have traced this epidemic, which eventually killed five hundred thousand Europeans, to 1870, when hundreds of thousands of French conscripts carried variola from the countryside surrounding Paris to training camps and battlegrounds during the Franco-Prussian War. After permeating Europe, smallpox landed on North American shores in early 1871, churning through coastal ports before reaching Toronto, Chicago, and beyond. Throughout the Great Horse Flu's run, reports of this epidemic's growth often appeared in newspapers alongside updates on the epizootic's expansion.[38]

Although details of timing and geography clearly pointed toward European rather than Indigenous American origins for the smallpox outbreak, narratives linking the Marias Massacre to the epidemic nonetheless continued to reverberate in the Democratic press. The *Memphis Appeal* offered an especially sweeping and forthright spin. "The frightful scourge," it pronounced in late October 1872, a month after the epizootic first appeared outside Toronto and less than a week before voters went to the polls to choose between President Grant and his opponent, *New York Herald* editor Horace Greeley, "is the terrible result of Grant's famed Indian policy," which it decried as "shaped first by Sheridan and thieves, and then by smallpox."[39]

A Good Many Animals

Just days before Grant's second inauguration, Walkup added a new riff on the fake news that opposition papers had been bandying about for years. From the start of the epizootic, reliable authorities traced it to the countryside north of Toronto. With precious few exceptions, newspapers, magazines, and government reports all hewed fast to this version of the outbreak's origins.[40]

Walkup's assertion that the Great Horse Flu began with Piikani ponies looted by US cavalry forces after the Marias Massacre drew on and amplified the first deviation from this consensus to enter wider circulation. In mid-February 1873, the *Helena (MT) Weekly Herald* published an article based on a recent interview with a "gentleman" who was visiting Montana's territorial capital from Fort Benton, the same post through which Baker's troops had apparently trafficked some of the robes they stole from Issokui-omachkan and his people. The Helena editor paraphrased this visitor's "opinion that the disease known as the 'epizootic' originated among the ponies of the Peigan [*sic*] Indians." The paper's unnamed informant went on to explain that "last spring these ponies (up in the British possessions) were all sick with a disease that had every symptom" associated with the epizootic. "A good many animals," the man from Benton continued in a charge that reached readers in other parts of the United States via wire services and newspaper exchanges, had perished "for want of proper care." The horse plague, the Montana journal contended, then spread from the Piikani homelands to eastern Canada via "the ponies of the tribes further east."[41]

A few weeks later, Walkup redoubled his smear campaign against Phil Sheridan by melding this Montana hearsay to the spurious smallpox tales that he and other Democratic editors had been spinning for more than a year. A hardened politician and newsman, Walkup surely understood that his attack on the lieutenant general—and, by extension, on Grant and the Republicans—would gain more traction if it squared with narratives already familiar to his readers. Walkup's charges, though, may also have gained fuel from credible doubts regarding the fate of the ponies cavalrymen stole from Heavy Runner's village.

Three of Issokui-omachkan's children—Comes with Rattles, Spear Woman, and Last Gun (who sometimes referred to themselves as William Upham, Emma Miller, and Dick Kipp, respectively)—later petitioned the US Senate for $75,000 to "reimburse" them, as one Montana senator explained in 1916, for Heavy Runner's "death and for property taken from him at the time of the Baker massacre." The affidavits presented in support of these heirs' unsuccessful claim offered conflicting accounts of how many horses US cavalrymen had driven off. Bear Head described this equine booty as a "great herd"; Baker's guide Horace Clarke, the métis son of Scots American fur trader and rancher Malcolm Clarke and his Piikani wife, Coth-co-co-na (Cutting Off Head Woman), placed the soldiers' haul at thirteen hundred; and another métis guide, Joseph Kipp, reckoned that US cavalrymen had pilfered "something like Five thousand head." Most other Piikani survivors, though, numbered the stolen ponies in the hundreds.[42]

None of these affidavits detailed what happened to the horses US cavalrymen had rustled. Other sources, though, reveal a three-step process by which officers and American settlers claimed Piikani ponies for their own. First, military leaders permitted settlers to recover horses they could show to be their "proved property." Next, several officers chose one or more of the remaining ponies for their own use. Finally, more than three months after the massacre, Colonel Régis de Trobriand auctioned off roughly 250 horses at Fort Shaw, the closest military post to Kiaayoai'tahtaa. Although de Trobriand snubbed this lot as "poorly looking animals," he also touted their sale as "a remarkable success." In a report to a superior, Trobriand smugly added that the "proceeds" from the auction would "more than cover for the government the expense of the expedition" against the Piikani village.[43]

Despite Trobriand's snipe about the ponies' homely appearance, there is no indication that the animals stolen by US troops were suffering from influenza when they were sold off, nor did these details jibe with the *Helena Herald* account on which Walkup based his screed.[44]

The Great Horse Flu reached Auburn, California, in the second week of April 1873. By then, the pair of short articles that Joseph Walkup had laid out along the *Placer Herald*'s inner fold had surely faded from many readers' memories. A century and a half later, though, Walkup's back-to-back articles on *American Progress* and the epidemiological aftermath of the Marias Massacre cast a clearer light on both the epizootic and its expansion westward.

Look past the triumphalist whitewash of Gast's chromolithograph, and this "beautiful picture" takes on new connotations. The processes of conquest and colonization that *American Progress* so vividly celebrated hinged on the violent, ongoing dispossession of Indigenous peoples. This all-too-human drama continued to unfold in landscapes profoundly shaped by nonhuman entities ranging from telegraph lines and railroad networks to horses and invisible pathogens. As for the tales Walkup and his Democratic allies spun about Native American massacres, smallpox, and the Great Horse Flu's increase, this exercise in conspiracy mongering drew deceptive, politically charged connections between federal misdeeds, the Grant administration's embattled policies toward Indigenous Nations, and infectious diseases. In so doing, it jumbled beyond recognition the tangled but very real ties between the epizootic, settler invasions of Indigenous homelands, and American Reconstruction.

CHAPTER 7

EPIZOOTIC OFFENSIVES

Mexico and the Southwest's Indigenous Borderlands

In March 1873—a month that began with the *Placer Herald* hailing John Gast's *American Progress* and blaming Phil Sheridan for the Great Horse Flu—the epizootic extended its grasp deep into Mexico. Human-made boundaries proved incapable of containing either the novel influenza virus or the hosts on which it preyed. When the scourge crossed political borders, though, the contexts in which it did its work shifted, as a closer look at this stage of the outbreak shows.

Once the epizootic reached the Rio Grande in late 1872 or early 1873, it took just a short swim or ferry ride for infected equines to introduce the malady to Mexican soil. Thereafter, the Great Horse Flu often behaved in familiar ways—replicating rapidly, sickening new hosts with astounding efficiency, gumming up equine-powered economies, exacerbating social inequities, and compelling humans to reconsider their understandings of influenza and how best to treat it. Significant differences between Mexico and the domains the epizootic had already struck, though, meant that these dynamics often assumed new shapes south of the border.

Mexico had just endured a wrenching quarter century of political turmoil, civil unrest, and military conflict. Although it had started to recover from these convulsions, the republic's markets remained stagnant and heavily focused on local or regional exchange. "Half of all federal highways" in Mexico, one historian explains, were "suitable only for beasts of burden." Many other roads remained "so narrow and broken that they could be passed only by pedestrian traffic." Mexicans leaned more heavily on burros to carry people and goods from place to place than their northern neighbors did. Given donkeys' versatility and surefootedness, this was a sensible move, but it also exacerbated the outbreak's impacts because the novel influenza virus killed asses at much higher rates than mules or horses. A final point of divergence distinguished the Great Horse Flu's south-of-the-border history: Mexicans worried more than *norteamericanos* about the risks that equines killed by the epizootic posed to human health.[1]

During the same months in which the Great Horse Flu swept toward the Valley of Mexico, it also invaded territories that the United States had wrested from its southern neighbor through the Mexican-American War (La intervención estadounidense en México) and the Gadsden Purchase. One might expect that the outbreak's attacks on the Southwest's settlements and US Army posts would have spelled trouble for a brutal winter campaign that Lieutenant Colonel George Crook and his forces had been prosecuting for several months against Dilzhę́'és (known to Americans as Tonto Apaches) and Yavapais. US troopers and their Indigenous auxiliaries in Arizona Territory, though, seamlessly transitioned to fighting afoot. Denied the use of pack animals and cavalry mounts, American cavalrymen nonetheless stepped up their attacks. Even as the Great Horse Flu lingered, Crook and his troops compelled their enemies to surrender in April 1873.

After this much-ballyhooed triumph, the epizootic took a diabolical turn. Now confined to reservations, the Dilzhę́'é and Yavapai survivors of Crook's exterminationist assaults suffered a devastating outbreak of the same malady that Joseph Walkup had maliciously—and mendaciously—traced to Piikani horses. Although the novel influenza virus struck only glancing blows at Native Americans' herds, the story of one of the deadliest, most lopsided, and least-known campaigns of the Indian Wars shows that the Great Horse Flu afforded Yavapais, Dilzhę́'és, and—by extension—other Native peoples no respite from the relentless onslaught that *American Progress* simultaneously trumpeted and concealed.

¡Viva *la Epizootía*!

Oaxacan-born physician and veterinarian Gustavo Ruiz y Sandoval later claimed that the Great Horse Flu struck "the border states of Coahuila and Nuevo-León" in January 1873, "causing great damage." When the epizootic invaded northern Mexico's "fields and the cities," Ruiz y Sandoval asserted, it "hardly "spar[ed] any of the horses that are so abundant in those regions," not even those "in the wild state." By February, the outbreak had engulfed much of the "northern half of the Republic." In addition to complicating Mexico's long-running counterinsurgency against Chiracahuas and other Apache (Nde) nations by "dismount[ing] many regiments of cavalry," the epizootic hampered overland trade throughout the US-Mexican borderlands.[2]

Tortuous topography, ecological diversity, poor transportation infrastructure, and lack of economic integration all help to explain the chaotic patterns the Great Horse Flu assumed after crossing into Mexico. The epizootic did not strike Tamaulipas, bordering southern Texas, or Zacatecas, 380 miles (611 kilometers) northwest of Mexico City, until April, several weeks after clobbering the national capital. Durango, nearly 180 miles (290 kilometers) west of Zacatecas, did not report its first cases until August, while the epizootic took until December 1873 to reach Guaymas, Sonora's busiest port. In stark contrast to the United States, where only Key West remained untouched, several stretches of Mexico, including eastern Veracruz state and the Yucatán in the east and Acapulco and Baja California in the west, never reported any cases.[3]

As one branch of the Great Horse Flu ground toward the Gulf of California, the outbreak's main salient steamrolled through the Mexican heartland, afflicting horses, donkeys, and mules from San Luis Potosí, Guanajuato, Sinaloa, and Querétaro in the north to Guerrero in the south, and from Veracruz on the Gulf of Mexico to Michoacán on the Pacific. It reached Puebla and Michoacán in mid-March, killing eighteen police horses in the former city. A week later in Pachuca, capital of Hidalgo state, one could "hardly find a single horse that is not infested with that terrible evil."[4]

By all accounts, the epizootic struck Mexico City hardest of all. Horses employed in drawing stagecoaches (*diligencias*) allegedly introduced the novel influenza virus to the capital from the borderlands to the north. The Great Horse Flu's "appearance," Ruiz y Sandoval claimed, "was so rapid that in a single day it spread to nearly four hundred animals" in the city's *diligencia* stables. On March 6, José Maria Lugo, professor of external pathology at

Mexico City's veterinary college, paid a visit to these flu-stricken steeds at their stables, where he found "a very considerable number of sick animals who all seemed to be suffering from the same disease." The malady, Lugo noted, typically began with a "tenacious" cough that was "dry in fits and starts" and "accompanied by a kind of moan." Within three days of showing these initial symptoms, "a limpid and perfectly clear liquid" began running "from both nostrils and sometimes from the mouth" of flu-stricken horses, swiftly becoming "more and more purulent." Other worrisome signs of complication often followed: edema and diarrhea in some patients, and fever and shortness of breath in many others.[5]

Virtually every horse, donkey, and mule who came "in contact with the sick" swiftly fell ill. By March 7, "all the horses and mules" employed by the Mexican postal service "on the line from the interior of the Republic to the northern borders" had reportedly contracted "a strong cough that prevents them from walking with the usual speed." A Mexico City veterinarian expressed his "fear that the epidemic will also be established in our capital" after attending to thirty flu-stricken horses and perusing "several reports" on the epizootic from American veterinarians, courtesy of the US consul. Nineteen horses had already perished from the scourge by the time the federal district's public health council appointed a team of veterinarians to investigate the outbreak and advise the public on how best to contain and combat it. The commissioners spent a week examining ailing animals before issuing their findings. Although the healers confessed that "the causes of this condition are still obscure to us," they declined to "advise anything" by way of treatment. In the end, the team reassured district residents that influenza could be expected to kill just 1 or 2 percent of "attacked animals." Soon the Great Horse Flu had saturated this metropolis of nearly a quarter million people while also invading "all the surrounding towns."[6]

Mexico City's pharmacies touted "an effective remedy that has given results in the North against this disease." Local veterinarian Manuel Fonte boasted that "of four hundred and fifty-seven sick animals that are under his care, only four have died." Many other Mexicans, though, entrusted their equines' well-being to folk medicines, including various herbs as well as spring water hauled hundreds of miles by horse or mule from Agua Santa, Chihuahua.[7]

As the epizootic tightened its grip, the same dynamics the outbreak had triggered in Canadian, American, and Cuban cities repeated themselves in Mexico's largest and most powerful metropolis. Mexico City's press printed "news of the best medicine found in the United States and Cuba against the epizootic." Postal service suffered "serious disturbances." Construction on the Mexican Railway to Veracruz stalled. Street railways reduced service, and the thoroughfares on which wealthy citizens typically flaunted their blooded horses and ornate carriages grew empty and—in one observer's florid phrase—"extremely sad."[8]

As usual, the Great Horse Flu's burdens fell heaviest on the poor. Rising prices on "basic necessities" threatened Mexico City's most vulnerable inhabitants with starvation and indigence. The clearest connections between inflation and the epizootic stemmed from the capital's widespread reliance on donkeys, who reportedly "succumbed in greater proportion" throughout Mexico "than horses and mules." In one district of San Luis Potosí state alone, 609 burros succumbed, compared to 20 mules and 224 horses. Ruiz y Sandoval attributed the virus's heavy toll on donkeys to pneumonia; as had been true in North America, this life-threatening complication "was noted with some frequency" in Mexico's burros, rendering the epizootic "very serious in these animals." A Mexico City newspaper complained that "prices of various items that come to the market on the back of a donkey," including vegetables and charcoal, were skyrocketing. "There being many sick donkeys," the same article explained, "less cargo is brought in than before, which causes shortages, and the drivers have to recoup something on what they sell to compensate for their higher expenses." Another of the capital's journals interviewed a vendor who explained that oranges had become "'very scarce . . . because the little burros . . . burst.'" The vendor's comments led the reporter who quoted them to remark that "the poor classes fast on Lent, but not out of devotion." Hunger persisted even after the Great Horse Flu relented because prices on many foodstuffs and other goods remained high even after most of the city's equines recovered.[9]

Although Mexico City's epizootic encounters largely followed Canadian and American precedent, inhabitants of the Mexican capital perceived the corpses of equines killed by the epizootic as much more menacing to human health than *norteamericanos* had. *El Siglo Diez y Nueve* warned in mid-March that the carcasses piling up in streets and alleyways were generating "pestiferous miasmas." Given "the present warm season," it continued, the foul vapors emanating from dead equines threatened to spawn "a typhoid plague" among the capital's citizens. The paper thus urged the district government to "bury the corpses of beasts at all times for the same reasons that cause the corpses of rational beings to be buried": to protect the living from contamination and contagion. Less than a week later, though, another article claimed that Mexico City's byways were filling up with "the cadavers of animals killed by the epizootic," sparking complaints that these "dead bodies" were "exhaling miasmas" capable of sickening humans. When the local government balked at the huge expense of burying hundreds or thousands of expired equines, *El Monitor Republicano* urged officials to incinerate these corpses instead. A day later, after district officials learned that "the prevailing epizootic ha[d] invaded cattle and sheep" too, they ordered "that animals that show symptoms of epizootic disease not be killed on the trail" into the capital "for the consumption of the city." The governor of the Federal District soon directed the veterinarian at Mexico City's massive public slaughterhouse complex "to prevent," as *La Voz de México* put it, "the meat of diseased cattle from being sold." Residents of outlying neighborhoods, though, "complain[ed], and with justice, that in those districts there is no manager to watch over and prohibit the sale of meat from animals damaged or killed by the epizootic. They add," reported *El Monitor Republicano*, "that they have already seen and even eaten some of that meat, and that they fear for their health." There is no record of anyone having contracted influenza by eating the flesh of flu-stricken livestock. Yet in Mexico City the epizootic so frequently coincided with or immediately preceded localized outbreaks of human influenza that Mexicans, like North Americans before them, began grumbling that they, too, were ailing from *la epizootia*.[10]

After leaving the Valley of Mexico, the Great Horse Flu ran up against the imposing Sierra Madre del Sur, which slowed its advance. The outbreak then nearly stopped altogether on reaching the Sierra Mixteca, known in Nahuatl as the "land of the clouds" and one of Mexico's least populated, most impoverished regions. Despite these obstacles, Ruiz y Sandoval claimed that the novel influenza virus "successively invad[ed]" Morelos and northern Oaxaca state in April and May. In June and July, it convulsed the city of Oaxaca, introduced, he averred, "by a single horse that contracted the disease on a hacienda located a few leagues from the town," before "radiating from this center" to "other locations in the State." The scourge caused "almost no deaths" among Oaxaca's horses, but it did "some damage to the donkeys" on whom that city's overwhelmingly Indigenous inhabitants relied.[11]

There Is No Room for You

As one salient of the Great Horse Flu pushed deep into Mexico, another struck the borderlands between the United States, Mexico, and the Southwest's Indigenous Nations alongside violent invasions by settlers and soldiers. The result was untold suffering for the several thousand men, women, and children of the Yavapai and Dilzhę́'é nations.

These neighboring peoples pursued similar lifeways in overlapping homelands bounded by the Lower Colorado River, central Arizona's fractured mountain ranges, the Gila River Valley, and the red-rock highlands jutting skyward from the Mogollon Rim. Historically, the Verde River (a stream that Apaches referred to as Túńlíníchoh, "big river," or Túchoh ńlį́į́, "big water flowing"; Yavapais called it 'Há Ktáya) marked what Maurice Crandall, a historian and enrolled member of the Yavapai-Apache Nation, calls "an informal boundary" between Yavapais, who primarily lived west of the Verde, and Dilzhę́'és, who mostly stayed to the river's east. From time immemorial, Crandall explains, his people enacted a shared vision of "the Verde Valley and Red Rock Country" as "our 'spiritual heartland,'" with Yavapai origin stories tracing their emergence into this world to 'Há Kskyáywa (Montezuma's Well), a stunning pool of water surrounded by sandstone walls south of present-day Sedona.[12]

Outsiders had long considered this region remote and impassable. Dilzhę́'és and Yavapais, by contrast, made themselves at home throughout expansive territories encompassing nearly twenty thousand square miles. "Families relocated frequently," one historian notes, "as they followed the ripening sequence of wild plant foods" on an "annual round" that cycled between winter camps in lowland river valleys, canyons, and deserts and warm-season abodes at higher elevations. Agave (also known as mescal), game animals, and crops including maize, squash, beans, watermelons, pumpkins, and sunflowers raised on floodplain plots in the Colorado and Gila River Valleys all played key roles in sustaining Yavapai and Dilzhę́'é kinship groups. Aha Macav peoples (known to Americans as Mohaves), who lived just to the Yavapais' west and often traded and allied with them, recalled their neighbors' steadfast expressions of sovereignty over the lands that sustained their bodies, communities, and spiritual relationships: "We are scattered over the country," the Aha Macav remembered the Yavapais having told them. "We have taken all the springs; there is no place for you to stay. Everywhere our tribes have made monuments of trees or brush to claim the land. There is no room for you."[13]

Spanish conquistadors made no incursions into the homelands the Yavapai and Dilzhę́'é held dear until the 1580s. Subsequent efforts to colonize northern New Spain rippled slowly but surely into what would later become Arizona—especially after the 1690s, when Jesuits established missions for Akimel and Tohono O'odham peoples (also known as Pimas and Papagos, respectively), whom Crandall refers to as "our traditional enemies," just a few days' journey from Dilzhę́'é and Yavapai territories. Although Europeans or Mexicans almost never set foot in the Verde Valley or Red Rock Country before the 1800s, these outsiders' plants, pathogens, weapons, and animals nonetheless made steady inroads. Equines, which the Yavapais may have first acquired by raiding Akimel O'odham villages but which they also began to purloin together with cattle and other stock from Spanish missions and ranches, featured prominently among the new arrivals. Yet keeping horses, mules, and donkeys fed, watered, and sheltered in dry and mountainous homelands usually proved more trouble than it was worth. As an American soldier later observed of Dilzhę́'és and Yavapais, "horses captured by them are generally eaten." The same fate commonly befell burros, "esteemed" by members of these nations "as a delicacy," especially when young and tender.[14]

Tribal elders Mike Harrison and John Williams recount that soon after their Yavapai ancestors first encountered Mexicans building a church and planting crops near Tucson, these newcomers earned their trust. "After that," Harrison and Williams say, "the chief called them *haiko hanna*. That means 'good white people.' The Mexicans were the white people who didn't kill us." Mutual toleration flourished in no small part because northward migration from Sonora, always halting under Spanish rule, nearly stopped altogether after Mexico achieved independence in 1821.[15]

Soon after pressure from the south abated, though, an onslaught bore down from the east. Starting in 1826, US-based fur trappers and traders, followed by California-bound argonauts, pushed in. Having acquired paper claims to well over half a million square miles of territory from Mexico in 1848's Treaty of Guadalupe Hidalgo, US federal authorities launched far-reaching campaigns to bring the Southwest's Indigenous Nations to heel. After allies of the Yavapais attacked Americans at the all-important Yuma Crossing on the Colorado River in 1852, US forces skirmished with Yavapais while forging powerful alliances with the Akimel O'odham and another long-standing Yavapai and Dilzhę́'é foe, the Piipaash (also known as Maricopas). Life became still more perilous for Dilzhę́'és and Yavapais starting in the late 1850s, when American miners, stock growers, and town-builders all began setting sights on their homelands.[16]

Yavapais and Dilzhę́'és did their utmost to endure and, when possible, resist. Yet each bid to fend off invaders brought additional reprisals and repression. By the time the epizootic pressed against their territories, Dilzhę́'és and Yavapais stood square in the crosshairs of a formidable American army of extinction.

I Must Have Horses

The novel influenza virus crossed from New Mexico to Arizona in early March 1873, just days after Joseph Walkup circulated his vicious lies about Piikani ponies, Phil Sheridan, and the epizootic's origins. As the Great Horse Flu raced across northern Mexico, it also struck the embattled Dilzhę́'é and Yavapai homelands via the Butterfield Stage Route, the main artery for communication and commerce between El Paso and San Diego.

By March 8, the *Arizona Miner* of Prescott, which invading miners had established just eight years before at a place Yavapais knew as 'Wíi 'Kwáth

Sk'íra ("gray pointed rocks," a reference to the granite formations that mark the area's landscape), and which a US soldier described in 1872 as a town of "about one thousand people" who were "full of energy and enterprise," complained that "the epizootic, or animal pestilence, has attacked several horses and mules" at Fort Whipple. This nearby US Army post served as the headquarters for Lieutenant Colonel George Crook. After graduating from West Point in 1852, Crook earned a deserved reputation as a dauntless Indian fighter. During the Civil War, Crook's corps formed part of Sheridan's Army of the Shenandoah. Crook's successes in 1864's Valley Campaign earned him a promotion to brevet major general. On learning of the epizootic's arrival at his Arizona outpost, Crook immediately dispatched couriers to notify his troops that influenza "has broken out among [the] Government herd at Prescott." Equines on several ranches in the surrounding countryside also fell ill, and newspapers described the equine malady as "prevail[ing] to an alarming extent" at every US Army post in the territory.[17]

The outbreak struck as Crook and his men were prosecuting a ferocious counterinsurgency campaign against Dilzhę́'és and Yavapais. An 1868 *Overland Monthly* article titled "The Apache Race" described the targets of Crook's assaults as "undoubtedly the most nomadic in existence," adding that the "absolute personal license and freedom from all control, which are the highest prized rights of the Apache proper, form also the most insuperable bar to any permanent relations between them and the American government." In the late 1860s and early 1870s, federal officials, intent on reining in Indigenous autonomy so that miners and other settlers could unlock what George Crofutt later extolled as "the great treasure chamber of our country," established several Indian reservations in Arizona, including the Rio Verde Reserve, established in 1871 in the heart of Yavapai and Dilzhę́'é country. Federal efforts to provide food, shelter, and security drew many Native people to the Verde and other reservations. Hardly any Dilzhę́'és or Yavapais, however, would willingly agree to forsake either their traditional lifeways or the homelands that had nurtured their people since time immemorial.[18]

Starting in September 1871, Yavapais, Dilzhę́'és, and other Apaches embarked on a yearlong uprising. Purloining more than five hundred head of cattle and large numbers of horses and mules in more than fifty raids, they killed several dozen Americans and Mexicans. Indigenous resistance, the *Army and Navy Journal* complained in 1872, had "more than decimated and altogether impoverished the civilized population of Arizona and Southern New Mexico." In the process, Apache and Dilzhę́'é attacks tarnished the United States' reputation. "English, French, and Russian officers and people have come to regard these unwhipped horrors," the *New York Herald* grumbled, "as evidence of the inability of this government to protect its frontiers."[19]

Crook endeavored to restore faith in American progress by forcing Dilzhę́'és and Yavapais into submission. In November 1872, Crook divided his forces into five separate commands, then ordered each to hunt down any Yavapais and Dilzhę́'és they found beyond the boundaries of the reserves the government had set up on several small corners of their homelands. By the time the epizootic reached Fort Whipple, Crook had sortied seven additional commands to hunt down Dilzhę́'és and Yavapais and confine any survivors on reservations.[20]

Crook embraced horses and mules as essential adjuncts in Indian warfare. Soon after assuming command over the Army's Department of Arizona in 1871, Crook detailed to a *Denver News* correspondent the essential roles he expected equines to play in his efforts "to suppress these raids and murders by the Apaches" (Americans, following Mexican and Spanish precedents, often employed this term as a catchall). "I must have horses," Crook blustered, "for infantry would be of no service in these mountains, and then I must have large pack trains, and the citizens must not be surprised [if] it takes a year to get ready; but when I do get ready I will give these Apaches no rest until they submit."[21]

Crook supplemented forces from the Twenty-Third Infantry with units from the Fifth Cavalry, including some soldiers who had fought under

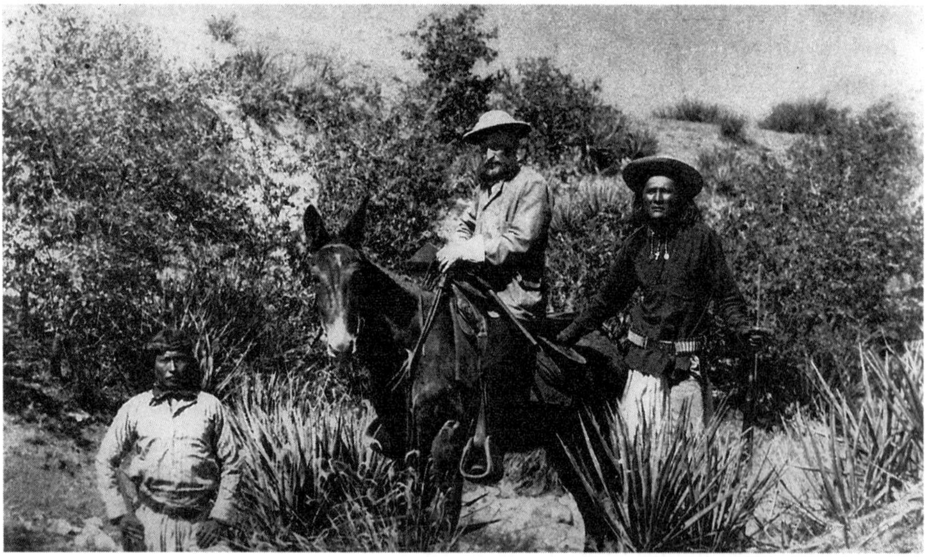

This photograph captured two essential contributors to Crook's Grand Offensive: mules and Native American scouts. "General Crook and the Friendly Apache, Alchise," in John G. Bourke, *On the Border with Crook* (New York: Charles Scribner's Sons, 1891), 241. Courtesy of the Sharlot Hall Library and Museum, Prescott, AZ.

Sheridan—and probably at least a few who had gunned down Piikanis at Kiaayoai'tahtaa. The commander knew that his success against Dilzhę́'és and Yavapais hinged on his capacity to supply food, fodder, ammunition, and other necessities to his troops as well as the Native auxiliaries Crook and his officers engaged to scout for them. Crook's longtime aide-de-camp and future biographer Captain John Gregory Bourke aptly noted that his boss had "made pack-trains," mule-powered outfits responsible for maintaining communication lines, "the great study of his life." To make his pack-trains "as nearly perfect as they ever have been or can be," Crook sought out experienced Chilean, Peruvian, and Mexican packmasters in California and Arizona mining camps, where these experts in equine-driven logistics continued to perfect methods handed down from packer to packer over decades or even centuries. With characteristic single-mindedness, Crook set about learning the tricks of the packers' trade and adapting them to provision multiple troop commands dispersed across a vast, remote region notorious for climatic extremes, disorienting deserts, deeply incised canyons, lofty plateaus, and mountain fastnesses.[22]

Crook recognized that to achieve this objective, he had to swap out "the ill-assorted collections of bony giants and undersized Sonora 'rats'" that had previously populated the corrals of Arizona's army posts and replace them with mules that "in weight, size, and build," Bourke explained, "were of the type which experience had shown to be the most appropriate." Crook then "kept himself posted as to what was done to every mule," insisting that each creature enjoy care "equal[ing] almost that given to the average baby." Crook's compulsive efforts enabled his force of 150 mules, subdivided into three separate trains as his troops entered the field, to haul an average of 320 pounds per animal, almost twice the maximum weight specified in army regulations.[23]

The Great Horse Flu's arrival jeopardized the mule-powered circulation of supplies, information, and orders between Crook's field commands, army posts, and the settlements that supplied the US Army with beef, produce, and other necessities. It also threatened the cavalry campaigns Crook had unleashed against Dilzhę́'és and Yavapais. With the army's horses and mules "suffering much from the epizootic," quartermasters hastened to buy up any "Indian ponies" who remained unaffected by influenza. But the Americans' Indigenous allies—O'odham, Piipaash, Havasu Baaja (Havasupai), and others—were too poor in horses to satisfy the military's wants. With the novel influenza virus "crippling the resources of the Department [of Arizona] in horses and mules," Bourke recalled that he and his fellow troops felt that they had little choice but "to abandon our animals, and take our rations and blankets upon our own backs, and do the best we could."[24]

Once the horse plague compelled Crook's armies to climb off their horses and wage war afoot, the invaders' assaults on Yavapais and Dilzhę́'és grew slower and more laborious. Yet despite their animals' ailing condition, this scorched-earth campaign hardly missed a beat. "In a very few weeks," Bourke brusquely recounted of the bloodletting that followed, "the good results became manifest, and the enemy showed signs of weakening."[25]

Regarded as Hostile and Punished Accordingly

Nearly two decades after these ruthless search-and-destroy missions, Crook bragged that his genocidal campaign had "finally closed an Indian war that has been waged since the days of Cortez." Crook's Grand Offensive (also known as the Big Scout and Tonto Basin War) brought glory to the lieutenant colonel and his men. It also prompted a hearty if short-lived outpouring of unvarnished praise for the Grant administration's controversial Indian policy. For Yavapai and Dilzhę́'é peoples, by contrast, this brutal campaign brought desperation, hunger, and death, leaving a legacy of suffering and dispossession that continues to reverberate today. Nearly half a year of relentless pursuits, lopsided fights, and merciless massacres killed between five hundred and a thousand Yavapais and Apaches and resulted in captivity for hundreds more at a time when these groups had a combined population of just a few thousand people.[26]

The US Army's success at harrying and starving so-called hostiles into submission became abundantly evident when "the last of the Apaches" surrendered to Crook at Camp Verde on April 7, 1873. "Had it not been for their barbarities," Crook later huffed, "one would have been moved to pity by their appearance." The Dilzhę́'és and Yavapais who capitulated to US forces on that fateful day, Crook recalled, "were emaciated, clothes torn in tatters, [and] some of their legs were not thicker than my arm."[27]

During the ceremonies and parlays that followed, the Dilzhę́'é leader Eschetlepan expressed the depths of his people's despair: "We're are [*sic*] nearly dead from want of food and exposure." Two decades later, Bourke recounted that "squaws at the San Carlos Agency"—a reservation beyond the traditional boundaries of the Yavapai and Dilzhę́'é domains where the US government exiled these groups following a brutal 1875 forced march that resulted in hundreds of additional fatalities—"still periodically mourn for the death . . . of their people" in the lopsided assaults that typified the Grand Offensive from start to finish.[28]

Crook launched this campaign roughly a week after the Great Boston Fire. His General Orders No. 10 succinctly laid out the rationale and strategy behind these assaults. Any Dilzhę́'é or Yavapai who refused to relocate to a US Indian reservation, Crook warned, would "be regarded as hostile and punished accordingly." The orders vowed that "active operations will be kept up against the hostile Apaches of Arizona and pressed with all practicable vigor until they submit to the authority of the government, cease from hostilities, and remain upon their reservations."[29]

In November 1872, with the nights lengthening and autumnal storms moistening parched desert soils for the first time in months, Crook dispatched units of cavalry and infantry to chase down every Yavapai or Dilzhę́'é who had not yet complied with his edict. Those who remained off reservations, though, understood that obeying General Orders No. 10 meant submitting to confinement within just a tiny corner of their ancestral territories rather than maintaining the practices of movement, belonging, and mutual care that comprised the enduring material and spiritual foundations for Dilzhę́'é and Yavapai well-being. To each column of his troops, Crook assigned O'odham, Hualapai, Piipaash, and White Mountain Apache scouts, ostensibly commanded by a hodgepodge of Anglo, Mexican, métis, and mestizo trackers, traders, translators, and ruffians.[30]

Crook's Grand Offensive began with an unbroken spate of routs. On November 25, 1872, US forces killed eleven enemies and captured three at Red Rocks (also known as Hell Canyon). On December 7, near present-day Sedona, they killed thirteen more while securing three additional captives. During the following week, Crook's men killed twenty-five additional Dilzhę́'és and Yavapais and took six captives in separate engagements at Bad Rock Mountain and in the Mazatzal Mountains. In a pattern that prevailed throughout the rest of the campaign, each of these early fights proved utterly one-sided. US forces suffered a grand total of just two fatalities. Yavapai and Dilzhę́'é fighters, intent on fulfilling obligations to protect noncombatants and armed almost entirely with bows and arrows rather than firearms, faced insurmountable odds in defending their people against surprise attacks from much larger contingents of soldiers and scouts armed with Springfield rifles and other cutting-edge weaponry.[31]

By the time the Great Horse Flu began disabling army horses and mules in March 1873, Crook's forces had pursued Dilzhę́'és and Yavapais with a relentless brutality that made Crook and his men the toast of frontier settlements throughout Arizona and far beyond. US troops and Indian scouts wiped out dozens of rancherías (a term used throughout the Spanish borderlands to refer to Indigenous villages as well as the kinship groups who comprised them) and took hundreds of captives. By depriving Crook and his men of cavalry mounts and pack animals, the epizootic forced troopers to hunt down Yavapais and Dilzhę́'és on foot with only tenuous supply lines. For all this, though, the outbreak neither halted nor delayed the army's march to victory, as one of the deadliest engagements in the entire Grand Offensive shows.

On March 11, 1873, Indigenous fighters ambushed three white travelers on Yavapai lands outside the mining camp of Wickenburg. Although the attackers quickly dispatched their first two victims, they allegedly tortured the third by shooting over 150 arrows into his body before finally putting him out of his misery. Crook responded by ordering his forces to show no mercy to any Dilzhę́'é́s or Yavapais found off their reservations. US troops and Native scouts proceeded to stalk and slaughter nearly one hundred Indigenous children, women, and men while taking dozens of prisoners.[32]

The deadliest single attack in this broader set of assaults took place on March 27 near the summit of a mountain settlers called Turret Peak, in the rugged terrain of Arizona's Black Hills. This area had long comprised the homeland of a Yavapai band whom Apaches referred to as the "yellow pine bent backward people." Scouts under Major George Randall, though, assumed that some of those suspected of the Wickenburg murders had sought refuge in a local ranchería. The tip-off came from signal fires that this ranchería's inhabitants had lit to notify kinspeople after running off several army mules, a precious source of meat in a ravening season made hungrier still by Crook's dogged efforts to destroy Native caches of mescal, prickly pear, and other foods. After Randall's men began moving toward these smoke signals, an Indian scout, the general later recounted, "while prowling around and watching, caught a squaw." The scout then "brought her into camp, and by intimidation made her tell where her people were." American soldiers, who had repeatedly relied on this tactic of compelling captives to disclose their kinfolk's whereabouts, subsequently "took her along as a guide."[33]

Under cover of darkness, Randall's troops, their feet wrapped "with gunny sacks, so as to make as little noise as possible," tiptoed toward the ranchería. Having climbed a steep, rock-strewn incline, they followed the promontory's sole "mode of ingress" to ascend the "palisades" above. Just before dawn, Crook remembered, his forces "crawled up close to the Indians" and "fired a volley into their camp," then "charged with a yell."[34]

The villagers, recognizing that they were under attack from positions they knew to be "almost impregnable," swiftly "lost all presence of mind." In their panic to dodge the attackers, Crook later recalled in his autobiography, "some" of the defenders "jumped off the precipice and were mashed into a shapeless mass. All of the men were killed," the general purported, and "most of the women and children were taken prisoners." Newspapers claimed that at least twenty-eight Indians lost their lives at Turret Mountain.

US forces also captured at least seventeen additional women. Neither US soldiers nor Indian scouts suffered even a single fatality.[35]

By early April, virtually all Dilzhę́'és and Yavapais came to realize that surrender offered their best chance of survival. Before long, dozens of family groups and bands trudged toward US Army posts and pledged to comply with the draconian terms Crook had laid out in General Orders No. 10. When Eschetlepan led some three hundred Dilzhę́'és to surrender at Camp Verde in early April, Bourke later wrote, the leader explained to Crook that his people "had never been afraid of the Americans alone, but now that their own people were fighting against them"—a reference to Crook's White Mountain Apache scouts, as well as to the small but growing number of Yavapai and Dilzhę́'é captives whom army officers cajoled and coerced into scouting—"they did not know what to do; they could not go to sleep at night, because they feared to be surrounded before daybreak; they could not hunt—the noise of the guns," Eschetlepan noted, "would attract the troops; they could not cook mescal or anything else, because the flame and smoke would draw down the soldiers; they could not live in the valleys—there were too many soldiers." Dilzhę́'és and Yavapais "had retreated to the mountain tops, thinking to hide in the snow until the soldiers went home, but the scouts found them and the soldiers followed them."[36]

As Eschetlepan made clear, the US Army had made life as Dilzhę́'és and Yavapais had known it since time immemorial an impossibility.

All the Food They Wanted

The Grand Offensive made Crook an instant hero and earned him promotion to brigadier general. Arizonans, who had been bullish on Crook since he arrived in the territory two years earlier, showered him with praise. The *Miner* lionized him as "the Napoleon of successful Indian fighters and frontier strategists. He has made bad Indians fear him; has won the love of all good ones, and will, with proper aid and backing from [the] Government, soon put a stop to murder and robbery in this Territory." Crook's victory combined with the April 11, 1873, killing of two US peace commissioners by Modoc fighters near the California-Oregon border to push the Grant administration, which had been trying for years to convince American settlers of the merits of its so-called peace policy, into adopting a more hawkish stance toward Native peoples throughout the West. Soldiers increasingly pursued American progress through campaigns modeled after Crook's success at perfecting packtrains, enlisting Native auxiliaries, and waging hard war to terrorize and starve Indigenous Nations into laying down their arms.[37]

Americans hailed Crook's Grand Offensive for securing the defeat of Yavapais and Dilzhę́'és, yet the Americans' hold over the ensuing peace soon faltered. John Gast had pictured Indians in full retreat, but the West's Native peoples had no intention of disappearing or forsaking the homelands that had sustained them body and soul.

Hoomothya (also known as Mike Burns), a young Yavapai captive who scouted for Crook's forces, recalled that when Dilzhę́'és and Yavapais came in to Camp Verde to surrender, Crook had pledged to supply them with "all the food they wanted," as well as "blankets, calicos, some corn, and wheat and barley seeds to plant along the bottomlands" of the Rio Verde Reserve, which soon became home to more than a thousand Yavapais and Dilzhę́'és. The US government, though, ensured that violence would continue by failing to honor Crook's pledges. Insufficient and unfamiliar rations, the quality of which suffered due to collusion between corrupt Indian Office bureaucrats and grasping Arizona contractors, fueled roiling discontent. Oliver Chapman, the reservation's chief clerk, doled out just one "cupful of shelled corn" per family per day—"scanty food to live on," as Dilzhę́'és and Yavapais persistently complained. Military officers had Chapman dismissed, but his friends at the Bureau of Indian Affairs struck back by securing his appointment as the reservation's agent, the head civilian post on the Verde. "A few days after he took charge," William Corbusier, an army physician who befriended many Yavapais by learning their language, lobbying US officials on their behalf, and doctoring their wounds and ills, later remembered, "the wails of the women for food were often heard on the hills near by."[38]

Government officials' unending efforts to count, control, and punish Dilzhę́'és and Yavapais stoked further unrest on the Rio Verde Reserve. Crook, intent on implementing the system of demobilization, surveillance, and incarceration that he had threatened to impose in General Orders No. 10, notified all those who surrendered that "they should remain upon the reservation, and not leave without written passes." He also instructed that "so long as any bad Indians remained out in the mountains, the reservation Indians should wear tags attached to the neck, or in some other conspicuous place, upon which tags should be inscribed their number, letter of band, and other means of identification." Reservation officials subsequently compelled Yavapai and Dilzhę́'é men, women, children, and elders to wear thin brass plates around their necks.[39]

Each tag bore a unique code. A Yavapai leader whom Americans called Marshall Pete, for example, wore one reading "Mohave C-5" (Mohave, like Apache, was a common American misnomer for Yavapais). After Marshall Pete died, this tag passed to another leader, Ohwalla Siutawa. Erasing Indigenous names and cataloging Native peoples with numbers and letters stripped reservation inmates of their humanity; such practices also made it easier for

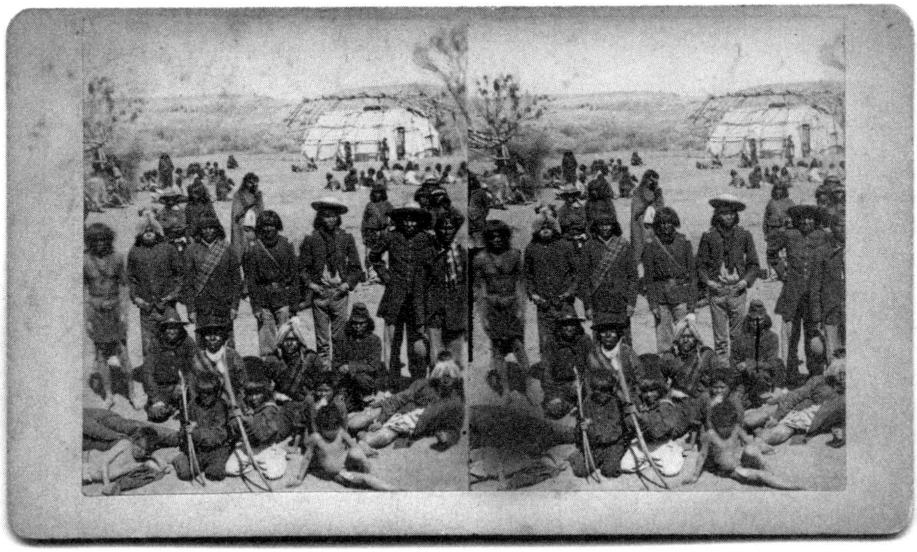

Dudley P. Flanders, a Massachusetts-born photographer headquartered in Los Angeles, probably took this stereograph in spring 1874 during a multimonth expedition that eventually yielded Flanders a catalog of more than one hundred Arizona photos. He titled it *Chiefs at Verde Reservation* and sold it in two sizes. It is likely that he first processed these negatives at Arizona's first photographic studio, run by Prescott's F. A. Cook. In early April 1874 Flanders advertised a five-day lecture series in the *Arizona Miner* that was illustrated with pictures he had taken in the local area, including one of "1500 savage Apache." Dudley Flanders, *Chiefs at Verde Reservation*, 1874. Collection of Jeremy Rowe Vintage Photograph—Vintagephoto.com.

the government to keep tabs on their whereabouts through daily roll calls. Chapman and his fellow agents almost invariably came down hard on Dilzhę́'és or Yavapais who left the reservation. They not only sortied troops to capture them but also sentenced those they brought back to the reserve in shackles to one-month terms that joined incarceration in the Verde's guardhouse with hard labor under the scorching Southwestern sun—"sometimes with a ball and chain," one historian notes, "to augment their suffering."[40]

Individuals, families, and bands responded to the injustices and deprivations of reservation life in different ways. On top of doing whatever they could to negotiate the terms of their confinement, Yavapais and Dilzhę́'és stepped up their involvement in wage work by laboring for settlers, the army, and the Indian Office. After establishing separate camps in the bottomlands bordering the Rio Verde, they also cleared dozens of acres of fertile, low-lying lands, sowed crops, and dug irrigation ditches to water newly planted plots of "corn, melons, and pumpkins" on their reservation, a ten-mile-wide strip stretching forty miles along the river.[41]

Even as some Dilzhę́'és and Yavapais sank roots into reservation soil, though, others continued to seek out alternative futures on other portions of their homelands. These refugees occasionally launched raids against Americans. Horses and mules easily ranked as the most popular booty, since they offered transportation as well as nourishment. For the most part, though, escapees did all they could to avoid settlers and soldiers.[42]

Crook and his forces responded to the flight of Yavapais and Dilzhę́'és from the Rio Verde and other reservations by launching additional strikes. In July 1873, US troops captured more than 200 "renegades" in a victory that led 200 other Dilzhę́'és to beat a hasty retreat to the Rio Verde Reserve despite the punishment they knew awaited them on their return. After another 160 men, women, and children lit out in October 1873, Indian scouts helped cavalrymen run down and kill 14 of these escapees. Only through additional onslaughts—the slaughter of 38 tribespeople at Four Peaks ('Wíi Kchása in Yavapai) in May 1874, for example, and 14 more at the headwaters of Cave Creek in September 1874—did the US Army eventually manage to extend to this reach of the Southwest the "blessings" George Crofutt hired John Gast to celebrate.[43]

Not in Condition to Resist

As the Dilzhę́'é and Yavapais stared down these challenges, infectious diseases added to their woes. Throughout summer 1873, army surgeon Corbusier later recounted, those seeking refuge on the Verde Reserve "all experienced much sickness, more especially those bands who were last to surrender." Because of the Grand Offensive, Yavapais and Dilzhę́'és alike "were exhausted from fatigue, sickness, and lack of proper food."[44]

Dysentery flourished in the reservation's crowded camps and fetid guardhouses. Underfed, malnourished, and beset by cramping, diarrhea, and dehydration, the inmates of the Rio Verde Reserve, as Corbusier recognized, "were not in condition to resist" malaria, which thrived in the wetland ecosystems where government officials forced Dilzhę́'és and Yavapais to rebuild their rancherías. Corbusier later described the Verde's mosquitos as "numerous and vicious; if one slept out a night or two without protection," the doctor asserted, "he would come down in about 11 days with violent chills and fever." "In some camps," Hoomothya remembered of his people's first horrific summer on that same reservation, "family after family fell dead . . . . Some died of chills and fevers, and some died of blood passes [i.e., dysentery] or malaria fever."[45]

Dilzhę́'és and Yavapais tried to protect themselves from dysentery and malaria by relocating their camps to higher, healthier ground. These moves came too late, though, to prevent a final cruel irony. In a development that

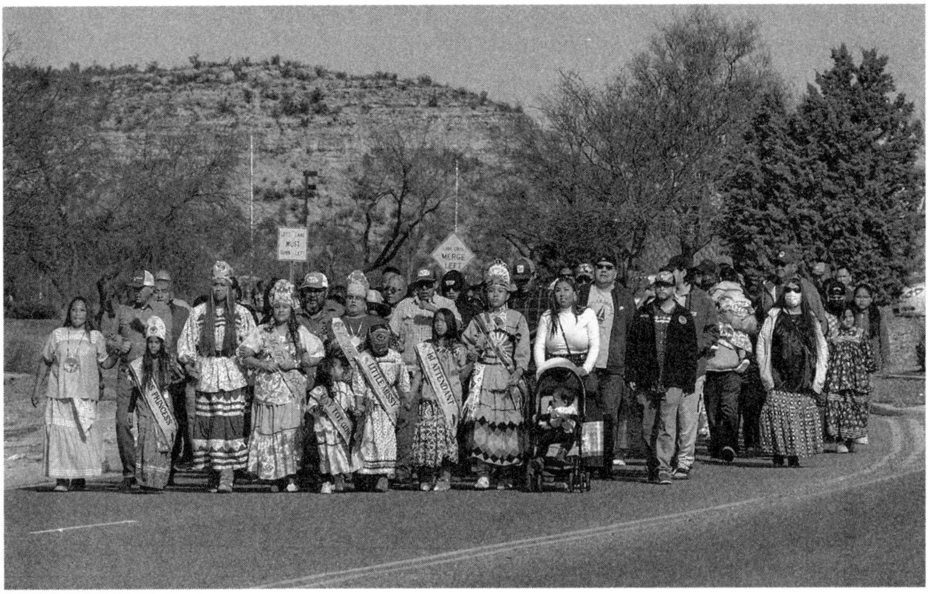

Yavapai and Apache tribal members march on Exodus Day, a yearly event to commemorate their peoples' forced relocation in 1875 from the Verde Reserve to the San Carlos Apache Reservation—and their ancestors' return to the Verde Valley in 1900. Exodus Day Commemoration, February 24, 2024. Courtesy of Daulton Venglar / Larson Newspapers.

flipped Joseph Walkup's barbed fable about the Great Horse Flu's Indigenous origins on its head, the novel influenza virus apparently lingered on in Yavapai and Dilzhę́'é homelands, then leapt from equine to human hosts. Corbusier noted that in September 1873, the inmates of the Rio Verde Reserve "were seized with the epizootic, at that time epidemic among the horses." Influenza subsequently joined malaria and other afflictions in causing "much . . . sickness among the Indians." "Deaths were so frequent," the doctor later lamented, "that the bodies were left in their oowas [the brush shelters in which many Yavapais lived], which were burned over them, or they were left to mummify in the dry air, as there were not enough well Indians to cut and carry the wood with which to burn the dead, as was their custom."[46]

In the decades that followed this cataclysm, Dilzhę́'és and Yavapais managed to survive imponderable ordeals. These included an arduous 180-mile forced march to the San Carlos Reservation in 1875 spurred by federal efforts to close the Rio Verde Reserve. Of the roughly 1,400 people forced to abandon their homes at gunpoint—and in direct contradiction to the agreement Crook had made with Eschetlepan and others when they surrendered in April 1873—around 375 people perished. After this deadly exodus, Yavapais and Dilzhę́'és endured decades of ongoing displacement before some managed to return to portions of their ancestral lands. There they rebuilt lives for themselves and their kin. Today, the descendants of the bands that Crook and his men hounded so mercilessly are spread across several tribal nations—most notably, the San Carlos Apache Tribe, the Tonto Apache Tribe, the Yavapai-Apache Nation, the Yavapai-Prescott Indian Tribe, and the Fort McDowell Yavapai Nation. In the epizootic's wake, Indigenous peoples refused to accept the destinies that Americans, Canadians, and Mexicans were attempting to foist upon them. Far from vanishing into the sunset, Piikanis, Yavapais, Dilzhę́'és, and other Indigenous peoples continued to carve out abiding places for themselves, as their descendants continue to do today.

After the Civil War, Americans cast the West as a promised land where Confederates and Yankees could bury their differences, rediscover their commonalities, and reunite to pursue shared goals premised on extinguishing or at least displacing Native nations. Tracking the Great Horse Flu's uneven expansion into Indigenous homelands and settlement hinterlands through Walkup's *Placer Herald*, Gast's *American Progress*, and Crook's Grand Offensive reveals some of the devilish mechanisms through which epidemiology, violence, politics, and culture combined in the late 1800s to transform Indian Country into US territories and states.

The work of reunifying and reconstructing the American nation, however, involved not just settlers and Native peoples but also migrants from the opposite shore of the Pacific. After Radical Republicans wrested control over Reconstruction from President Andrew Johnson in 1866, they embarked on an ambitious program to define, expand, and defend the rights and responsibilities of former slaves. Endeavoring to codify the "new birth of freedom" that Johnson's predecessor, Abraham Lincoln, had famously foretold, the Radicals often invested these rights in "persons" rather than the narrower category of "citizens."

The epizootic reached San Francisco Bay the same week that hundreds of Dilzhę́'és and Yavapais surrendered to George Crook. There it soon took an unexpected turn. After some of the city's Anglo inhabitants hired Chinese San Franciscans and harnessed them in place of flu-stricken horses, a public furor erupted. This resort to human draft power inspired local politicians to pass discriminatory ordinances designed to harry the city's Chinese population without violating the new colorblind jurisprudence Radical Reconstruction had instituted. Chinese San Franciscans responded by challenging their people's dehumanization. Whether American courts would endorse their claims to personhood, though, remained an open question.

CHAPTER 8

CELESTIAL STEEDS

Human Haulage and Anti-Chinese Racism in San Francisco

As early as November 1872, San Franciscans feared that the Great Horse Flu had reached the city by the bay. Reports of the epizootic catapulting to the Pacific Shore, however, proved premature. Not until April 1873 would the novel influenza virus begin to infiltrate the most populous metropolis west of New Orleans and north of Mexico City.

Newspapers detailed the epizootic's invasion of this city of around 190,000 humans and 9,200 equines alongside dispatches documenting Crook's assaults against Yavapai and Dilzhę́'é camps, as well as the subsequent surrender of Eschetlepan and his people. Meanwhile, reports that Kintpuash (known to Americans as Captain Jack) and other Modocs had killed two members of a US Peace Commission some 350 miles northeast of San Francisco hit newsstands on Sunday, April 13. Two days later, the *Alta California* claimed that the US Army's orders to retaliate and "exterminate the Modocs" were "universally approved by our citizens." The next day, the same paper proclaimed that "the fiercest denunciations were breathed against the devilish treachery of the Indians."[1]

The most revealing drama precipitated by the Great Horse Flu's arrival in San Francisco, though, involved Chinese American laborers, not Indigenous fighters. After the epizootic laid their horses low, Anglo businessmen enlisted Chinese Americans to replace flu-stricken equines. A three-act drama ensued, exposing submerged entanglements between human burden-bearing, racial subjugation, and struggles for dignity that bridged the Pacific World and resonated deep into the twentieth century.

Act I saw the novel influenza virus convulse the city and immobilize most of its horses. Act II began when builders hired Chinese Americans to heft supplies over their shoulders using baskets suspended from bamboo or wooden carrying poles. Several small retailers and the US Postal Service soon joined a few of San Francisco's largest and most influential firms in scaring up Chinese American men to pull wagons and drays. In the best-documented instance, onlookers harassed a team of Chinese San Franciscans as they strained to deliver dairy products and other foodstuffs to customers' homes. This dehumanizing spectacle extended from San Francisco's notoriously steep streets to its scandalously sensationalistic newspapers—and thence to readers throughout North America via wire service jibes. One local journalist, for instance, mocked Chinese Americans who strained to keep the wheels of commerce turning as "Celestial steeds." Act III began with Chinatown leaders reprimanding a labor contractor from their community for helping a local lumberman to hire laborers to draw his dray; "prominent Celestials," as the *San Francisco Bulletin* reported, sent "threatening letters" to Ah Quong, attacking him for "degrad[ing] his nationality by inducing men to hire out as beasts of burdens [*sic*]."[2]

The merchants who led San Francisco's large, diverse, and stratified Chinese community had good reason to lash out at Ah Quong, for the Great Horse Flu had exacerbated their preexisting vulnerability to local laws that used Chinese burden-bearing as a pretext for legal harassment. Anti-Chinese activists had recently established themselves as a major force in San Francisco politics by capitalizing on grassroots hatred among the city's white population. As English artist and correspondent William Simpson remarked while visiting the city on an early 1870s round-the-world journey, "John Chinaman has the whole population against him . . . . If I should have a 'Massacre of Chinese' from anywhere in that locality served up as part of my breakfast news any morning," Simpson concluded, "I shall not be in the least surprised."[3]

As the epizootic receded, surging racism and nativism led San Francisco's Board of Supervisors, the municipality's lawmaking body, to enact a new wave of ordinances targeting Chinese San Franciscans. These measures reflected competing imperatives. On the one hand, most of the city's lawmakers were intent on currying their constituents' favor and fanning the flames of anti-Chinese animosity. Yet members of the Board of Supervisors also understood that any law explicitly mentioning race would face stern challenges under the Civil Rights Acts of 1866 and 1870, as well as the Fourteenth Amendment to the US Constitution, the linchpin of Radical Reconstruction, which pronounced that "no State shall . . . deprive any person of life, liberty, or property, without due process of law; nor deny to any person within its jurisdiction the equal protection of the laws."[4]

Despite the statutory and constitutional protections Radical Republicans had recently established, the Chinatown leaders who reprimanded Ah Quong understood that the Board of Supervisors was hell-bent on restricting their people's mobility, earning power, and freedom. Racist stereotypes casting Chinese Americans as mere animals had long helped to justify their people's oppression, so these "prominent Celestials" took pains to contest the new ordinances the supervisors had enacted. Ultimately, though, the struggles unleashed by the epizootic's stint in San Francisco marked but one skirmish in a larger, longer-lived struggle. In overseas Chinese communities as well as in China itself, the plight of men who performed horses' work triggered uncomfortable questions and raging conflicts about the implications of human burden-bearing for justice, belonging, and equality.[5]

Something Remarkable

The flu struck San Francisco on Wednesday, April 16. The next day, "a good many" of the city's hack horses could be "plainly heard" coughing. Soon the epizootic tore like wildfire through San Francisco's livery stables. By Friday, April 18, "over a thousand" horses had fallen ill. The "rapidity" with which the epizootic "spread all over the city" struck the *Chronicle* as "something remarkable." A week later, "the alarming prevalence of the horse disease" led the same paper to concede that "whatever hopes were at one time entertained that the distemper would be mild in type and limited in extent" had been "utterly routed" by this "epidemic, the ravages of which are being hourly increased." Knowledgeable observers forecast a total shutdown of horse-powered transportation. With an estimated three-fourths of the city's equines infected by April 26, San Franciscans faced the unwelcome prospect of carrying on without horses and the power these creatures placed at human disposal.[6]

The ensuing disruptions resembled those the Great Horse Flu unbridled all along its route from Canada to California. People unfortunate enough to injure themselves or fall ill faced "great suffering and danger . . . as physicians, having their horses laid up, are obliged to do all their visiting on foot, and consequently cannot make the requisite haste in cases of great emergency." Steamships had little choice but to cast off from San Francisco Bay with "lessened cargoes," with "many shippers not willing to incur the extra expenses demanded for drayage." Mailmen, "newspaper carriers," and express company messengers "whose routes are in the suburbs" suffered from "the greatest hardship," lamented the *Chronicle*, as the outbreak forced them "to walk several miles over badly formed roads."[7]

Thousands of conductors, drivers, teamsters, draymen, and other workers faced joblessness due to the outbreak. The Central Pacific Railroad also discharged "a large number of men employed at their freight depots, in consequence of the small amount of freight offering." Unemployment rippled outward from the transportation sector. "The spread of the horse disease," one newspaper alleged, "caused between 5,000 and 10,000 men to be idle. Not because there is not work to do," it clarified, "but because it cannot be done without the assistance of animals."[8]

Yet as had been the case throughout its transcontinental run, the epizootic brought opportunity alongside disorder. Newspapers did brisk business running ads for flu remedies and veterinary manuals. Growers of carrots and dealers of bran—foods often prescribed for ailing equines—reaped bonanzas alongside sellers of asafetida and other common remedies, with prices tripling or quadrupling. Even a tony art dealer made hay, taking in more than $16,000 from a midweek auction, thanks to a "large attendance of wealthy merchants" whose usual business had been disrupted "by the prevalence of the epizootic."[9]

Horse workers also benefited, at least temporarily. One-way fares for hacks, which middle- and upper-class San Franciscans considered de rigueur for weddings and funerals, skyrocketed from a few dollars to "$15, and even $20" a trip. "The rates of drayage have been doubled," another article noted, "and some draymen whose horses are well enough to be used, are making very high wages"; tariffs climbed "as high as $10" for trips that ordinarily fetched 75 cents or less, allowing some to rake in $40 or even $50 a day, several times more than they typically brought home in an entire week. The promise of profit joined the possibility of paralysis to lure some laborers into forcing their animals to stay on the job even after the creatures showed clear signs of sickness. Farmers seemed similarly willing to risk their horses' well-being, with dozens "drawn hither" from San Francisco's outskirts, as one *Chronicle* writer observed, "by the large prices paid for drayage." With "nine out of ten horses that are being worked" reportedly "suffering from the prevailing disease," reformers leapt to their defense. Officers of the San

Francisco Society for the Prevention of Cruelty to Animals arrested several draymen for working flu-ravaged horses, warning reporters that "more [arrests] will be made as occasion may require."[10]

As in the East and Midwest, oxen provided a less objectionable, more reliable alternative than sick equines. Starting on Friday, April 25, Levi Strauss & Company introduced the "first ox team" to hit San Francisco's streets in many years. This famous firm, described in an 1872 directory as "importers and jobbers" of "clothing and dry goods," was just weeks away from patenting the metal-riveted denim work clothes that later made Levi's a household name. "Attached to a heavy truck," Levi Strauss's bovines made "slow work at best" of hauling clothing and dry goods to and from the company's Battery Street headquarters. Later the same day, "several yoke" of oxen began drawing large loads for other firms, including Wells, Fargo & Company, which brought in oxen from Sacramento and San Mateo in accordance with a contingency plan managers had hatched months before. San Francisco's bovine renaissance, one journalist wistfully noted with a nod back to the overland migrations that had led hundreds of thousands of humans and oxen from the Midwest to California over the preceding decades, "recall[ed] tender memories of childhood to the many Missourians in our midst."[11]

These ponderous beasts kindled frustration alongside fond memories of frontiers past. Even "one day's working on the cobble pavement" of San Francisco's thoroughfares inevitably inflicted "great pain" on unshod bovines—and could even "permanently disable them." Oxen, another journalist complained, "are not plenty, not swift of foot, and not easily managed except by one accustomed to their use." Tender-footed, plodding, and needful of drivers possessing an increasingly obsolete skill set, oxen proved a poor solution for the woes the epizootic had wrought.[12]

San Franciscans, like people in most places previously afflicted by equine influenza, also resorted to manpower to keep the wheels of economic and cultural life churning. "Handcarts," as the *Examiner* pronounced eight days after the outbreak began, were "doing a splendid business," with a "job wagon . . . seen being drawn along Kearny street last evening by two frisky young men, who had hitched themselves into the harness." Yet a crucial difference soon became evident. Elsewhere in North America, nativism, anti-Black racism, and class conflict had greeted the deployment of men and adolescent boys to draw wheelbarrows, wagons, fire engines, streetcars, and other conveyances. Only in San Francisco, though, would the recourse of human draft power become so closely associated with a single social group.[13]

In a city where anti-Chinese racism raged, the replacement of beasts of burden with Chinese American men aggravated long-running but recently resurgent struggles over belonging, discrimination, democracy, and the law.

The resulting conflicts exposed the volatile conflicts that San Francisco's diverse peoples were waging over how best to reconcile mass immigration from China with sectional reunion, emancipation, and the transformed conceptions of rights, personhood, and justice that Radical Republicans were attempting to enshrine as guiding principles for a reconstructed America.

Immigrant Burdens

Chinese San Franciscans began doing the work of flu-stricken horses a little over a week after the epizootic reached the Golden Gate. Grocers, an April 24 wire service item noted, had started to "hire Chinamen with pack baskets to transport their goods." "Unable to obtain express wagon teams" for hauling supplies to worksites because of the horse flu, "house painters, carpenters, and others" in the building trades likewise began to "engage Chinamen with poles and baskets to convey their burdens from point to point." The irony, as most Chinese San Franciscans would have understood, was that just two years earlier, the city's Board of Supervisors had outlawed baskets and poles, a burden-bearing technology that migrants from southern China had introduced to California. Such "behavior-based laws" resulted from increasingly virulent campaigns by the city's white majority to discourage additional Chinese from coming to the United States by turning the screws on San Francisco's Chinese immigrant community.[14]

That community, like most others in the city, dated back to the gold rush. On Christmas Day 1848, the Hudson's Bay Company's San Francisco agent sent a parcel of this glittering metal to Hong Kong as payment for goods imported from Hawai'i. Two weeks later, one of the British trading enclave's English-language papers reprinted a Honolulu journal's astonishing report: Six thousand miners, the Hawai'i paper claimed, had already extracted $4 million worth of gold from the American Fork River and other Sierra Nevada streams. "The discovery of gold in California to such an unlimited extent," the American missionary Samuel Wells Williams remarked from Guangzhou in late March 1849, "has thrown our community into the same ferment as elsewhere. . . . The stories we hear are wonderful; the El Dorado seems at last to have been found." Word of this treasured land raced from European and American trading outposts bordering the South China Sea to towns and villages in the adjoining countryside. After a harrowing, monthslong voyage from Shanghai, an initial party of fifty Chinese gold-seekers landed in California, which Chinese speakers called Gam Saan (金山, Gold Mountain), in fall 1849.[15]

Most of these emigrants, like those who soon followed in their footsteps, originated in Guangdong, an Oregon-sized province surrounding Hong Kong, Macao, Guangzhou, and other treaty ports. Since the 1780s, Guangdong's population had skyrocketed from 16 million to 28 million (the 1850 census enumerated just over 23 million people in the United States, which was more than forty times larger in area). Rough terrain, poor soil, and other factors made it impossible to farm all but a fraction of Guangdong's lands. Even in locales where agriculture prospered, landowners often favored high-value cash crops such as indigo, tobacco, sugarcane, citrus fruits, and even mulberry bushes for silkworm production over rice or other staples capable of sustaining the province's fast-growing populace.[16]

For centuries, people from this hilly, strife-torn domain had struck out for foreign shores in hopes of expanding their mercantile operations and seeking out better—or at least better-paying—jobs. Cantonese-speaking emigrants and sojourners from Guangdong had long predominated in many of Southeast Asia's overseas Chinese communities. Starting in the mid-1800s, though, a succession of droughts, floods, famines, political upheavals, and conflicts combined to drive hundreds of thousands more to embark for foreign shores. An 1893 gazetteer recalled the cumulative toll that the First Opium War (1839–42), the Taiping Revolution (1850–64), the Punti-Hakka Clan Wars (1855–67), and other wars had exacted on Sunning (Xinning, later known as Taishan), which sent more migrants to Gam Saan than anyplace else in China and is even today nicknamed "First Home of the Overseas Chinese": "The fields in the four directions were choked with weeds. Small families found it difficult to make a living and often drowned their girl babies because of the impossibility of looking after them."[17]

In a diaspora that fanned out to destinations ranging from Singapore to Sarawak and Melbourne to Manila, San Francisco ranked as an especially desirable port of call. After just a few hundred Chinese disembarked in San Francisco in 1849, more than 2,700 reached the city in 1851, and 20,000 in 1852. Many Guangdongese were inspired to leave for barbarian lands across the Pacific because they wanted to replicate the successes of their countrymen, thousands of whom returned to China bearing undeniable evidence of California's golden promise. "Once the handful of pioneers somehow made an amount of money that they considered to be a fortune at gold mountain in California," Pyan Ling, one of the first Chinese American women social scientists in the United States, explained, "their relatives, friends, and acquaintances then clamored to follow in the footsteps of the lucky pioneers . . . . The Chinese overseas, therefore, tended to bring in his relatives and friends from his village in China to his new home overseas."

Taishan and many of the other villages participating in chain migrations to California were located in a single district, Sze Yup (四邑, Four Counties), west of Guangzhou in the Pearl River delta; nearly all the rest clustered in adjoining Sam Yup (三邑, Three Counties).[18]

Guangdongese migration to Gam Saan slowed precipitously in 1853, rebounded somewhat in 1854, then dipped again until the late 1860s. Migration to California flagged because of anti-Chinese violence in the gold regions, discriminatory state statutes that levied exorbitant taxes on Chinese American miners, and the exhaustion of California's richest, most accessible placer deposits. In 1855, 1864, 1866, and 1867, more Chinese left Gam Saan than arrived there. But then the Central Pacific Railroad's 1868 decision to hire thousands of Chinese laborers fueled a three-year upswing that swelled San Francisco's Chinese-born population and sparked escalating anti-Chinese sentiment. By the time the Great Horse Flu struck San Francisco in spring 1873, Guangdongese immigration during the preceding twelve months approached or possibly even exceeded the record levels of 1852.[19]

Disembarking on San Francisco's piers, newcomers from China hefted their baggage onto waiting wagons, then rode atop or ran alongside these horse-powered vehicles for the two-mile journey to Chinatown. Even though many migrants spent just a night or two in San Francisco before decamping for railroad construction camps, placer mines, or other worksites and business opportunities, Gam Saan nonetheless remained the Western Hemisphere's most populous and powerful overseas Chinese community.[20]

Estimates of the city's Chinese-born population in the early 1870s varied wildly, from ten thousand to forty thousand or more. According to the 1870 census, Chinese San Franciscans accounted for at least 8 percent of the city's overall population. The acceleration of immigration starting in 1872 pushed that figure over 10 percent by the time the epizootic invaded. In San Francisco as in the rest of the United States, Chinese American demography skewed overwhelmingly young and male. Men outnumbered women by thirteen to one, and more than 83 percent of Chinese San Franciscans were in their teens, twenties, or thirties.[21]

Despite demographic commonalities and shared origins in the Pearl River Delta, Chinese San Francisco was neither homogeneous nor harmonious. Migrants pursued a range of occupations and met with varying degrees of success. By 1870, several of San Francisco's Chinese American merchants—members of one of the lowest-ranking social strata in Guangdong's Confucian social order—had accumulated property exceeding $10,000 in value. Most migrants, though, barely scraped by. The average Chinese migrant to San Francisco was a common laborer whose desperation meant that he

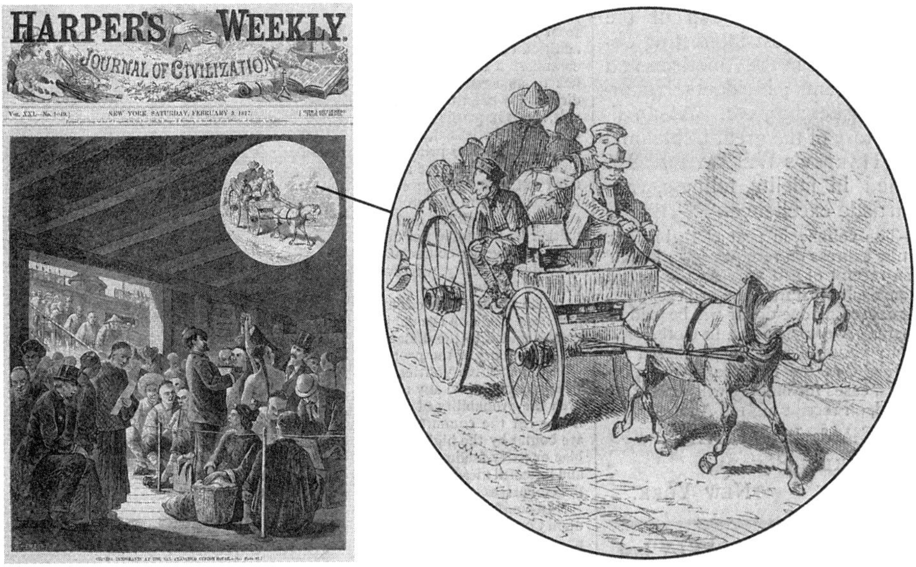

The inset from this 1877 *Harper's Weekly* cover shows newly arrived Chinese immigrants venturing by wagon from San Francisco's piers to Chinatown. Paul Frenzeny, "Chinese Immigrants at the San Francisco Custom-House," *Harper's Weekly*, February 3, 1877. Courtesy of University of Colorado Libraries.

"had no likes or dislikes in a job; he took whatever job [was] available to him without considering the working conditions or even the wage scales." Chinese sources documenting the lives of those who came from Guangdong to California "do not indicate that they were homeless drones or criminals or slaves. They were mostly poor, ignorant, and uneducated, but they were free."[22]

Disparities in wealth, status, ethnicity, region of origin, language, religion, and other factors threatened to divide Guangdongese migrants, but dense organizational networks nurtured community among Chinese San Franciscans. As the pioneering early twentieth-century sociologist Mary Coolidge observed in *Chinese Immigration* (1909), "Every Chinaman is enmeshed in a thousand other relations with his fellows." Most such "relations" emanated from what historian Yong Chen calls "the most significant Chinese American social institution," *huiguan* (會館, literally translated as "guildhall").[23]

Known to Anglo San Franciscans of the early 1870s as "companies," huiguan are usually referred to by scholars today as "home district" or "native-place" associations. San Francisco's six huiguan represented migrants from different parts of Guangdong. Organized and led by merchants, supported by membership dues, and patronized by virtually all Chinese San Franciscans, these voluntary associations offered an array of benefits and services. The Sze Yup Company, for instance, aided the sick, insured proper burial for members who perished in Gam Saan (and, in many instances, the subsequent repatriation of their bones to home villages in Guangdong), and met newly arrived emigrants from the Four Counties at the Pacific Mail Steamship Company docks with hired drays to haul their belongings to the huiguan's ornate Stockton Street lodge.[24]

Each huiguan, as Augustus Loomis noted in 1868, also served its members by "help[ing] them to settle disputes whether with their own brethren, with different clans, or with people of other nations," while also providing counsel "to manage for them when they f[e]ll into the hands of officers of the law" or became embroiled in civil suits. In 1862, huiguan leaders created "a general body of government" or "Congress" known as the Zhonghua Huiguan (中華會館), which non-Chinese often called the Chinese Six Companies. Among other functions, the Six Companies sought to resolve conflicts between home district associations while safeguarding and advancing the Chinese American community's interests before San Francisco's press, the public, and government officials and legal tribunals in Qing China, South China's trading enclaves, and the United States.[25]

Unbeknownst to Chinese San Franciscans or their neighbors, the epizootic's intensification soon spurred "prominent Celestials"—a label that almost certainly referred to huiguan leaders—into damage-control mode after some of their countrymen began bearing and drawing burdens that ailing horses could no longer pull.

Merely a Matter of Persecution

The men hired to heft lumber, provisions, and other materials in late April 1873 probably ranked among Chinatown's large and growing contingent of common laborers. Such workers presumably arrived in San Francisco already versed in bearing loads in baskets that hung from carrying poles fashioned from wood or bamboo.

In the early 1830s, American missionary Reverend David Abeel wrote from Guangzhou, Guangdong's capital, that it was "necessary" for visitors to that city's streets "to catch the warnings, and watch the motions of the porters, who carry all moveable bodies upon their shoulders, and who constitute no inconsiderable portion of the moving multitude. Their burden is suspended to the ends of centre of bamboos," Abeel noted, "and transferred, however balky and ponderous, to any distance and with much dispatch." Benjamin E. Lloyd's *Lights and Shades in San Francisco* (1876) cast carrying poles as wonders rather than hazards. "Chinese peddlers," he observed, "with their baskets or panniers suspended from either end of a bamboo pole, throng" San Francisco's fish and vegetable markets. "How skillfully they arrange their stock in the capacious baskets!" Lloyd marveled. "There are trays, boxes, and bags, apparently thrown in without reference to classification, but placed with wonderful compactness . . . and everything arranged in order." Chinese San Franciscans regularly used carrying poles to transport loads weighing 150 pounds or more at what Lloyd described as "a rapid, swinging gait, puffing and panting, but never slacking their pace."[26]

Years before the epizootic struck, San Francisco's Board of Supervisors had seized upon these contraptions in an early effort to harass Chinese San Franciscans without violating state laws, federal statutes, or the Fourteenth Amendment. In late 1870, municipal lawmakers enacted a so-called Basket Ordinance. Their intent was clear to all: to discourage potential migrants from Guangdong and neighboring provinces from migrating to Gam Saan. "As this is the only manner in which Chinamen convey goods from point to point," the Basket Ordinance was, as the *Alta California* griped, "merely a matter of persecution." This ordinance comprised just one part of a broader campaign by municipal and state lawmakers to badger Chinese Americans and discourage their countrymen from setting out for California. Anti-Chinese fervor reached fever pitch in San Francisco in the late 1860s and early 1870s, triggered by the return to the city of thousands of Chinese Americans, many of whom had been laid off following the completion of the Central Pacific Railroad. The Board of Supervisors capitalized on swelling racism by lobbing a barrage of discriminatory ordinances at Chinatown and its inhabitants. Such measures, though, had to remain racially neutral on their face; otherwise courts could strike them down as unlawful or unconstitutional.[27]

Heeding their constituents' pleas to discourage further migration to Gam Saan while taking care not to run afoul of the colorblind jurisprudence Radical Republicans were busily writing into American law, San Francisco's all-white lawmakers weaponized subtler markers of difference. The Basket Ordinance made it a misdemeanor "for any person to carry baskets suspended on polls [*sic*] across their shoulders and walk on the sidewalk." The supervisors' universal language cloaked the measure's specificity: Although the ban applied to "any person," only Chinese San Franciscans used carrying poles.[28]

Police swiftly arrested those who violated this new prohibition. All those hauled into court for bearing baskets on San Francisco's sidewalks were men

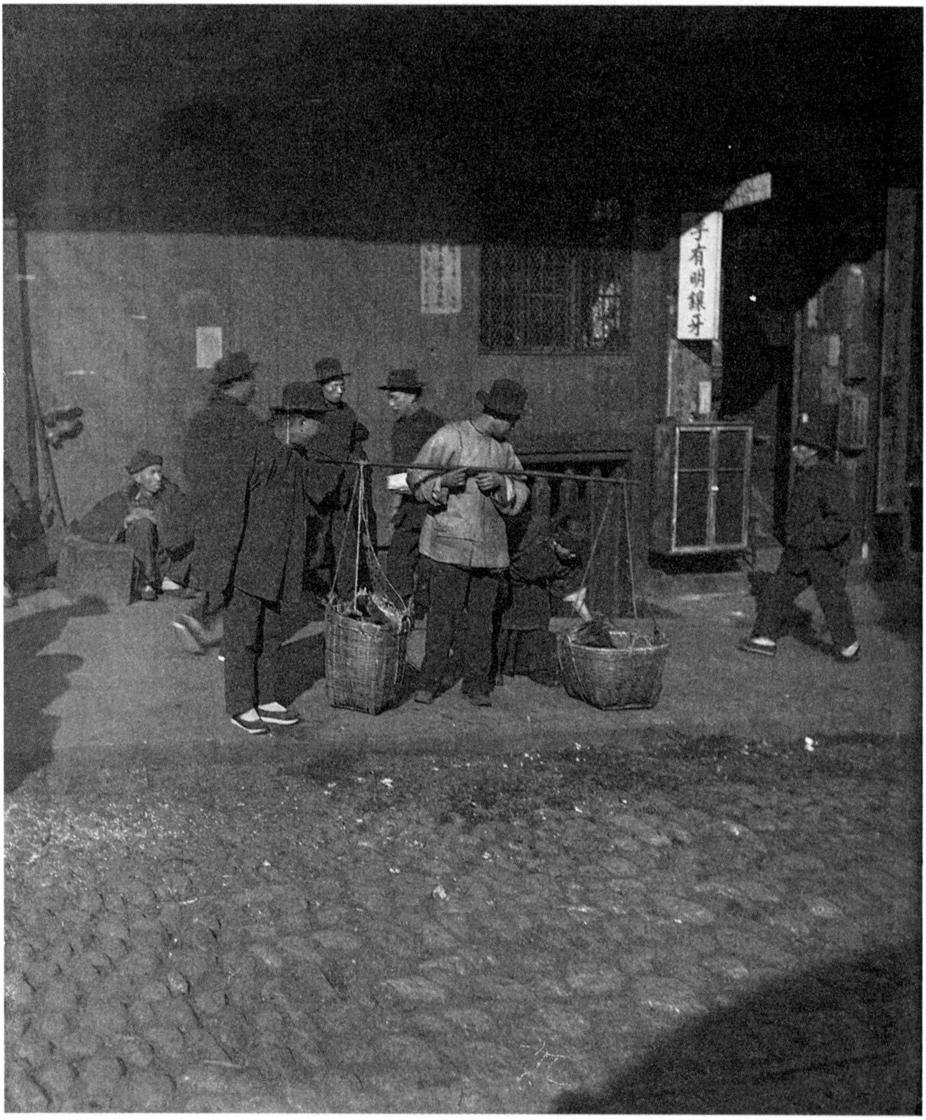

Arnold Genthe captured hundreds of photographs of Chinatown between his 1895 arrival to San Francisco as a tutor to an aristocratic German family and his 1911 departure for New York. This image shows that carrying poles remained in use decades after the Board of Supervisors attempted to outlaw their use on the city's sidewalks. Despite the title, the peddler's baskets are filled with chickens, not vegetables. Arnold Genthe, *The Vegetable Peddler, Chinatown, San Francisco*, 1896–1906. Genthe Photograph Collection, Library of Congress Prints and Photographs Division, Washington, DC.

of Chinese descent. A few pled guilty and received fines of five dollars each. Several others, though, "forfeited their bail" and "propose[d] to test the legality of the ordinance."[29]

In the ensuing legal challenges, a man identified only as Ah Wong (also known as Ah Wang) served as lead plaintiff. None of the available sources explain how Ah Wong, who probably worked as a peddler or common laborer, could afford counsel. Presumably the Six Companies, the huiguan representing migrants from Ah Wong's home district, or possibly both stepped in to fund his defense and appeal. Chinatown leaders certainly would have recognized the Basket Ordinance as a frontal assault on their community. At the very least, the regulation made it harder for Chinese San Franciscans to move possessions and goods along the city's pedestrian thoroughfares. Perhaps even more significant, though, the measure threatened to expose the Chinese American community's susceptibility to anti-Chinese measures that made no outward mention of race or color. Keen to these risks, Chinatown power brokers, intent, as the *Alta California* noted, on "using all the means of the law to have the matter fully tested," may well have resolved to retain an attorney for Ah Wong.[30]

On arraignment before Judge Alonzo Sawyer's police court, Ah Wong "answered through Nathan Porter." Porter, like the other legal aces whom huiguan leaders hired to protect their countrymen's civil rights, boasted impeccable credentials. A former Rhode Island legislator and San Francisco district attorney from 1861 to 1868, Porter assailed the Basket Ordinance for exceeding the supervisors' authority, accused lawmakers of failing to "state facts sufficient to constitute cause of action," and complained that the measure specified no penalty for its violation.[31]

After Judge Sawyer, evidently swayed by Porter's multipronged defense, ruled in Ah Wong's favor, the city appealed. Porter broadened his attack on the Basket Ordinance before Judge Elisa McKinstry of the Twelfth Judicial District. In addition to casting the law as reaching "beyond the power of the supervisors," Porter also assailed it as "racially discriminatory." Chinese American plaintiffs won a surprising number of victories in huiguan-funded legal campaigns, but efforts to strike down the Basket Ordinance ultimately failed. In *People v. Ex parte Ashbury*, McKinstry brushed off Porter's bid to question the law's constitutionality. In upholding the ordinance, McKinstry declared it a legitimate expression of the supervisors' statutory responsibility to protect public thoroughfares from obstructions and other nuisances.[32]

Two years after McKinstry sent Ah Wong back to jail, the Great Horse Flu threatened San Francisco's building tradesmen with shutdowns just as the spring construction season began to bustle. An unknown number of

Chinese San Franciscans stepped in to save the day by freighting goods and supplies by basket and pole. Some of these laborers probably exploited a glaring loophole lawmakers had left when framing the Basket Ordinance: Carrying baskets on sidewalks risked arrest, but the supervisors neglected to extend the ban to city streets. Policemen, though, also seemed to have refrained from enforcing the measure after the epizootic struck, perhaps because they understood that barring baskets from San Francisco's sidewalks would inflict layoffs and lost profits on the white skilled tradesmen and small proprietors who dominated the city's construction industry.[33]

Meanwhile, many Anglo-owned firms were already replacing flu-stricken horses with Chinese American pullers. On Thursday, April 24, several dozen laborers hired in Chinatown began straining to draw "some of the wagons used in the transportation of the mails between the Postoffice [*sic*] and the ocean steamers" moored in San Francisco Bay. A wire service report reprinted in British Columbia's *Daily Colonist* quipped that even the most ardent defenders of San Francisco's embattled Chinese American population "entered no objection to this proceeding, and as there are no cases of epizootic among the Chinamen it will probably prove successful as a temporary expedient."[34]

A Novel Team

Elsewhere in the United States, boys and men had responded to the Great Horse Flu by drawing carts, wagons, sleighs, fire engines, streetcars, and other conveyances. Onlookers and the press greeted these displays of human draft power with combinations of gratitude, dismay, and delight. In San Francisco, too, the sight of people doing horses' work prompted surprise and mirth. Yet on the Pacific Coast, the carnivalesque spectacle of species hierarchies turned upside down swiftly assumed xenophobic overtones.

The city's newspapers largely ignored the many instances in which non-Chinese workers stepped in for flu-stricken horses. Instead, the press fixated on cases in which Anglo business owners engaged Chinese American laborers to pull wagons, drays, and other wheeled vehicles. The best documented example involved N. B. Terwilliger & Co., which sold butter, cheese, eggs, honey, poultry, "and other products" from a double storefront just a few blocks northeast of Chinatown. According to the *Chronicle*, orders at Terwilliger & Co. piled up "thick and fast" after the Great Horse Flu brought San Francisco to its knees. Proprietor Napoleon Bonaparte Terwilliger complained to the *Examiner* that he was "greatly inconvenienced by the sickness of his horses" because he was now "unable to deliver goods in time for his many customers." When patrons groused "that their butter had given out, or the cheese was all used up, and they wanted more immediately," Terwilliger sent out "boys running with packages." Yet these boys—newspapers did not identify them by race or ethnicity—"could not carry enough at a time, and were all day making the rounds."[35]

On Saturday, April 26, Terwilliger, "distracted with the contemplation of the distress which was being felt by his many customers" when "the delivery of their regular supply" failed to show up at their doors, marched to Chinatown, "went at once to the head of one of the Chinese Companies," the *Examiner* recounted, "and explained to him the predicament in which he found himself." Terwilliger indicated his desire "to engage ten strong, able-bodied coolies." Soon the "head" (it is unclear if the "Company" this man oversaw was a huiguan or a mercantile firm) "led out" several of his countrymen so Terwilliger could "select the ones which he thought would answer his purpose." The retailer picked out ten Chinese Americans, each of whom impressed the imperious Terwilliger as "sound of wind and limb, and possessed of much bottom." These were highly desired traits in thoroughbreds and draft horses—and, prior to the Civil War, in African Americans being sold at auction. The *Alta California* similarly hailed a quality that enslavers had prized in human chattel when it described the men chosen by Terwilliger as "likely."[36]

Next, the members of this ten-man team "were driven down to the stables" behind Terwilliger & Co. and "without much more ado hitched into the delivery wagon." Terwilliger's "steeds," the *Examiner* marveled, "attracted more attention than any establishment which ever traversed our thoroughfares." The *Alta California* claimed that so many bystanders gathered to gawk at the man-powered wagon that policemen had to close the street "for a few minutes at the Grand Hotel and in front of Washington Market at the start." Spectators barred the wagon's progress until a cop "cleared the way . . . from the throng crowding around to gaze on the novel team." Although the *Examiner* alleged that the Chinese American laborers' "docility and good temper was generally admired," the *Chronicle*'s coverage revealed the nativist dimensions of the furor that confronted these men at every turn. As the ten-man team trundled Terwilliger & Co.'s "large wagon, filled with boxes" through the streets, "crowds of boys" began "following this remarkable turnout, hooting at the Celestials, and the spectacle," the *Chronicle* tutted, "produced great merriment wherever it went."[37]

Newspapers, as these quotations reveal, vied to contrive the most outrageous account of this wagon's voyage. Journalists and editors competed to entice readers fired up by the anti-Chinese crusade that had gripped the city since the late 1860s by waxing eloquent about the dehumanizing metamorphosis of Chinese San Franciscans into mere draft animals. The *Alta*

California titled its article about these unnamed wagon-pullers "Celestials in Harness," while their rivals at the *Examiner* began their story on this affair by riffing on the same trope:

A NOVEL TEAM
Enterprise of a Business Firm—One of
the Effects of the Epizooty—Celestial Steeds

The body of these articles proceeded to develop this animalizing theme. Terwilliger's Chinese American pullers, the *Examiner* wryly proclaimed, initially seemed "a little skittish in the harness, being inclined to kick and pull unevenly; but after a time they settled down to their work, and a better driving team is not now to be found anywhere." The laborers, the same article continued, had been "thoroughly broken to harness by the time they had drawn the wagon half a mile." Eventually the team managed to maintain a six-minute "gait," the *Examiner* declared, then added that "it is thought that their trainer will be able to work them down into the 'forties'"—a standard winning time at Bay Area trotting tracks of the era, at least before the Great Horse Flu postponed many races—"before the end of the season."[38]

White San Franciscans had long likened their Chinese counterparts to insects (ants, bees, locusts, and so forth), vermin (especially rats), or small livestock (particularly sheep and swine). Such stereotypes denigrated the migrants' habits and culture, obscured their individuality, and undermined their claims to manhood, belonging, and citizenship. Animals loomed in anti-Chinese ideology not just as abstract metaphors but also as embodied markers of exoticism and inferiority. Non-Chinese onlookers repeatedly impugned Chinese Americans by accusing them of feasting on "mice and rats, animals considered filthy and disease-carrying," as well as dogs and cats, "animals that are domesticated but not raised for food" in Western societies. Casting Guangdongese migrants as eaters of pets and pests reinforced the "menacing, swarming, pestilential animal images" that scholar Claire Jean Kim argues "became stitched indelibly into the body of the Chinese."[39]

The cover of an 1874 issue of *Thistleton's Jolly Giant (The Critic)*, a satirical magazine that prided itself as San Francisco's most virulently anti-Chinese publication, vividly illustrates how white San Franciscans amplified cultural differences into species distinctions. An accompanying note explained that the artist, Prussian immigrant George F. Keller, "is a believer in Darwinism; he has made a careful study of this subject and in proof of the theory of which Darwin in the originator." Keller's cartoon "show[ed] conclusively that John Chinaman has had his origin in a Monkey; from thence to a Chinaman, and eventually into a pig." Another *Thistleton's* article from 1874 spat of the Chinese, "We know that one out of every ten white men in this city is unemployed at the present time, in consequence of these filthy animals working at starvation prices." Bestial tropes, in short, served to underscore the supposed impossibility of assimilating migrants from China into the US polity and the perceived necessity of stopping additional Guangdongese from making new homes for themselves in Gam Saan.[40]

Like these items from *Thistleton's*, racist representations of Terwilliger's wagon-pullers trapped the West Coast's Guangdongese migrants in what Kim calls "a borderlands between human and animal, a fraught zone of ambiguity, menace, and transgression." White Californians "never" depicted Chinese Americans "as fully human to begin with, so they did not have this status to lose. They were always already animal or animal-like." The *Alta* jested that at the end of six hours of lugging the merchant's heavy wagon through San Francisco, "the "Celestials were then taken out" of their harnesses, "rubbed down, and blanketed"—the customary end-of-day routine for workhorses—"to be used again on Monday if the horse disease does not abate . . . . Terwilliger & Co.," it concluded, "were greatly praised by the bystanders for their enterprise and ingenuity in utilizing the Celestial element."[41]

The *Examiner* went even further in animalizing Chinese American wagon-pullers. Terwilliger & Co., it declared, "deserve great credit for the enterprise which they have shown in the present emergency. Well may we ask," it concluded, "have they not found a solution for the Chinese problem?" If this loaded question offers any indication, the Great Horse Flu's surprising consequences inspired at least some Anglos to extol the virtues of reducing Chinese San Franciscans to a horselike destiny of toil and degradation.[42]

The day after Terwilliger enlisted a Chinatown labor contractor to hire pullers to draw his delivery wagon, several other white-owned businesses followed suit. On Sunday, April 27, the Central Pacific, which had imported fifteen thousand to twenty thousand Guangdongese during the late 1860s to extend its tracks through the Sierra Nevadas and the Great Basin, responded to epizootic-related downturns in freight traffic by laying off many drivers at its San Francisco depot, then "hitched chinamen [*sic*] to their idle drays." Terwilliger's other imitators also included Henry Stivers, who lived and worked just around the corner from Chinatown. With the help of a Chinese American labor contractor known as Ah Quong, the lumbermen followed the lead of his neighbor Napoleon Bonaparte Terwilliger by hiring twelve men to pull his dray.[43]

Wire service reports titillated readers throughout the West with accounts of this broadening resort to Chinese American muscle. "Some queer sights are to be seen on the streets of San Francisco during the prevalence of the

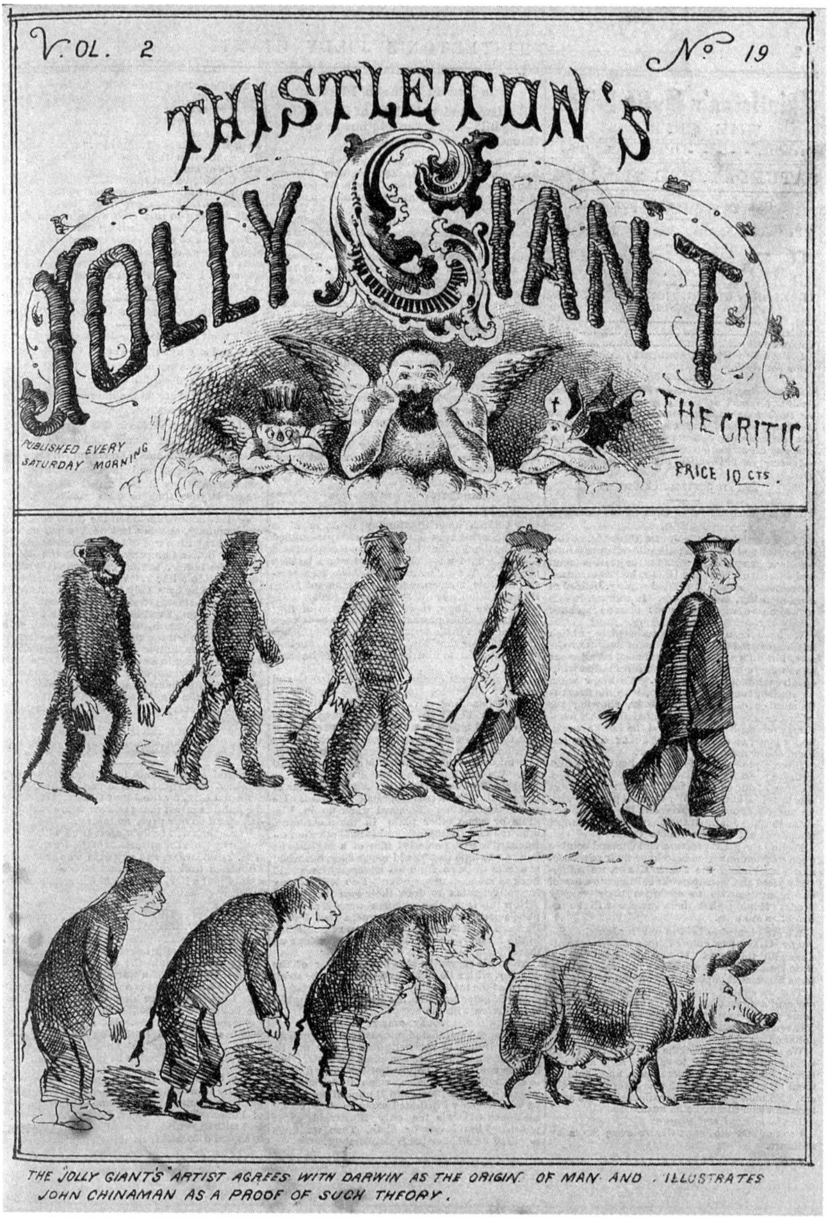

This 1874 cover from *Thistleton's Jolly Giant (The Critic)* cast Chinese San Franciscans as occupying a middle stage in an evolutionary sequence leading from monkeys to pigs. The illustration's caption explained that the magazine's "artist agrees with Darwin as the origin of man and illustrates John Chinaman as a proof of such theory." By likening Guangdongese migrants to animals, San Francisco's virulent anti-Chinese movement took aim at Chinese San Franciscans' claims to belonging and personhood. George Frederick Keller, *Thistleton's Jolly Giant (The Critic)*, February 21, 1874, cover. Courtesy of the San Francisco History Center, San Francisco Public Library.

epizootic," quipped the *Idaho World*. "A butcher named Terwilliger," the *World* continued (gamely if misleadingly), "recently hired ten Chinamen, harnessed them up to his wagon, and the Mongolian team did a good day's work." The *Dakota Republican*, meanwhile, embellished dispatches from San Francisco with common tropes deriding Chinese migrants as anonymous, interchangeable, and irredeemably foreign: "JOHN CHINAMAN lessens the horrors of the epizootic in San Francisco," it jibed, "by assuming the role of 'Melican man hose,'" and other papers got in the act by publishing their own pidginized renditions of "American man horse."[44]

Degraded His Nationality

While the viewpoints of Anglo journalists, editors, lawmakers, attorneys, judges, and anti-Chinese activists are comparatively easy to recover, existing sources offer no insights into the feelings of those who strained at the epizootic's height to haul Terwilliger's wagon, Stivers's dray, and several other vehicles. Nor do they shed light on how other Chinese San Franciscans responded to their compatriots' service as replacements for flu-sickened horses. A brief but suggestive item published nearly three months later in the *Evening Bulletin*, though, reveals that powerful Chinese San Franciscans objected to the reduction of their fellow Guangdongese to mere draft animals.

"Prominent Celestials," this July 31 article contended, had recently sent "threatening letters" to "Ah Quong, the business manager of a Chinese house on Sacramento street, who furnished a dozen Chinamen to Henry Stivers to draw a dray during the prevalence of the epizooty." The *Bulletin* went on to summarize these Chinatown leaders' beef with Ah Quong. "The cute fellow," the *Evening Bulletin* paraphrased the charge these "Prominent Celestials" had leveled against their countryman, "*degraded his nationality by inducing men to hire out as beasts of burdens* [*sic*]."[45]

This terse mention raises questions that the available evidence cannot resolve: Who was Ah Quong, and what did he think of the "threatening letters" he received? Did the labor contractors who supplied Chinese American laborers to Terwilliger, the Central Pacific, and other employers face similar recriminations? Although the *Bulletin* article offers no clear answers to these queries, it does open our eyes to the intriguing possibility that huiguan heads may well have sought to make an example of Ah Quong to advance their long-running campaign to mitigate the reputational, political, and legal hazards presented by Anglo San Franciscans' ongoing efforts to animalize their Chinese neighbors.[46]

We can better understand the Chinatown leaders' complaint by placing it in a fuller context. The controversies the Great Horse Flu provoked in San Francisco spoke to the submerged links between two broader debates about human draft power that reverberated through China and diasporic Chinese communities. One of these reached back to the legal battle over the 1870 Basket Ordinance but grew sharper in the epizootic's wake as the Board of Supervisors took up a string of purportedly colorblind but unmistakably anti-Chinese ordinances. Across the Pacific, meanwhile, a second and longer-running set of disputes was just gaining traction. After rickshaws reached Shanghai and Guangzhou from Japan in the early 1870s, then spread to the streets of numerous other major Chinese and Chinese diasporic cities, critics of colonialism and capitalism lashed out at these human-powered vehicles. Common threads of concern about the dangers of allowing men to labor like animals linked these episodes to the rebuke Chinatown leaders directed against Ah Quong.[47]

Historians have spent decades detailing how the figure of "the coolie" stoked ferocious worldwide arguments over race, labor, rights, and citizenship, yet they have almost completely ignored one of the term's original and enduring meanings in Chinese, English, and other languages. In 1834, the American missionary David Abeel observed that "one class" of porters were "called by the Chinese, 'horses without tails.'" These animalized laborers, Abeel explained, served as "the bearers of men of some distinction and wealth, who generally appear abroad in sedan chairs," so they were commonly referred to as "chair coolies." William Speer, one of California's leading defenders of Chinese immigrants, alleged in 1870 that "coolie" derived from *quli* or *kŭlì* (कुली), a Hindi term (originating in Turkic) that "signifies simply a porter or bearer of burdens"—a meaning still prevalent today.[48]

This usage persisted in nineteenth- and twentieth-century Chinese and Chinese overseas communities. With growing numbers of Chinese laborers disembarking in the Americas, South Africa, the Pacific World, and beyond, variations on *kŭlì* popped up in English, French, Spanish, and other tongues. Such loanwords, the prolific Indian intellectual Vijay Prashad points out, "entered the European lexicon in the context of imperialism to index a person of inferior status who simply labors for hire." Thereafter, "to be called a coolie" meant "to be denigrated, and to be considered at best as a laborer with no other social markers or desires."[49]

Even as the Chinese diaspora was freighting additional baggage onto this term, Chinese speakers continued to associate *kŭlì* labor with human burden-bearing, as long-running controversies over rickshaws demonstrate. Between the late 1800s and mid-1900s, the travails of the "rickshaw coolies" who labored to pull these newfangled contraptions spurred scathing condemnations, popular insurgencies, and government prohibitions.

Known in Japanese and Chinese as 人力車 (*jinricksha* in the former language and *rénlìchē* in Mandarin, terms variously translated as "man-powered carriage" or "human-powered vehicle"), rickshaws consisted of two large wheels joined by a stout axle and topped by a cab for carrying passengers or freight, with two long shafts projecting forward at shoulder height. First invented in Japan in the late 1860s by an American missionary, these novel conveyances were introduced to Shanghai and Guangzhou in 1873 and 1874. By the close of the 1880s, rickshaws and the men who pulled them clogged the streets of Hong Kong, Singapore, Beijing, and many other large Chinese cities and major Chinese diasporic destinations. In Guangzhou and other treaty ports bordering the South China Sea, these "man-powered carriages" soon eclipsed sedan chairs, presumably forcing many of the "horses without tails" mentioned by Abeel to pull rickshaws instead. By the dawn of the twentieth century, rickshaws were also displacing carts and wagons in northern China, where equine-powered vehicles had long predominated over sedan chairs and other human-powered conveyances.[50]

Laborers who had hitched their livelihoods to horse- and mule-drawn vehicles lashed out at rickshaws and the men who pulled them. Beijing's mule carters responded with particular aggression. A British consul described how a group of carters conspired to purloin several rickshaws in the 1880s, not long after these vehicles "rapidly supplanted" their equine-powered competitors from the Qing capital's streets. Dragging "the horrid foreign things, which degraded men to the level of animals," to the banks of a nearby canal, they cast them into the water. Beijing's dwindling ranks of muleteers continued to rage against the rickshaw kŭlìs who undersold them. "Why don't you drive carts?," a British official who arrived in Beijing in 1909 overheard one carter shout. "You prefer to drag them. *You would be like animals or beasts of burden although you could easily be men*." As these quotes show, the fears of emasculation and degradation that San Francisco huiguan leaders had expressed in their 1873 allegation that Ah Quong had "*degraded his nationality by inducing men to hire out as beasts of burdens*" echoed across the Pacific and far into the future.[51]

Intellectuals and revolutionaries grew even more incensed at the plight of rickshaw kŭlìs after the Qing dynasty's 1911 fall. As competition from trams, trucks, motorcycles, and automobiles mounted, rickshaws remained a potent embodiment of Chinese subordination both at home and abroad. "We talk about democracy and humanism, about everyone being treated equally and having an equal opportunity," proclaimed *New China* in 1919. But if "a rickshaw puller is a human being the same as we," this journalist implored, "how can we then sit in a rickshaw with the puller working him like an ox or a horse in the rain and the mud?!"[52]

A famous 1936 novel, *Camel Xiangzi* (later translated into English and published as *Rickshaw Boy*), offered an even more pointed exploration of dehumanization. The title character of this widely read work—Xiangzi, a puller who answered to the nickname "Camel"—railed against the daily debasement he and his fellow rickshaw pullers suffered. "Men have separated themselves from the animals," Camel groused, "but now drive their own kind back among the beasts." Straining to draw passengers and goods like the two-humped beast of his nickname, Xiangzi worried that "he was being transformed into an animal . . . . He had stopped thinking and, therefore, the human being in him was destroyed."[53]

Stripped of intellect and self-respect, kǔlìs like Camel had good reason to descend into despair. Not just in Beijing but also in Shanghai and beyond, their "visibly pathetic condition . . . epitomized both the continued role of backbreaking human labor in a mechanizing society and the poverty of the workers under exploitation by bosses, Chinese and foreign." Critiques of labor that reduced men to mere beasts, in short, cast the crises of Chinese workers and the Chinese nation as inextricably intertwined.[54]

Rickshaw kǔlìs of the early twentieth century, like Chinese San Franciscans at the Great Horse Flu's height, repeatedly joined ranks to defend their interests. Instead of battling in court against discriminatory ordinances, though, pullers waged dozens of strikes that unsettled commerce and everyday life on dozens of occasions in Chinese cities and overseas Chinese communities alike. They also played a prominent role in the Guangzhou Uprising of 1927, a Soviet-sponsored revolt in which peasants and workers temporarily wrested control over one of China's largest cities. As the *South China Morning Post* noted, "ricksha [*sic*] men" ranked "among the most bloodthirsty assailants during the Communist coup." After World War II, Chiang Kai-shek's Nationalist government ordered pedestrian rickshaws—and, with them, a species of kǔlì labor that had long galled many Chinese—to be phased out within three years. After the Chinese Revolution of 1949, Mao Zedong extended Chiang's ban.[55]

These prohibitions became law more than seven decades after huiguan leaders in San Francisco attacked Ah Quong for procuring laborers to drag Henry Stivers's lumber wagon. Vast geographic, temporal, and ideological distances separated post–Civil War San Francisco from post–World War II China, yet human burden-bearing triggered similar apprehensions in both realms. When Chinese American labor contractors and Anglo business owners collaborated to replace flu-addled horses with kǔlìs in a city where Guangdongese migrants faced mounting challenges to both their presence and their personhood, they unwittingly presaged disputes that would resonate across the Pacific for decades to come.

Barbarous Orders

The "threatening letters" that Chinatown leaders directed at Ah Quong in July 1873 marked just one front in the larger battle huiguan leaders were waging to protect themselves and their community from a legal strategy the Board of Supervisors had instigated with the 1870 Basket Ordinance. Ah Quong's critics alleged that the contractor was playing into the hands of San Francisco's ascendant anti-Chinese movement by enabling Stivers replace ill horses with able-bodied Chinese American men. A rant against "John Chinaman" in the May 3, 1873, issue of *Thistleton's Jolly Giant* concisely summed up the nativists' case: "He underlives us, he undersells us. He steals from us, and he will eventually drive us from our land and start a Celestial Kingdom here on his own account."[56]

Just a few weeks after this diatribe reached print, municipal lawmakers considered a trio of new ordinances that Robert Goodwin, the supervisor who drafted them, forthrightly described as "local legislation to discourage the immigration of Chinese, who are coming here now at the rate of two thousand a month." The first ordinance Goodwin proposed, explained the *Alta California*, sought "to prevent the shipment to China of the remains of deceased Chinamen." Many Guangdongese placed great importance on having their bones returned to their ancestral homes, a desire Goodwin sought to exploit by proposing steep fines starting at one hundred dollars for unearthing bodies from "'any cemetery or graveyard within the city and county'" without written permission from San Francisco's coroner.[57]

The next regulation the supervisors discussed, the Queue Ordinance, was equally hateful. "One of the most spiteful and vindictive of all official measures directed against the Chinese during their residence on American soil during the nineteenth century," this measure targeted the long braids Guangdongese men wore to signify their manliness and loyalty to the Qing emperor. Goodwin's measure required San Francisco's jailers to shave inmates' hair close to the scalp. Everyone understood that this provision sought to punish Chinese San Franciscans who had determined to resist the Basket Ordinance and other discriminatory ordinances. As they refused to pay court-mandated fines for violating these municipal regulations, Chinese San Franciscans filled San Francisco's jails, making it difficult or impossible for policemen or judges to continue enforcing anti-Chinese laws. The Queue Ordinance aimed to neutralize this tactic by forcing Chinese San Franciscans to make an impossible choice between keeping their queues to uphold cultural imperatives or prolonging their campaign to resist discrimination under the law.[58]

The third and final ordinance taken up by the Board of Supervisors sought to reform San Francisco's laundry licensing regulations by pegging fees for a mandatory permit to the number of horses these proprietors used to pick up and deliver linens, clothing, and other items. The supervisors set quarterly license fees at two dollars for laundries employing one horse, four dollars for laundries using two or more, and fifteen dollars for laundries that relied entirely on manpower. As Goodwin and his fellow supervisors well understood—and as the epizootic had recently highlighted—the hundreds of laundries operated by Chinese San Franciscans overwhelmingly utilized carrying poles instead of horses. This Laundry Ordinance, like the others Goodwin presented, was at once racially neutral on its face and rottenly bigoted to its core.[59]

The Board of Supervisors gave all three measures a second reading in early June 1873, tabling the burial measure but passing the Laundry and Queue Ordinances over strenuous objections from several members. A. B. Forbes, for instance, lambasted these laws as "barbarous orders . . . , which breathe a spirit only worthy of savages." For their part, Chinese American merchants and huiguan officers threatened to "ask for the abrogation of the Burlingame Treaty [the 1868 compact assuring amity and trade between the Qing emperor and the United States], the return of all Chinese to China, and the ouster of all Americans there." Mayor William Alvord refused to sign either of the regulations the supervisors had approved.[60]

A few weeks later, the supervisors abandoned the Queue Ordinance (the board enacted a similar measure three years later), but they mustered sufficient votes to pass the Laundry Ordinance over Alvord's veto. An outraged Forbes deplored the heavy fees the city would now demand from the proprietors of laundries that lacked horses as "contrary to the constitutional law of our land, illiberal and unjust both in letter and in spirit, and unworthy of a place on the records of any civilized and enlightened nation." The Six Companies went on to challenge the ordinance on behalf of San Francisco's Chinese American laundrymen, leading California's Supreme Court to strike down the law in 1874. Decrying the measure as "unequal in its operation and deal[ing] in odious and unjust discrimination," the state's highest court made it clear that its chief objection was the law's deleterious impact on the white and African American women who operated most of the city's other horseless laundries.[61]

The concerns that impelled huiguan leaders to reprimand Ah Quong foreshadowed broader disputes over human burden-bearing that would soon ripple throughout other diasporic Chinese communities as well as in

China itself. Chinatown leaders, though, undoubtedly placed the labor contractor's actions in the immediate context of the Laundry Ordinance, the Basket Ordinance, and the Board of Supervisors' larger push to clamp down on Chinese immigration by hectoring Chinese San Franciscans.

Better Angels?

"Dis-ease": The term means "to disorder, trouble, and unsettle." This is what pathogens do to the organisms they infect. It is also what contagions inflict on communities, ecosystems, societies, species, and polities, as the epizootic's Western travels demonstrate.

The tangled tales that the Great Horse Flu helped to weave as it pressed from the Missouri River to the Pacific Ocean reveal how the outbreak's westward expansion further complicated the already tricky business of Reconstruction. *American Progress* pointed toward a harmonious and united future. Blazing this forward path, though, entailed additional bloodshed, confinement, and oppression—not only for Native Americans but also for Chinese immigrants and others. In these ongoing struggles, the colorblind jurisprudence enshrined by Radical Republicans afforded a modicum of protection, as did appeals to what Lincoln memorably called "the better angels" of human righteousness, inclusive nationalism, and the rule of law. Yet as Chinese San Franciscans, Yavapais, Dilzhę́'és, and others faced down the relentless gales of the Americans' escalating onslaught, these seemed like thin reeds indeed.

CHAPTER 9

OTHER WORLDS TO CONQUER

Closing Throes and Enduring Legacies

After shaking up San Francisco, the Great Horse Flu entered what appeared to be its final phase. The epizootic, the *Minneapolis Star Tribune* remarked in early May 1873, "had completed its grand tour of observation," having "finally reached the western extreme of this continent. . . . We are anxious," the *Star Tribune* speculated, "to know where it will go now. Will it still continue its course westward and visit its ravages among" the Pacific Ocean's "sea horse" population, the Minnesota paper wondered, "or will it turn back eastward and revisit us all once more with its merciless devastation"? The epizootic, "like Alexander[,] may sigh for other world's [*sic*] to conquer, but it is to be earnestly hoped that its yearnings will not lead it to retrace its old route."[1]

As the Great Horse Flu's subsequent adventures showed, the scourge neither plunged into the ocean nor reversed course. Instead, it continued to expand after splitting into two main fronts. The first began turning northward as the outbreak crossed Central California. In May, the scourge permeated the Golden State's northern reaches while attacking such far-flung locales as Walla Walla, Washington; Emmitville, Idaho; and Oregon towns including Salem, Corvallis, and Portland. In Hillsboro, outside Portland, an account described the malady as "so mild as to not materially interfere with work." Salem recorded zero fatalities, and even though "nearly all the horses" who toiled alongside sixty men to excavate an irrigation ditch near Salem showed clear signs of flu, "still they work right along." Milder symptoms for horses and their kin translated into less severe disruptions for humankind than in San Francisco or the East.[2]

The epizootic prolonged its northward push in June, striking "about half the horses in Olympia," Washington, by the third of that month and afflicting "nearly every horse" in Lewiston, Idaho, a few weeks later. Although the malady nearly disappeared from newspaper columns in July and August, it continued churning northward. It invaded British Columbia in September, sickening horses and hindering the "movement of passengers and freight" in the Okanagan Valley and the Fraser Canyon and Caribou mining regions. By month's end, "all the horses and mules" on Vancouver Island were reportedly "laid up with it."[3]

As it had throughout its conquests, the Great Horse Flu also reportedly beset other creatures on the Pacific Coast, including cattle, turkeys, dogs, hogs, and humans. "Everybody, his friends and their horses," noted a correspondent from Witter's Springs, California, "have got the epizootic here." In Pendleton, Oregon, a newspaper alleged that "the men and the horses have the epizootics [*sic*] all together." Montana's Cedar Creek gold diggings suffered an especially nasty outbreak. Over the previous four years, more than a thousand miners had invaded this rollicking district within the homelands of the Salish, Kootenai, Kalispel, and other Indigenous Nations. By late October, though, it became nearly impossible "to get enough men to work" the area's placer deposits "owing to sickness."[4]

The Great Horse Flu's southern salient, meanwhile, squeezed through the Isthmus of Tehuantepec, Mexico's narrowest stretch, then struck Chiapas on the Pacific and Tabasco on the Gulf of Mexico in late September and early October. Mexican medical and veterinary expert Gustavo Ruiz y Sandoval confessed that the last report of the epizootic he could uncover dated to November 1873, when "it was causing havoc in Guatemala." New York City's assistant sanitary inspector Adoniram Brown Judson, though, discovered from his correspondence that Corinto, on Nicaragua's Pacific shoreline, was "the last point at which its presence is reported." If the outbreak pushed any deeper into Central America, neither Judson nor Ruiz y Sandoval managed to learn of its presence. The virus does not seem to have penetrated Costa Rica, the Isthmus of Panama (which remained under Colombian control until the 1900s), Caribbean islands beyond Cuba, or South America, nor did it cross the seas to trigger large-scale outbreaks in Europe, Asia, Africa, or Oceania.[5]

The epizootic's ostensible disappearance led Ruiz y Sandoval, writing in January 1874, to claim that the malady had gone "extinct." Yet the novel influenza virus, its variants, and their descendants lived on. Indeed, contemporary reports and recent scientific studies concur that these pathogens probably continued to circulate.[6]

Back in the United States, more pressing concerns overshadowed the Great Horse Flu and nudged it out of the headlines. Flu-like symptoms nonetheless continued to affect equines and other creatures. Many new cases were restricted either to animals who had never fully recovered, or those who somehow eluded the scourge on its first pass. In a growing number of locales, though, equines struck by the Great Horse Flu's initial wave seem to have suffered from second bouts of influenza. In January 1873, for instance, residents of Morrow County, Ohio, alleged that "the horses that got well of Epizootic are attacked with greater violence now by the same disease." A month later, a horse in Finchford, Iowa, was purportedly "sick with the epizootic the second time. It is not a relapse," the correspondent insisted, "but a bona fide second attack of the old complaint." These and similar reports from localities scattered across the United States strongly suggest that the novel influenza virus continued to spawn new variants different enough from their forebears to go undetected by host immune systems. "The fact of a horse having once had it," as the *Shippensburg (PA) News* gravely observed, "is no safeguard against its return."[7]

Widespread accounts of what the *Chicago Weekly Post* called "modified epizootic" kindled worries that the equine scourge was "bound to have another run." Wire services related a rash of fresh flu cases in New York City, Philadelphia, and other parts of the Northeast in June 1873, leading the *New Orleans Times-Picayune* to fret that "this recurrence of a disease so general and fatal among horses" would again damage "the vital interests of the entire country." Fortunately for equines and humans alike, this alarming disease cluster failed to spread beyond the Atlantic Seaboard, and most victims experienced only mild symptoms.[8]

Thereafter, anxieties that the epizootic was poised to rear its ugly head periodically flashed across newswires. Yet rather than mushrooming to epizootic proportions, such cases remained "sporadic"—that is, uncommon and scattered. An editor in Kansas probably captured the situation in most of the United States when he observed in autumn 1873, "Occasional cases of epizooty are reported in different portions of the State, but no general outbreak is feared." In most respects, the outbreak had run its course—or so it seemed.[9]

The Great Horse Flu deserves a more central role in the stories we tell about both US history and the history of disease. By contributing to a deep depression that began in fall 1873 and wreaked havoc for years to come, the epizootic helped to sidetrack Reconstruction. No less important, hindsight reveals that the epizootic constituted a crucial if underacknowledged epidemiological milestone. Scholars have long lionized the 1870s as the decade in which germ theory and the bacteriological revolution took root. Yet from the vantage point of a world continually pummeled by AIDS, COVID, avian influenza, and a host of emergent scourges, the Great Horse Flu helps us to discern a second and more troubling trajectory. Dreams of conquering disease flourished between the late nineteenth century and the late twentieth, yet with every passing decade, humanity now seems sure to suffer from an expanding assortment of maladies—especially viruses—that gain force by circulating between human and nonhuman hosts. Unraveling the unbroken threads that connect us to the epizootic offers insights into not just our collective past but also our present—and possibly even the future.

Had the Lesson Been Heeded?

At first glance, the Great Horse Flu seemed more like an anomaly than a turning point. It produced no lasting downturn in equine populations and no discernible improvement in animal welfare, nor did it do anything to hasten the replacement of horses, donkeys, and mules by steam-powered machines. In these respects—though not, as we will soon discover, in others—the epizootic changed remarkably little.

By the time the outbreak exhausted itself, influenza and its complications had killed well over one hundred thousand horses, donkeys, and mules—and quite possibly a half million or more. Yet North America's herds soon recovered and then some. Despite the huge death toll flu and its complications had levied, the US Agricultural Census documented a 45 percent increase in the nation's horse population between 1870 and 1880, outstripping the human population increase of 30 percent. Even the two census regions where horse populations grew most slowly—the North Atlantic and South Central—reported a climb of 16 and 47 percent, respectively. Canadian herds showed slower but nonetheless impressive growth: The number of horses counted by agricultural census-takers grew nearly 27 percent between 1871 and 1881. US populations of donkeys and mules experienced even greater gains, increasing 61 percent over the 1870s in the nation overall and notching substantial increases of 20 and 50 percent, respectively, in the two slowest-growing regions, the Northeast and the West. Such numbers, alas, reveal only so much. Neither Cuba nor Mexico compiled agricultural censuses in the 1870s. American and Canadian statistics, moreover, leave out the large numbers of horses, donkeys, and mules who resided in towns, cities, and ranching regions, as well as among Indigenous Nations and in the West's unmanaged herds. Despite these unknowns, it nonetheless seems abundantly clear that populations of horses, asses, and mules largely rebounded from the Great Horse Flu and then some.[10]

Herds grew, which may have been good news for North America's equines. Yet humans continued to treat these animals just as poorly as they had before the epizootic. During and after the Great Horse Flu's peak, more than a few commentators claimed to have seen the light of humanitarianism. "The value of the horse was made particularly impressive a few months since when the horses were attacked with the epizootic," proclaimed a guest at the annual meeting of the Ladies Branch of the Buffalo Society for the Prevention of Cruelty Toward Animals in March 1873. "When we awoke one morning and found that the baker did not come, the milkman failed to arrive, and the butcher could not carry his meat, it was then we realized at once the usefulness of the noble steed."[11]

Borrowing a page from Charley Bucephalus, this speaker cast the Great Horse Flu as a blessing in disguise because of the golden opportunity it presented for humans to mend their wicked ways. When the outbreak relented, though, people soon reverted to old habits of neglecting, abusing, and otherwise mistreating the equines they claimed as their own. "Folks rather thought this horse epidemic, would learn some folks something," a Pennsylvania editor bewailed with down-home folksiness in mid-January 1873. Just weeks earlier, with the epizootic raging, he and many of his neighbors had confidently predicted that this scourge would "teach them the importance—not to say humanity—of properly caring for the horse—less abuse—less over-driving and overloading in the future. Had the lesson been heeded?" the editor pointedly asked. The breathlessness with which he delivered his verdict hinted at the depths of his disappointment: "Witness the every day feats of fast driving;—note the overloaded carts, wagons and sleighs passing along—the poor brutes slipping, sliding and scratching over the icy streets—refused even the luxury (necessity) of being properly rough shod;—look at the horses on a bitter cold day," he insisted, "standing in every square, smoking with perspiration—*unblanketed* . . . . Don't ask," the downcast newsman chided, "whether anybody has learnt a lesson of humanity from the epizootic scare."[12]

Henry Bergh understood better than most just how resistant the general population remained to this "lesson." In November 1873, Bergh stepped up before a "goodly" audience in Buffalo and delivered a lecture titled "Our Speechless Slaves." Bergh intended his address, which was sponsored by the local Society for the Prevention of Cruelty to Animals and introduced by former US President Millard Fillmore, to drive home a crystal-clear thesis: "An animal was not a machine, as some contended, but has passions, feelings and emotions."[13]

Bergh recounted the extent to which Americans and their neighbors relied on equine energies, then questioned the common notion, influentially articulated by René Descartes's *Discourse on Method* (1637), that animals were mere mechanisms, devoid of souls, self-consciousness, and the capacity for reason. Bergh's slant, though, leaned more on impression than reason. Indeed, he devoted most of his talk to recounting a "remarkable dream he once had, in which he believed himself dead, and on his way to another sphere of existence stopped at what proved to be a paradise of animals." During this nocturnal excursion to a spiritual realm populated by animals who were not just sentient but also sentimental, Bergh told his fellow reformers that "an ox related to him its misfortunes on earth; also a horse, and lastly a cow." All three beasts "graphically told" Bergh about their travails; taken together, these creatures' litany of woes, the humanitarian lamented, "reflected severely on the 'superior creature,' man."[14]

Although Bergh and other anticruelty activists continued to hold up an unflattering mirror to humankind's mistreatment of horses and other favored animals, their critiques fell on deaf ears. Amid deepening economic woes—triggered, as we soon will see, in no small part by the Great Horse Flu—nearly everyone continued to believe that lavishing additional care or kindness on equines was an inconvenient and unaffordable luxury. With so many humans suffering, the American anticruelty movement lost steam. Canadian animal welfare organizations also "found the 1870s difficult," one historian notes, "and most folded after a few years for lack of funding," while Cuba and Mexico saw no organized campaigns to better the lives of horses or other work animals until the 1880s and 1900s, respectively. Bergh's dream awaited first a new century, then a new millennium. In many respects, it still waits.[15]

One of the chief reasons the epizootic inaugurated little lasting change in animal welfare was that the economic significance of horses, mules, and donkeys as "living machines" continued to grow long after the Great Horse Flu wound down. Indeed, equine populations in most of North America continued to expand until the World War I era. The epizootic exposed the deep dependence of the continent's humans on the motive power of horses and their cousins. During the outbreak's peak, this vulnerability led many innovators, technophiles, humane reformers, and commentators to envision a future in which steam-powered devices made animal power—and, with it, cruelty toward animals—obsolescent. Reasonable observers, though, knew that so sweeping a technological transition required innovations that would take many more years to develop, refine, and implement.

Most authorities pinpointed urban transit systems—especially street railways—as the obvious place to start replacing equines with machines, yet epizootic-spurred experiments with steam-powered streetcars made little headway. The City Railway of Louisville, Kentucky, garnered effusive praise in 1872 by introducing a Remington engine capable of reaching speeds of up to six miles an hour. "Noiseless, smokeless, warmed by steam, and fitted up in handsome style," exclaimed a *Courier-Journal* reporter, "one rides in this car as comfortably as in a Pullman, and wonders how people ever could endure the rattle and clatter and dirt and dust and cold and general misery attendant upon a trip in the old-fashioned horse-car." The success of Louisville's trial sent the *Commercial* into paroxysms of frustration regarding the status quo: "In this inventive age, when steam has been fettered and devoted to such wide and multifarious purposes, it is absurd to place our entire dependence on muscle"—especially that of flu-prone beasts. Such experiments led the *Chicago Evening Mail* to prophesy that "the day is not far distant when steam will take the place of the slow-paced, irregular, epizootic horse power, now used to convey our hundreds of thousands to their homes, and if the city can hasten the time by official action, and at the same time get the benefit of it, we should all be glad to see it."[16]

Yet far from embracing steam-powered streetcars, municipal governments instead reverted to blocking their adoption. In New Orleans, for instance, the mayor justified the wholesale return of horse- and mule-drawn cars to the city's vaunted street railways by claiming that fossil-fueled engines had been "found to be fraught with great danger to life and property." It hardly helped that all the old problems that had hitherto hampered the introduction of steam-powered streetcars—heavy costs, concerns over smoke and clatter, fears that such machines would terrify pedestrians and equines alike, and so forth—persisted.[17]

Into the 1890s and sometimes beyond, horses and mules continued to power nearly all of North America's street railways. Change proved slower still in smaller towns and rural regions. US horse populations did not reach their peak until the late 1910s at more than 25 million; Canada's horse population grew until 1921, when it topped out at 3.5 million; and the number of mules in the United States expanded until 1925, peaking at nearly 6 million. Reliable statistics on donkey numbers in North America are lacking.

The same holds true for equines of every kind in Mexico and Cuba. Given the later introduction of electrified transit and internal combustion engines to Latin America, it seems safe to surmise that equine populations did not reach their apex in these countries until even later in the 1900s. Despite optimistic forecasts throughout the year of the horse plague, neither mechanization nor humanitarian reform made lasting gains.[18]

Everyone Remembers

In late 1872, as New Orleanians' tussle with the Great Horse Flu was finally letting up, the *Times-Picayune* lamented that the Crescent City continued to labor under "a considerable deficiency." More than a month after the largest, most disruptive outbreak of equine influenza in North American history reached the Lower Mississippi Valley, the *Times-Picayune* forecast that the epizootic would "soon be remembered only as a strange and unaccountable visitation, which for the time being had its sway and worked out its mission of disease and death." As this journalist foresaw, time's passage would indeed go on to dim and distort recollections of the epizootic. Yet contrary to such predictions—and despite the outbreak's admittedly slight effects on mechanization, humanitarian reform, and equine demography—the epizootic proved harder to forget than anyone expected.[19]

The Great Horse Flu undoubtedly ranked as one of the most peculiar disease events ever recorded. This fact alone, though, hardly guaranteed it an enduring place in human recollection. The so-called Spanish flu of 1918–20, after all, which killed some 675,000 Americans, half a million Mexicans, more than 50,000 Canadians, and at least 7,200 Cubans, soon became a "forgotten pandemic," vanishing from public memory even as millions mourned their losses. Unlike the "public amnesia" that prevailed in this pandemic's wake, the Great Horse Flu remained an active element in American memory until an unexpected chain of historical transformations finally dislodged it.[20]

Historians have long grasped the far-reaching significance of one of these transformations—the early twentieth-century decline of equines as prime movers. Scholars have proven less attentive, by contrast, to two epidemiological developments: first, a growing rejection of a centuries-old truism that cast human influenza and equine influenza as similar or identical disorders stemming from a common cause, and, second, an epochal shift from horses to hogs and poultry as the key intermediaries through which novel flu variants passed from wild birds to human hosts.

Even after the Great Horse Flu petered out in late 1873, the outbreak's scale, duration, and inscrutability lent it ongoing purchase. French-born, New York–based veterinary surgeon Alexandre Liautard took it as a given in

1881 that "everyone remembers the epizootic of 1872." Nearly twenty years later, a Pennsylvania newspaper echoed this assertion. "It isn't so long ago," the *Wilkes-Barre Sunday Leader* reasoned in 1897, "that the average man of thirty cannot remember the 'epizootic.' It tackled man and brute alike," the paper noted, "and wasn't particularly averse to encircling the neck of an old hen, as hundreds of fine fowl died from its effects."[21]

Into the early 1900s, older folks continued to regale newspaper readers with stories about the Great Horse Flu's ravages. When a transit strike paralyzed electric railways in 1900, for instance, the *St. Louis Globe-Democrat* published an interview in which "Uncle" Dan Larkin reflected on the standstill Missouri's largest city had experienced "way back in '71 [*sic*], when the

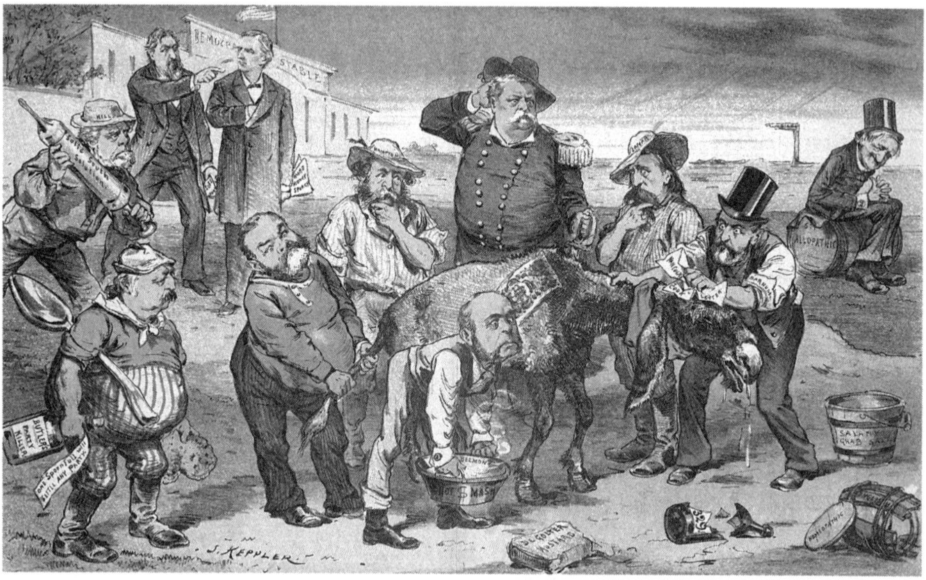

Austrian-born cartoonist Joseph Ferdinand Keppler created this wry political commentary two weeks before the 1880 elections. Keppler, a leading figure in reviving *Puck* and turning it into perhaps the preeminent satirical magazine in the United States, portrayed the Democratic Party as a flu-stricken donkey. Hapless party leaders surround the forlorn beast, with Democratic presidential candidate General Winfield Scott Hancock (in his Union uniform) scratching his head confusedly. Note the barrels in the background, which are labeled "Allopathic" and "Homeopathic." The donkey is gulping a draft of "Butler's Party Killer" tonic and receiving an enema reading "solid south solution." As this cartoon shows, the epizootic remained current in American memory for years to come. Joseph Ferdinand Keppler, "A Strange Case of Epizootic," *Puck*, October 20, 1880. Courtesy of the Bert Hansen Collection of Medicine and Public Health in Popular Graphic Art Medical Historical Library, Cushing/Whitney Medical Library Repository, Yale University.

epizootic laid up the horses and mules." In 1907, Indianapolis's "'oldest inhabitant'" told the *Star* about the time the epizootic "seized upon the horses of Indianapolis and other cities and the affairs of the city were wholly at rest for a period of almost a month . . . . Like the sun and the moon which stood still at the command of Joshua in days B.C.," this Indianapolitan elder continued, "business, church affairs, politics, society and almost every branch of industry that makes the city's life teem with activity remained transfixed while veterinarians battled with the plague that threatened to keep the city practically dead for months, winning in the end only a partial victory on account of the deaths of hundreds of the city's most valued animals."[22]

Recurrent outbreaks of equine influenza also explain why Americans continued to remember the Great Horse Flu. With the malady retracing its old route from the Atlantic Seaboard to Pittsburgh in 1875, for instance, the *Dispatch* reassured readers that "nothing as serious as 1872 is anticipated." As cases of equine influenza spiked upward once again in 1880, the *Hartford Courant* observed that even though "the distemper at present prevailing among horses in this section has many features in common with the great epizootic of 1872," the new outbreak had "thus far . . . show[n] no such severity."[23]

New equine flu outbreaks kept epizootic memories relevant. Yet a pair of hypotheses—that influenza among humans and equines stemmed from the same underlying cause, and that the malady could be communicated from the one to the other—also supported recollections of the Great Horse Flu. This became especially evident during the so-called Russian flu of 1889–92, a multiwave outbreak first reported in the eastern reaches of the tsar's domains. When Boston's city physician investigated a sudden eruption of respiratory illness at one municipal institution in December 1889, he remarked that these inmates' "symptoms vividly recalled those which marked the horses when the epizootic raged so extensively here in 1872." This healer was hardly alone in equating human influenza with its equine counterpart. Consider, for instance, how Mexico City's *Two Republics* fretted that the Great Horse Flu's past foretold the Russian flu's prologue. "Do I think it will come here?" it asked near the end of 1889, then answered: "Why not? The epizootic did, and that was nothing more than a 'horse influenza.'"[24]

Memories of the epizootic also remained current because the American economy remained heavily dependent on equine exertions into the early twentieth century. An 1895 article in the *Knoxville Journal and Tribune* confidently envisaged that "in a decade every man can become his own charioteer and the days of trouble caused by lame horses and epizootic will have become a thing of the past." And yet even six years later, this brave new world had yet to materialize. "Many people will remember the epizootic of 1874 [*sic*]," declared a *Boston Globe* report on a 1901 "horse epidemic" in metropolitan

New York that one veterinarian described as "the most serious outbreak of disease among horses" since the Great Horse Flu. "What changes," this article marveled, "have come to the horse since then!" After conceding that "rapid transit has dispensed with him a measure since electricity came so generally to the front," the *Globe* reminded readers that "neither the trolley nor the automobile has yet succeeded in displacing the horse." A week later, a rival paper parroted this moral: "When the horse gives out," the *Evening Transcript* affirmed, "it is demonstrated that we are still a long way from dispensing with his services. In fact, so much has business increased . . . that the lack of horseflesh seems to have as paralyzing an influence upon business as it ever did."[25]

The Great Flu Pandemic, like the Russian flu and recurrent equine influenza before it, recalled memories of the Great Horse Flu. "The present epidemic of Spanish influenza," a *Hartford Courant* reporter noted in October 1918, "calls to the minds of many of the older generation a severe plague among horses in the early '70s . . . popularly known as 'epizootic.'" "Horses died everywhere," the same writer continued, "in stables and often in the streets, and there were no known cures for the disease." This journalist summoned up the equine outbreak of the early 1870s to highlight an especially significant similarity between the epizootic and "the present human epidemic." As eyewitnesses attested, most fatal cases during the Great Horse Flu's reign "occurred after a secondary infection which bore the same relation to the first infection that pneumonia bears to influenza proper in the present plague."[26]

With the influenza pandemic's second wave loosening its stranglehold over the United States in late 1918, recollections of the 1872–73 contagion spurred "health authorities" to advise continued vigilance. "The fact is being recalled," one wire service item remarked, "that when the 'epizootic' made its appearance it seemed to have run its course, but a recurrence was even worse than when the disease first appeared." A few days later, the *Cincinnati Enquirer* reported that US Department of Agriculture (USDA) experts were "apprehensive" that "horse influenza or epizootic" might soon break out. "Nearly every war of modern times," these veterinary authorities pointed out, had caused "a disease manifestation among the world's horses." Although "influenza among horses" was supposedly "under better control in all parts of the country" than ever before, the same report nonetheless warned that "unlike certain other infectious diseases, one attack of influenza does not grant a lasting immunity." Incessant viral evolution, we now understand, meant that the pathogens responsible for both the Great Horse Flu and the Great Pandemic ceaselessly generated new variants, some of which differed so significantly from their progenitors that they could easily infect hosts who had already survived one or more bouts with influenza.[27]

Almost Exclusively a Human Virus

Yet even as the Great Pandemic rekindled epizootic memories, it was also nudging researchers toward a new forgetfulness. The Great Horse Flu became less relevant as experts revisited a pair of intertwined premises that had stood fast since the Great Horse Flu's transcontinental run nearly half a century earlier: that equine and human influenza were similar or even indistinguishable diseases, and that flu readily circulated between human and equine hosts. In 1918, the USDA took direct aim at the first of these assumptions: "The serious epidemic of influenza affecting the human family," it asserted, "has no relation to the disease of the same name which affects horses." Major George A. Soper of the US Army's Sanitary Corps extended this critique to the second presumption in explaining why a growing number of authorities were questioning old beliefs in the likeness of equine and human influenza. "Descriptions of influenza in horses and some of the circumstances under which it is transmitted," Soper explained in a 1919 article in the *New York Medical Journal*, "so closely resemble what is known of influenza in man as to suggest that the two diseases are identical." But this popular wisdom, Soper contended, could no longer stand up to scientific scrutiny: "That they are not identical, and that neither may be transmitted to the other, are facts which have long been believed by epidemiologists and are now confirmed." A Tennessee newspaper put a simpler spin on this budding scientific consensus: "Horses have influenza, too; but it is of a different sort from that which people have."[28]

Why did early twentieth-century medical and veterinary experts come to see an impassable divide between human and equine influenza? Several factors led many North Americans to draw new distinctions between diseases their forebears had perceived as identical or at least closely related. Veterinarians and other equine healers no longer diagnosed "influenza" as narrowly as their forebears had. By the early twentieth century, they applied the term not only to "shipping fever" (so named because it tended to infect horses in holding and transportation facilities) but also to several other discrete syndromes that also tended to produce flu-like symptoms in infected equines. As Soper argued, "By some, influenza ["in the horse"] is not believed to be a single disease, but a group of diseases." Veterinarians would later equate shipping fever with bacterial pleuropneumonia; they also discovered that several types of equine herpesvirus could cause fever, coughing, nasal discharge, and other common symptoms long associated with equine influenza.[29]

Heaping additional doubt on the notion that human and equine influenza were twins, or at least close cousins, was the failure of repeated experiments to communicate the Great Flu Pandemic to nonhuman animals (including equines) by inoculating them with biological material taken from human influenza victims. A 1919 *New York Tribune* article told how scientists had "found it impossible to transfer the complaint" that had afflicted hundreds of millions of people "to any of a long list of animals; monkeys alone showed a toxic effect," the *Tribune* maintained, "but true influenza did not develop." It is difficult to reconstruct why researchers proved unable to sicken laboratory animals by exposing them to the virus responsible for the Great Pandemic. In any case, though, these findings served to undermine centuries-old perceptions of influenza as a species-jumping infection.[30]

The growing conviction that human and equine flu were fundamentally different disorders, however, also drew momentum from sweeping changes in influenza's disease ecology. Virologists now speculate that at some point in the early 1900s, swine and domesticated poultry replaced equines as the main "mixing vessels" for flu. Although this oft-used metaphor threatens to obfuscate more than it reveals, it nonetheless captures the crucial role that nonhuman animals play in the virus's evolution and epidemiology. Wild waterbirds, as we have seen, have always served as the primary natural reservoir of genomically diverse influenza A variants. Avian strains, though, almost never strike human populations directly. Instead, they ordinarily afflict people only after hybridizing with human-adapted strains through viral reassortment within the cells of domesticated animals.[31]

We know very little about how, when, and why poultry and swine displaced equines as the key go-betweens for novel flu strains to reach human hosts. All available evidence, though, indicates that this process reached its culmination in the years leading up to the Great Pandemic. The most likely driver of this landmark change was the displacement of horses and their cousins in the transportation sector by internal combustion engines. A pair of leading evolutionary biologists, Martha Nelson and Michael Worobey, explain that "after centuries of influenza epizootics in equines, the 20th century marked a rapid decline in use of horses for urban transport and farm work." As horses and their kin receded ever further from the central roles they had long held in human economies, human-equine contact grew less intimate as well as less frequent, especially in metropolitan areas. As a result, the circulation of flu viruses between humans and equines apparently slowed or stopped.[32]

Nelson and Worobey summarized the implications of this evidence in a 2018 article in the *American Journal of Epidemiology*. "In addition to representing one of the greatest disease events in human history," they argued, "the Spanish flu pandemic may also mark a turning point in the ecology of influenza and the increasing importance of swine as reservoir hosts, a trend that accelerated during the second half of the 20th century." Researchers suspect that the H1N1 variant responsible for killing millions of humans, which had "avian origins," first spread to hogs in Iowa in 1919. From that time to the present, highly pathogenic avian flu variants have reached humankind chiefly via pigs or domesticated birds. To cite an especially notable example, H1N1 virions leapt from hogs to humans in Mexico in early 2009, sparking an outbreak that eventually killed nearly three hundred thousand people worldwide.[33]

By the time the pathogen responsible for causing influenza was finally isolated beneath an electron microscope in the 1930s, it "was believed to be almost exclusively a human virus." This doctrine held fast until the 1950s, when "closely related viruses were discovered" to be responsible for causing influenza in "horses, pigs, and birds." Virtually every person alive during the Great Horse Flu had perished by the time these discoveries confirmed the discarded nineteenth-century assumption that flu among humans and equines resulted from the same agent.[34]

By Virtue of Its Communicability

Some of the lessons the Great Horse Flu imparted regarding how best to treat influenza in horses and humans alike began taking root in the 1870s, though their fuller realization awaited twentieth-century medical, veterinary, and scientific discoveries. Minimalist interventions—ample rest, blanketing, clean bedding, and the like—met with widespread success against the epizootic. As a result, the outbreak added additional momentum to the longer-term shift away from heroic medicine, and toward more rational therapies for influenza and similar complaints.[35]

As for the patterns by which the Great Horse Flu expanded across space and time, these ended up affording exceptional opportunities for investigators to probe the outbreak's course as well as its underlying causes. The epizootic revived long-running debates between those who conceptualized influenza as atmospheric in nature and those who argued that it was infectious or contagious. By late 1872, though, it became apparent that equine influenza often spread against or askance observed wind currents. Traipsing across geographic and climatic barriers without missing a beat, it could even expand its range in multiple directions at once.

The scourge's subsequent movements further undermined the long-standing perception that influenza could reach new hosts through the movements of air masses and weather systems. In an 1873 address to the American Public Health Association, Adoniram B. Judson, a veteran of the Union army surgical corps who worked for the New York Health Department and would later go on to a distinguished career in orthopedic surgery, attacked the widespread notion that flu was "in the air." "The irregularities in time and place, in the appearance of this disease," he pointed out, "are so numerous and surprising that they cannot be classified or brought into harmony with . . . the laws which govern the phenomena of any of the recognized atmospheric conditions . . . . Epizoötic influenza spreads from city to city, and from country to country," Judson emphatically concluded, "by virtue of its communicability, and regardless of atmospheric conditions."[36]

In Judson's view, the Great Horse Flu's behavior flew in the face of anticontagionist arguments, yet debates over influenza's epidemiology raged on. With germ theory still very much in its infancy, scientists, physicians, and veterinarians had much to learn—not just regarding the flu, but also about infectious disease more generally. The limited research on the epizootic of 1872–73 attracted little attention, though it may have played a minor role in casting doubt on atmospheric theories of disease causation. In retrospect, it even seems that some students of the Great Horse Flu were grasping toward a synthesis resembling our present-day understanding of how influenza virions spread from host to host. Judson, for instance, admitted that "the apparently sudden seizure of all the horses in a city, or limited neighborhood, renders it possible that within narrow limits it infects through the atmosphere." A January 1873 *Medical Times* article offered a more expansive version of Judson's middle-of-the-road proposition. Influenza, it argued, was "not communicable by ordinary contact." Instead, the author proposed that the malady reached new hosts via "morbific germs" that "float in the atmosphere." No one, alas, seemed capable of identifying the pathogen in question. Judson confessed that "the darkness which surrounds the origin of this epizootic is impenetrable in the present state of our knowledge of the preservation and revitalization of disease germs," while Mexico's Gustavo Ruiz y Sandoval, who approached influenza as both a physician and a veterinary surgeon, conceded in his 1874 thesis on the epizootic that the argument he had mustered in favor of influenza's contagious nature was "too little to constitute the last word on the question."[37]

Influenza virions continued to elude direct human detection until the 1930s. It then took many years of additional research to confirm and elaborate on the prescient insights the Great Horse Flu had offered into influenza's etiology and epidemiology. We now know that the virus spreads not only through direct contact but also via the airborne transmission of flu-bearing aerosols and droplets. North Americans of the early 1870s, it turns out, may have inclined toward a fuller, more intricate, and more complex sense of infectious diseases in general—and influenza in particular—than scholars have generally recognized.

Financial Epizootic

Ultimately, the epizootic's greatest consequences were economic and political rather than epidemiological. Given the considerable losses the epizootic inflicted—the destruction of the immense quantities of wealth and capital embodied in the creatures the scourge killed and permanently debilitated as well as the rolling blackouts of equine-powered production and exchange that pummeled nearly every stretch of the northern Americas for weeks at a time—the outbreak's longer-term financial impacts merit a closer look. By contributing to a wrenching depression that was global in scope but nowhere more intense than in the United States, the Great Horse Flu helped to initiate what historian Eric Foner calls "the first great crisis of industrial capitalism." Deepening into the "longest period of uninterrupted economic contraction in American history," the grinding depression that ensued exacerbated poverty, aggravated class conflict, "rudely disrupt[ed] visions of social harmony," triggered "the greatest reversal of partisan alignments in the entire nineteenth century," hammered the final nails into the coffin of Southern Reconstruction, and—in all these ways—derailed the crucial postwar project of national healing, reconciliation, and consolidation.[38]

The trouble began nearly a year after Andrew Smith observed his first cases of epizootic in the Three Townships north of Toronto. In September 1873, the banking house of Jay Cooke & Co. collapsed. European investors, buffeted by financial wobbles in Vienna and Berlin, had balked at buying up the $50 million allotment of Northern Pacific Railroad bonds Cooke had pledged to sell to fund that company's construction across the Northern Plains. Cooke's bankruptcy, observed New York City attorney George Templeton Strong in his diary, foretold "the general smash that must come before long." Indeed, other investment firms soon faltered and failed. "The epizootic," one newspaper declared, "has raged most fearfully among the banks of New York." Two days later, Strong noted that the New York Stock Exchange, intent on containing the crisis, "had closed its doors"—and kept them closed for nine more days. Perhaps, like a horse suffering from the epizootic, all the financial system needed was a warm blanket and a little rest. Yet despite the Exchange's unprecedented precautions, the crisis could no longer be contained.[39]

The ready metaphor the Great Horse Flu provided for disruption and contagion gained new currency as the alarm spread. An Illinois newspaper joked that "horsemen call the panic the 'financial epizootic,'" while a Missouri newspaper quipped that "the disease broke out simultaneously in Kansas City, Atchison and Leavenworth," and banks in St. Joseph, Missouri, suffered "a gentle attack of it" soon after. The "suspension of the Banks of the whole country," the *Bristol (TN) News* lamented on September 30, "seems to be about as common as was the Epizooty, a year or less ago." A few days later, the *Chicago Tribune* noted that "the panic . . . possesses many features in common with the epizootic visitation of last year." The tumult that had "paralyzed business" in the Windy City, the *Tribune* expounded, "originated in the same place" as the Great Horse Flu (the Northeast), "swept in the same direction (westward)," and "has caused a tremendous run (at the banks instead of the nose) . . . . In all these respects, and several others that might be noted," the *Tribune* concluded, the two rapidly spreading outbreaks produced "almost an absolute identity of effects." Subsequent events showed that what one small-town Missouri paper called "the great bank epizootic" was just getting started—but unlike the Great Horse Flu, this contagion of economic malaise prevailed for many years to come.[40]

Most economists and historians attribute the Panic of 1873 to three intertwined factors: the overheated, highly speculative, and wildly corrupt expansion of North American railroads, which had doubled the extent of their track networks since 1865; declining European demand for the bonds that railroad corporations relied on to finance construction; and contractionary monetary policies pursued by governments on both sides of the Atlantic, particularly the US Coinage Act of 1873, which demonetized silver and caused its price to plunge. Although the Coinage Age was passed in April, its effects remained relatively mild until late summer, the season when "country banks recalled" their deposits from New York banks "to pay harvest-related expenses" in one of the many rhythms that continued to bind seemingly abstract financial markets to natural fluctuations in daylight, climate, and the life cycles of domesticated plants and animals.[41]

Once this seasonal fluctuation was superimposed on the monetary tightening resulting from the Coinage Act, "money panic," as one Kansas correspondent put it, "swept like another epizootic through the land." Because of extreme "stringency in the New York money market," the failure of Jay Cooke & Co. quickly drove many other banks over the edge. Reserves shrank dramatically and interest rates soared, bringing Wall Street turmoil to Main Streets throughout North America.[42]

By October, a crisis that started in the rarefied circles of high finance had grown into "a world depression of unprecedented severity." By the mid-1870s, half of all US railroad corporations entered receivership. New construction virtually stopped, iron and steel production nose-dived by 45 percent, thousands of businesses shuttered their doors, and millions of people lost their jobs and slipped into poverty. This same depression had much milder effects on Mexico, which only began to recover from the disruptions of the Wars of the Reform during the late 1870s, and Cuba, which remained mired in the Ten Years' War with "its economy," one prominent historian notes, "on the verge of collapse." Canada, by contrast, suffered on par with the US; "the period 1873–1879," one scholar explains, "was unambiguously one of recession." Manufacturing stagnated, joblessness surged, and so many people departed Canada—mostly for the United States—that the confederation's population declined.[43]

The epizootic, though, served not just as a metaphor for the fast-spreading depression but also as one of its underlying causes. In December 1873, a *Rocky Mountain News* correspondent bemoaned that Chicago's economy had been buffeted "within the last two and a half years" by "the most adverse circumstances"—specifically, the Great Chicago Fire of October 1871; the "great fire" that destroyed sixty-five acres of Boston's wealthiest commercial property thirteen months later; and "the epizoot," which ensured that "for a whole month not a stroke of business was done here." In this correspondent's telling, Cooke's collapse represented but "the last turn at the wheel" for an economy that was already teetering toward the abyss. Two years later, Chicago's *Inter Ocean* published an article titled "The Panic of 1873." After identifying the "reduction of protective duties" by Congress and "the contraction of the currency" in the late 1860s and 1870s as two key drivers of the downturn, it proceeded to examine several "minor contributory causes," including "the great fires in Chicago and Boston, which destroyed immense amounts of the accumulations of industry," and "the epidemic of horse-disease, which for weeks seriously impeded and embarrassed business." This succession of disasters, the *Inter Ocean* asserted, "disordered the whole situation of trade." In the *Inter Ocean*'s estimation, then, the Great Horse Flu ranked as one of the "important wheels" driving "the general movement toward a panic" and the convulsive depression that followed.[44]

To the extent that the epizootic helped to precipitate this economic crisis—directly by disrupting equine-powered economies and indirectly through its contributions to the Great Boston Fire—it helped to thrust the United States into a new historical era. By bringing postwar economic growth to a dramatic halt, the depression unleashed wrenching social and political conflict. Industrial production had increased by 75 percent between 1865 and 1873 but flatlined once the Panic struck. Commentators have long interpreted the Gilded Age—a period named after an 1873 novel coauthored by Mark Twain and Charles Dudley Warner—as an era of pivotal transformations. "Until the Panic of 1873," historian Mark Wahlgren Summers points out, "Reconstruction's collapse seemed nowhere near inevitable." As the depression deepened, though, long-standing internal divides within the Republican

Party intensified, and in the 1874 elections the party lost its majority in the US House of Representatives as well as numerous state legislatures. With Congress forced by hard times to pinch pennies, and ex-Confederates and other white supremacists stepping up vicious campaigns of violence and terror throughout the South, white voters soured on Radical Reconstruction. Federal support for African American civil, political, economic, and human rights consequently quavered, then collapsed altogether.[45]

Poverty, underdevelopment, and white supremacy wracked the unreconstructed South. Resurgent Democrats championed "Redemption"—the fight to reimpose white supremacy on African Americans. They also took advantage of grassroots anti-Chinese nativism to pass state and federal laws restricting Chinese immigration and harassing Chinese American communities. As for the North, it grew into what one historian calls "an industrial colossus with new values, new leadership, and new aspirations." Gaping divides of wealth and power set sections and social classes at each other's throats. As unemployment, poverty, and class divides all worsened, the discontent of laboring Americans erupted in New York's Tompkins Square riots in 1874, the massive 1877 railway workers' strike known as the Great Upheaval, and other mobilizations. Meanwhile, with crop prices plummeting by 50 percent or more, a powerful agrarian movement spearheaded by the Patrons of Husbandry (also known as the Grangers) prevailed on legislators in Illinois and other prairie states to slap tough new regulations on railroad companies and grain elevators.[46]

Although conflict convulsed economic, social, and political life throughout the depression of the 1870s, Americans of nearly every stripe nonetheless agreed that it was time to ratchet up the violent seizure of Indigenous peoples' remaining homelands. Phil Sheridan, George Crook, and other military leaders responded by prosecuting brutal campaigns against the West's Native peoples. Despite occasional reversals—most notably, the destruction of George Custer's cavalry at the 1876 Battle of the Greasy Grass by a combined force of Lakotas, Cheyennes, and Arapahos—assaults against Native American territory and autonomy accelerated, with settlers and the US Army killing off thousands of horses while inflicting widespread death and unfathomable suffering on Indigenous communities and nations. With nearly all Indigenous Nations now under the Americans' heel, the United States stood poised to turn its energies from continental conquest to overseas imperialism. It is impossible to know, of course, what might have transpired if the Great Horse Flu had never happened, yet there are sound reasons to believe that the epizootic played a subtle but significant part in driving these developments and reversals.

EPILOGUE

How will this end—for me, those I hold dear, and humanity more broadly? As COVID-19 erupted outward from Wuhan, China, then convulsed widening reaches of the planet in early 2020, this question began peppering my thoughts, as it assuredly did for millions of other people. In the months and years that followed, this question ballooned into an all-consuming preoccupation for public health officials, healthcare workers, media outlets, governments, and ordinary citizens across much of the world. Eventually, though, epidemiologists realized that COVID was here to stay. Like influenza before it, this bug has become a feature—an ineradicable component of the world we inhabit, the world that inhabits us.[1]

People who lived through the Great Horse Flu trod a similar path as an unprecedented crisis resolved into a new normal. Yet we should not forget that earthlings of the early 1870s populated very different material and mental universes than our own. To them, the epizootic constituted just one outbreak among an incessant barrage of infectious diseases. Smallpox continued to churn relentlessly through North America during the year of the horse plague. In 1873, another cholera pandemic—weaker than the two that preceded it, and also more skillfully managed through improved public health measures and more effective therapies—reached the Western Hemisphere from Asia. Yellow fever convulsed the Lower Mississippi Valley, malaria struck Yavapai and Dilzhę́'é survivors on the Rio Verde Reserve, and scourges including measles and whooping cough caused severe though mostly localized outbreaks.[2]

Only later in the 1870s, and especially in the 1880s and 1890s, would the scientific breakthroughs made by Louis Pasteur, Robert Koch, and others begin to resolve a startling succession of epidemiological mysteries. Scientific sanitation, the development of vaccines, the invention in the 1930s of the world's first viable antibacterial therapies (sulfa drugs), and the advent of mass-produced antibiotics starting with penicillin in the early 1940s led medical and veterinary experts to tout the conquest of infectious disease as an achievable goal. By the 1960s, humanity's triumph over epidemics, pandemics, and epizootics seemed not only possible but imminent and inevitable.[3]

After a long hiatus from public memory, the Great Horse Flu reappeared in a 1974 *Sunday Sun Magazine* article titled "The First Energy Crisis: When Horses Failed," in which *Baltimore Sun* reporter George A. Gipe sought to contextualize skyrocketing gasoline prices. Perhaps the most compelling reason to recall the epizootic today, however, has less to do with energy or economics and more to do with epidemiology. Although flu variants no longer circulate between horses and humans with much gusto, the outbreak of 1872–73 nonetheless offers a trenchant reminder of influenza's prowess. Despite widespread descriptions of COVID as a sort of supercharged influenza, the epizootic, like the Great Flu Pandemic of 1918–20, proved even more infectious and just as deadly as the outbreak that began in late 2019.[4]

When I reflect on the Great Horse Flu from the postpandemic (and probably prepandemic) vantage point of the present, I also see a second, less heralded, but possibly even more significant historical arc taking shape. Major epidemiological milestones on this alternative trajectory include the so-called Russian flu of 1889–92 (which some scientists have recently posited might have been caused by a coronavirus) and the Great Flu Pandemic of 1918–20. Starting in the second half of the twentieth century, hundreds of scourges, most of them viral, jumped across species divides to afflict human hosts—335 as of 2008, by one count, with COVID, a new H1N1 variant, and dozens of others emerging since that tally. The who's who of these novel maladies has grown from one decade to the next. At this writing, the most prominent in the viral division of these emergent zoonotic plagues include Ebola, mpox, Zika, West Nile, SARS, MERS, SARS-CoV-2, Nipah, Hendra,

HIV/AIDS—and, lest we forget, assorted types and variants of influenza A. The latest flu scare has centered on an H5N1 strain that has resulted in the culling of more than 166 million chickens, turkeys, ducks, and other domesticated fowl between 2022 and early 2025 in the United States alone. This same outbreak has spilled over to wild waterbirds, dairy cattle, house cats, and a small but growing number of human hosts. Most of the viral maladies that have emerged since the late twentieth century have originated either in ecosystems recently disrupted by human incursions or in facilities where nonhuman animals have been confined, slaughtered, or marketed. Meanwhile, illnesses that public health officials once believed that they could contain if not eliminate—cholera, tuberculosis, measles, polio, and many others—have evolved into novel forms that host immune systems are proving ill equipped to fight.[5]

The globalization of exchange and transportation networks has accelerated the pace at which infectious diseases can extend their ravages far beyond their points of origin. Twenty-first-century plagues, whether emergent or resurgent, are adeptly exploiting the niches and vulnerabilities opened by human dysfunction: warfare, poverty, biodiversity declines, healthcare disparities, natural disasters driven or exacerbated by global climate change, vaccine hesitancy, and more.[6]

The Great Horse Flu struck many observers in the early 1870s as a curiosity as well as a singularity. Scratch beneath the outbreak's outward oddness, though, and scarier lessons come into view. More than 150 years of change have refashioned the world into a place that time travelers from the year of the horse plague would scarcely recognize. Few humans depend on equines anymore, while humankind has never wielded more powerful tools and techniques for preventing, detecting, containing, combating, and recovering from influenza. But despite all these developments, this exploration of the epizootic affords precious little reassurance.

Throughout the COVID pandemic, experts and laypeople alike constantly referred to this scourge as a "super-flu." By tracing the Great Horse Flu, though, and placing this animal-centered outbreak in the broader context of influenza's long history as an inveterate killer of human beings, it seems abundantly clear that the novel virus that emerged from the countryside north of Toronto in September 1872 was far more infectious than SARS-CoV-2 ever became. A second point of resonance between the 1870s and the present—a startling lack of government capacity for tackling the outbreak—demands attention, too. The epizootic struck before the United States or its neighbors had established national institutions to protect human and animal health, while municipal and state responses failed to check the outbreak's spread. Epidemiological safeguards improved dramatically throughout the late 1800s and 1900s. As COVID spread outward from Wuhan, China, efforts by local, national, and international health agencies helped to slow the outbreak's spread and reduce its severity.

The failure to contain this scourge during its early stages, though, coincided with efforts by a significant minority of people in the United States and many other countries to weaken public faith in vaccination, quarantines, and other proven methods for combatting contagions. Even as millions of scientists, physicians, veterinarians, health workers, public officials, and others continue to wage heroic struggles against infectious diseases, it seems all but certain that the toll of infectious disease outbreaks on humans and other animals will climb in the years ahead—possibly sharply.

The Great Horse Flu eventually vanished. Yet with hard times deepening, political divides sharpening, and repression against Native Americans, African Americans, and Chinese Americans intensifying in the outbreak's wake, this was not necessarily a happy ending. It seems only right to conclude this book on a similar note.

The epizootic of the early 1870s suggests that we are just one reassortment event away from the next influenza epidemic or pandemic. No less concerning are devastating cuts in US federal funding for scientific and medical research; the American withdrawal from the World Health Organization; and recent changes to vaccine recommendations by the Centers for Disease Control. The story of the Great Horse Flu should open our eyes to the hazards that highly pathogenic influenza variants continue to pose for humans and many other creatures. It should also impress upon us the necessity of pressuring governments at all levels to confront the growing perils that flu and other emergent zoonotic diseases pose by reinvigorating evidence-based approaches to public health.[7]

ACKNOWLEDGMENTS

Writing this book has not been easy. Like most things worth doing, it has taken its toll and entailed considerable sacrifice. This project grew out of a more ambitious tome, tentatively titled *An Animals' History of the United States*. After laboring for many years, drafting several hundred pages, and learning a great deal, I began to despair that I had embarked on a fool's errand. Inspired partly by the positive reception a draft chapter on the Great Horse Flu received from the Newberry Library's History of Capitalism Seminar—and, more important, by the increasingly urgent tug that the outbreak of 1872–73 exerted on my attentions—I pivoted in the spring of 2018 to pursue a more focused book on the epizootic. I have not looked back.

Several grants and fellowships have facilitated my ongoing engagement with human-animal history while making it possible for me to research, write, and revise the volume that you hold in your hands. A Guggenheim Fellowship and a National Endowment for the Humanities Public Scholar Award provided time away from teaching and other material support for the larger project from which this book emerged. After I narrowed my focus to the Great Horse Flu, the University of Colorado Boulder's Center for Humanities and the Arts (CHA) extended a College of Arts and Sciences (CAS) sabbatical to a full year. CHA also provided a fine scholarly community—CHA director Jennifer Ho and faculty fellows Aun Ali, Cheryl Higashida, Rahul Parson, Stephanie Su, and Levi Thompson—that helped me continue to make progress even during pandemic lockdowns. A College Scholars Award from CAS afforded me another productive semester of research leave. Last but hardly least, a Grant for Scholarly Work in Biomedicine and Health from the National Library of Medicine (NLM)—Award Number 1G13LM013554-01, funded by the US National Institutes of Health—provided generous funding for research travel, graduate assistants, and summer salary. I am undyingly grateful to these agencies, foundations, and institutions for the trust they have placed in me and the enthusiasm they have shown for my work.

I am grateful to the many audiences that have listened to me present portions of this research. These have included the Utah Historical Society, Stanford University's History Department, the American Society of Environmental History, the Western History Association, the Labor and

Working-Class History Association, and CU-Boulder's Center for the Study of Origins (which is now sadly defunct). Participants in the Creatures of Capitalism Symposium, organized by Troy Vitesse and sponsored by Harvard University's Weatherhead Center, workshopped a precursor to chapter 2; I am most grateful for their constructive criticism. Although I was unable to attend Oxford University's "Contours of Endemicity" conference in 2023, the paper I wrote for that gathering later bore fruit in portions of chapter 9. A version of chapter 6 was previously published in the *Utah Historical Quarterly*; I am grateful to editor Jedidiah Rogers for his encouragement and insight on that piece, and to the *Quarterly* for permission to publish a revised take on it. A portion of chapter 9 appeared in *Modern American History*, which has graciously allowed me to draw on that article here. I would like to express special appreciation to the many colleagues who have read and commented on portions of this manuscript: Maurice Crandall, Jennifer Ho, Beth Lew-Williams, and the faculty and graduate students who participated in two different sessions of the CU-Boulder History Department's Faculty Seminar.

Several graduate students aided me immeasurably as research assistants, thanks to funding provided by the NLM as well as the CU-Boulder History Department's Graduate Research Mentorship program. Andrew Pace helped me with Spanish-language sources. Micaela Cruce was resourceful, astute, and persistent in tracking down materials on a variety of topics. Kerri Keller built a crucial foundation for the GIS and mapping components of this project. And Maggie McNulty proved indefatigable, efficient, and remarkably patient in bringing the cartographic components of this project to fruition.

Over the many years it took me to complete this book, colleagues and staff at CU-Boulder have supported me wholeheartedly. I appreciate the help, guidance, and problem-solving provided by CAS, the Department of History, the Center of the American West, the Division of Arts and Humanities, the Center for the Study of Origins, the Office of Contracts and Grants, the Research and Innovation Office, and the Center for Native American and Indigenous Studies. Among the many folks in these units to whom I owe thanks, I am especially grateful to Donna Axel, Tessa Brandt, Elizabeth Fenn, Susan Kent, Cherise Lamour, Ryan Lueck, Ted Lytle, Kellie Matthews, Tamar McKee, Brooke Neely, Paul Sutter, Tim Weston, Tony Wood, Marcia Yonemoto, and Phoebe Young.

My research was aided immeasurably by a fabulous cadre of librarians and archivists. Special thanks to those at El Archivo Histórico / Centro de la Documentación Institucional de la Secretaría de la Salud, El Archivo Histórico de la Facultad de Medicina, the Bancroft Library at the University of California Berkeley, the Beinecke Library at Yale, the Boston Athenaeum, the

John Hay Library at Brown, the Chicago History Museum, the Denver Public Library, the Hemeroteca Nacional de México, History Colorado, the Houghton Library at Harvard, the Huntington Library, the National Archives and Records Administration, the Sharlot Hall Museum Research Center, the Toronto Reference Library at the Toronto Public Library, the Thomas Fisher Rare Book Library at the University of Toronto, and the Wellcome Collection. The staff of the Interlibrary Loan and Rare and Distinctive Collections at the University of Colorado Libraries deserve special thanks.

Ryan Hall shared his copies of the Heavy Runner Records, which proved crucial in chapter 6. A fleet of scholars provided helpful responses to my queries. Seth Archer, Gordon Chang, Ryan Hall, Mark Honigsbaum, Reinaldo Funes Monzote, Louis Pérez, Andrew Robichaud, Rebecca Scott, John Harley Warner, and Michael Worobey all went above and beyond to share their time and expertise with me. Kathleen McDermott at Harvard University Press (HUP) offered counsel and support to me throughout this project's early years and subsequent germination. Chris Bebenek proved helpful in negotiating a release from my contract with HUP. Amanda Moon, Thomas Lebien, and their staff at Moon & Company have shared their wisdom in droves and supported me as my conviction in myself ebbed. Time and again, they reined me in and sharpened my focus. I could not be more grateful to the University of North Carolina Press for welcoming me and this book with open arms. Mark Simpson-Vos encouraged me, and Tara Jordan handled the logistical details with aplomb. Cate Hodorowicz has showered me with kindness; I could not be more appreciative of her professionalism, encouragement, and keen writerly eye. Two anonymous peer reviewers of the book offered support as well as clear directions on how to strengthen it. Christi Stanforth's copyediting kept me on the straight and narrow, and Matthew Somoroff masterfully shepherded this book through production.

Ari Kelman's friendship means the world to me, and I cannot thank him enough for all ways he has helped me over the years. I am especially grateful for the time and energy he devoted to critiquing the penultimate draft of this book with his trademark thoroughness, wisdom, and discernment. While I have not been able to implement all the excellent guidance he provided, this is nonetheless a much better book because of Ari's tremendous generosity.

My family and friends have put up with this book—and with me—for far longer than they might have wished. My Whittier Neighborhood crew is too large to list individually, but you know who you are and that I love you! A special shout-out to Luke and Lisa Daniel and Tim Habib and Rachel Hutson, who kindly offered up their homes for a pair of pivotal writing retreats. I would also like to give special thanks to David Beaton, Tommy Beaudreau, Karen Buelow, Tedd Buelow, Rachel Bygrave, MK Christian,

Cate Costley, Gabriel Goodliffe, Charles Jones, Alessandra La Rocca Link, John McClelland, Shawn Patrick, Sherri Sheu, and Grant Van Pelt. One of my oldest friends, Steve Wagner, earned my undying appreciation by stepping in to help me navigate some challenging contract complexities.

As I was gearing up to complete a full draft of this book, my dear friend Timothy Kirkland passed away unexpectedly. Losing Tim has been devastating, and this book is dedicated in part to his memory. Tim had the gift of gab, a love of good writing, and a talent for making people feel comfortable, valued, and adored. He was a wonderful friend and I miss him every day. Lori, Addi, and Charli have had to endure an impossible loss. They have nonetheless managed to continue loving me and my family boundlessly, for which I am grateful beyond words.

My in-laws, Jim and Sherry McMaster, have offered support and diversion. My sister, Melissa Delisi, and her family, Jamison, Landon, Finley, and Matthew Delisi, have had my back throughout. I am thankful, too, for my extended family—my aunts, cousins, and everyone else, in various parts of the US as well as the UK. My father, John Andrews, has always believed in and encouraged me. This book is partly dedicated to the memory of my mother, Martha Andrews, who loved me dearly and unfailingly supported me, my family, and my work. Tragically, she suffered a bad fall on the same day that I submitted the manuscript of this book. She died a few weeks later from her injuries. There is no way for me to express my gratitude for all she did for me, nor can I adequately convey just how much I miss her.

My children, Fiona Andrews and Santiago Andrews, have offered constant, much-needed reminders to pull my head out from research and writing to enjoy the present while planning for whatever the future may bring. I feel so fortunate that we are family, and I could not be prouder of either of you! Our dog Roxie's loving nature has offered comfort and joy ever since she came into our household during the COVID lockdown, not to mention insistent and enjoyable reminders to consider how nonhuman creatures have experienced and shaped human lives and human histories.

As for Amy Andrews McMaster, she has showered me with love, never lost faith in my abilities, and kept me rooted in my need for fun, adventure, and joy as we continue to make the life of our dreams.

NOTE ON SOURCES, MAPPING, AND COMPANION WEBSITE

This book draws heavily on research in text-searchable newspaper and periodical databases that make it easier than ever before to identify relevant materials from a huge number of publications from around the United States, other parts of North America, and the world beyond. These digitized repositories have enabled me to piece together the story of the Great Horse Flu, an event that drew considerable press coverage, but also one that rarely stayed in the news for more than a few weeks in any given locale. These databases, however, are no panacea. Many of them require costly subscriptions; some—most notably, much of the Hemeroteca Nacional de México's newspaper collection—can only be accessed in person; and all have quirks and foibles.

It is especially important for readers to know that although I have done my utmost to be thorough, existing databases provide access to only a relatively small proportion of the truly vast body of newspapers, magazines, and other periodicals that were published in the early 1870s. Locating relevant articles within these databases, meanwhile, can be difficult. Indeed, I have had to lean heavily on permutations of a single search term—"epizootic" and its variants ("epizoot," "epizooty," and so forth) as well as French and Spanish cognates—to identify articles deserving closer scrutiny.

Readers who go to the trouble of delving into this book's notes will find that I cite thousands of articles drawn from hundreds of publications in French, Spanish, and especially English. Two graduate researchers with Spanish skills, Maggie McNulty and Andrew Pace, helped with translations. For both French and Spanish, we employed Google Translate to accelerate translation and zero in on the most relevant passages. We then corrected and honed these translations. Rich as these digitized newspapers proved, they nonetheless constitute just a subset of the massive media coverage and expert commentary the Great Horse Flu generated throughout 1872 and 1873.

One benefit of the broad network of sources that these digitized newspapers and periodicals provide deserves fuller mention. Generous funding from the National Institutes of Health / National Library of Medicine enabled me to develop an innovative project to chart the Great Horse Flu's expansion in unprecedented detail. In partnership with two graduate student researchers, Kerri Keller and Maggie McNulty, I translated qualitative information from newspapers, periodicals, and other sources into a database tracking the first recorded mentions of the epizootic in more than 1,200 locations in Canada, the US, Cuba, Mexico, and beyond. Keller and McNulty then fed this data into a Geographic Information System (GIS). Using several additional tools, they generated maps and animations that track the outbreak's spread from its initial appearance until its eventual dissolution. Please see my website, www.thomasgandrews.com, to access this GIS as well as other materials for research and teaching.

NOTES

ABBREVIATIONS

AM	*Arizona Miner* (Prescott)
BE	*Brooklyn Eagle*
BET	*Boston Evening Transcript*
BG	*Boston Globe*
BS	*Baltimore Sun*
CE	*Cincinnati Enquirer*
CEM	*Chicago Evening Mail*
CEP	*Chicago Evening Post*
CT	*Chicago Tribune*
GPO	Government Printing Office (Washington)
HC	*Hartford Courant*
MR	*Missouri Republican* (St. Louis)
NOR	*New Orleans Republican*
NOTP	*New Orleans Times-Picayune*
NYH	*New York Herald*
NYT	*New York Times*
ODA	*Our Dumb Animals*
PH	*Placer Herald* (Auburn, CA)
PI	*Philadelphia Inquirer*
RC	*Report of the Commissioners Appointed to Investigate the Cause and Management of the Great Fire in Boston* (Boston: Rockwell & Churchill, 1873)
SFAC	*Alta California* (San Francisco)
SFC	*San Francisco Chronicle*
SFEB	*San Francisco Evening Bulletin*
SF Examiner	*San Francisco Examiner*
TG	*Toronto Globe*

INTRODUCTION

1. Andrew Smith, *TG*, reprinted as "Horse Epidemic in Canada," *Long Island Traveler* (Cutchogue, NY), October 17, 1872. For especially helpful descriptions of symptoms, see Choice [pseud.], "Dingman's Ferry," letter dated November 18, 1872, in *Port Jervis (NY) Tri-States Union*, November 29, 1872; "Local Paragraphs," *Memphis Appeal*, November 23, 1872; NYH, n.d., in "A Horseless City," *Louisville Courier-Journal*, October 29, 1872; "The Horse Disease," *New York Evening Post*, October 23, 1872; *Houston Age*, November 30, 1872,

quoted in "In Houston," *Dallas Herald*, December 7, 1872; NYH, n.d., in "Horseless City." The striking concurrence between present-day understandings of influenza and historical descriptions of the Great Horse Flu's symptoms, progress, and outcomes strongly suggests that a variety of the pathogen known since the early twentieth century as the influenza virus propelled this outbreak of equine sickness and suffering; see Gabrielle A. Landolt and Thomas M. Chambers, "The Clinical Features, Pathobiology, and Epidemiology of Influenza Infections in Horses," in *Animal Influenza*, ed. David E. Swayne, 2nd ed. (John Wiley and Sons, 2017), 511; and Kara M. Lascola and Lindsey Boone, "Equine Influenza," last modified 2024, in *Merck Veterinary Manual*, https://www.merckvetmanual.com/respiratory-system/respiratory-diseases-of-horses/equine-influenza.

2. "Epidemic Among Horses," NYH, October 19, 1872 ("farmers" through "market"); "Epizootic," *Ottawa (ON) Citizen*, October 21, 1872 ("progress").

3. "The City on Foot," *Buffalo Courier Express*, October 22, 1872 ("extent"); "Daily Gossip," BG, November 2, 1872 ("called upon").

4. "A City Without Means of Transit," NYH, October 30, 1872 ("singular spectacle"); "Hippo-Malaria," NYH, October 29, 1872 ("ominous" to "paralyzed"); "Business Stagnated Up the River," *New York Sun*, November 16, 1872; "The Horse Disease," CT, October 31, 1872 ("goods" to "penniless"); "Business Stagnated Up the River" ("draw sand"); letter dated October 31, 1872, in "New York," CT, November 7, 1872 ("theatre").

5. "The Canadian Horse Disease," *Prairie Farmer* (Chicago), November 2, 1872 ("no sooner"); "The New Horse Disease," *Minneapolis Star Tribune*, November 3, 1872 ("seemed to act" through "born"); "The Horse Epizootic," *Central City (CO) Register*, October 30, 1872 ("pitiless").

6. Report from New York, October 25, in "The Horse Disease," CT, October 28, 1872 ("lumbering districts"); "Equine Epidemic," HC, October 24, 1872 ("rare sight"); "The Horse Disease," CT, November 18, 1872 ("greatly hindering"); "From Orrville," *Holmes County Republican* (Millersburg, OH), November 21, 1872 ("serious obstacle"). On farmers avoiding town, see "Letter from Petersburg," *Richmond (VA) News Leader*, November 9, 1872.

7. "Hipporhinorrhea," CEP, November 2, 1872 ("all the horses" through "poor beasts"); "The Horse Disease," CEM, December 4, 1872 ("remarkably low"). For fatality figures, see "The Unharnessed Horse," CEP, November 9, 1872; "Convalescing Chargers," CEP, November 13, 1872; CEM, November 20, 1872; "The City in Brief," CT, December 1, 1872; CEM, December 11, 1872.

8. "Chicago Real Estate," *New York Evening Post*, November 21, 1872 ("dull"); "City Brevities," *Indianapolis Journal*, December 6, 1872 ("suburban"); "Financial and Commercial," PI, November 4, 1872 ("general depression"). On contractors' fears, see "The Horse Disease," *Chicago Inter Ocean*, November 4, 1872.

9. David M. Morens and Jeffery K. Taubenberger, "Historical Thoughts on Influenza Viral Ecosystems, or Behold a Pale Horse, Dead Dogs, Failing Fowl, and Sick Swine," *Influenza and Other Respiratory Viruses* 4 (2010): 334; David M. Morens and Jeffery K. Taubenberger, "An Avian Outbreak Associated with Panzootic Equine Influenza in 1872: An Early Example of Highly Pathogenic Avian Influenza?," *Influenza and Other Respiratory Viruses* 4 (2010): 375.

10. "Equipneupleurheunibus," *Memphis Appeal*, November 23, 1872; "Frituras," *Juan Palomo* (Havana, Cuba), November 24, 1872; *Herkimer (NY) Democrat and Little Falls Gazette*, November 27, 1872.

11. On etymology, see *Oxford English Dictionary*, "influenza (n.)," accessed June 2025, https://doi.org/10.1093/OED/9310051538. Discussions of responsible agents include E. P. Dyball, "'The Epizootic,'" *The People* (Concord, NH), November 21, 1872; Videx [pseud.], "Veterinary Department: Equine Epidemic Influenza," *Turf, Field and Farm*, January 17, 1873, 38–39; S. S. Rathvon, "Hippy-Zymosis," *Lancaster (PA) Evening Express*, February 11, 1873. For articulations of atmospheric etiology, see "Epizootic in Pulaski," *Pulaski (NY) Democrat*, November 7, 1872; "End of the Epihippic Wave," *Rutland (VT) Herald*, November 12, 1872; "Epizootic Maladies," *Nashville Union*, November 21, 1872.

12. On putative strain, see Michael Worobey, email to author, July 2, 2021. Chapter 1 unpacks the reasoning and evidence behind these claims.

13. James Law, "Influenza in Horses," in US Commissioner of Agriculture, *Report of the Commissioner of Agriculture for 1872* (GPO, 1873), 209. Unfortunately, an even more comprehensive later study did not hazard to speculate on the disease's overall prevalence. Adoniram B. Judson, "History and Course of the Epizoötic Among Horses upon the North American Continent," *Public Health Reports and Papers Present at the Meetings of the American Public Health Association in the Year 1873* (New York and Cambridge, MA: Hurd and Houghton and the Riverside Press, 1875). For rates of 50–75 percent in Chambersburg, Pennsylvania, where the outbreak had yet to peak, see *Valley Spirit* (Chambersburg, PA), November 27, 1872. An estimated three-fourths of horses in Providence and Newburgh were afflicted; "The Epizootic Extending," HC, October 28, 1872; "Epizootic," *Tri-States Union* (Port Jervis, NY), November 15, 1872. Along the Menominee River in Wisconsin, more than 75 percent of horses were affected by the time the outbreak's second week ended. "Menominee Items," *Green Bay Press-Gazette*, November 15, 1872.

14. "Newport," CE, November 19, 1872; "Hippo-Malaria," NYH, October 29, 1872; "Hipporhinorrhea," CEP, November 2, 1872; "The Epizootic," *Crawfordsville (IN) Weekly Journal*, December 12, 1872; *Columbus (IN) Republican*, November 21, 1872; "The Epizootic Plague," *Plattsburgh (NY) Sentinel*, November 8, 1872; "State News," *Bangor (ME) Whig and Courier*, November 21, 1872; "Cabot Items," *Montpelier (VT) Argus and Patriot*, December 26, 1872; "The Horse Disease," *Juniata Sentinel* (Mifflintown, PA), November 6, 1872; "The Epizootic Extending," HC, October 28, 1872.

15. On contemporary estimates of "less than 2 per cent" and "not over three per cent.," see "The Horse Epizootic," *Times* (London), December 2, 1872; and "Hipporhinorrhea," *Atlanta Constitution*, November 20, 1872.

16. Data Paddock, "USDA Horse Total, 1850–2012," accessed February 4, 2026, https://datapaddock.com/usda-horse-total-1850-2012/; Charles L. Flint, "A Hundred Years Progress in Farming," *Vermont Farmer* (Newport), January 9, 1874; US Commissioner of Indian Affairs, *Annual Report of the Commissioner of Indian Affairs for the Year 1873* (GPO, 1874), 347.

17. For a helpful meditation on continental categorization, see Martin W. Lewis and Kären Wigen, *The Myth of Continents: A Critique of Metageography* (University of California Press, 1997).

18. Quotes in this and subsequent paragraphs from "The Position of the Horse in Modern Society," *The Nation*, October 31, 1872, 277.

19. As Andrew R. L. Cayton astutely notes, "Calling for continental history is one thing. Writing it is another." "Writing North American History," *Journal of the Early Republic* 22 (2002): 107–8. Inspirations for a more continental approach include Herbert Bolton,

who cautioned against the dangers of nation-centered histories that had "raise[d] up a nation of chauvinists" and insisted that "much of what has been written of each national history" in the Americas "is but a thread out of a larger strand." Herbert E. Bolton, "The Epic of Greater America," *American Historical Review* 38 (1933): 448–49. See also Alan Taylor's trilogy, *American Colonies* (Viking, 2001); *American Revolutions: A Continental History, 1750–1804* (W. W. Norton, 2016); and *American Republics: A Continental History of the United States, 1783–1850* (W. W. Norton, 2021). Other helpful guideposts in this evolving historiography include Richard White, "Is There a North American History," *Révue française d'études américaines* 79 (1999): 8–28; Paul W. Mapp, "Atlantic History from Imperial, Continental, and Pacific Perspectives," *William & Mary Quarterly*, 3rd ser., 63 (2006): 713–24; and Frank Towers, "Conclusion: Continental History and the Problem of Time and Place," in *Remaking North American Sovereignty: State Transformations in the 1860s*, ed. Jewel L. Spangler and Frank Towers (Fordham University Press, 2020). For helpful critiques regarding the tendency of continental histories to reinscribe older imperialist paradigms, see Karen Dubinsky, Adele Perry, and Henry Yu, eds., *Within and Without the Nation: Canadian History as Transnational History* (University of Toronto Press, 2015); and Matthew Brown, "The Global History of Latin America," *Journal of Global History* 10 (2015): 365–86. Most other published studies on the Great Horse Flu are cited in the body of this book.

20. As Cayton notes, "Thinking in continental terms reinforces and deepens the intellectual preoccupations of American historians." "Writing North American History," 110.

21. Statistics from Frederic Hudson, *Journalism in the United States, from 1690 to 1872* (New York: Harper & Brothers, 1872), 774–75; and Mark Wahlgren Summers, *The Press Gang: Newspapers and Politics, 1865–1878* (University of North Carolina Press, 1994), 10.

22. Summers, *Press Gang*, 20 ("any respectable" through "'exchange'"); and Hudson, *Journalism in the United States*, 774–75 ("national teachers").

23. "Jay" [pseud.], "Letter from Boston," October 28, 1872, in *Belfast (ME) Republican Journal*, October 31, 1872 ("the newspapers"); Anon. to *Times*, October 25, 1872, in "The Horse Epidemic," *Times* (UK), November 6, 1872; "The Horse Disease," *Anderson Intelligencer* (Anderson Court House, SC), December 5, 1872. For a short overview of the scholarship on the broader implications of such sources, see Heidi J. S. Tworek, "Digitized Newspapers and the Hidden Transformation of History," *American Historical Review* 129 (2024): 143–47.

24. Charles E. Rosenberg, "What Is an Epidemic: AIDS in Historical Perspective," *Daedalus* 118 (1989): 1. David Steel anticipated Rosenberg's argument; see "Plague Writing: From Boccaccio to Camus," *Journal of European Studies* 11 (1981): 106.

25. Richard J. Evans, *Death in Hamburg: Society and Politics in the Cholera Years* (1987; repr., Penguin, 2005), 567.

26. Evans, *Death in Hamburg*, 367.

CHAPTER 1

1. James Law, "Influenza in Horses," in US Commissioner of Agriculture, *Report of the Commissioner of Agriculture for 1872* (GPO, 1873), 206–18.

2. "Influenza Epizooti [*sic*]," *Vermont Phoenix* (Brattleboro), November 15, 1872; "The Horse Disease," *Tri-States Union* (Port Jervis, NY), November 15, 1872; "The Horse Epizootic," *Central City (CO) Register*, October 30, 1872.

3. Alfred W. Crosby, "Virgin Soil Epidemics as a Factor in the Aboriginal Depopulation in America," *William & Mary Quarterly* 33 (1976): 289. For reports of previous outbreaks

among Canadian horses, see D. M. M'Eachern and Andrew Smith, *The Canadian Horse and His Diseases* (Toronto: J. Campbell, 1867), 162–64; and "Influenza in Horses," *Canada Farmer*, December 15, 1873, 448. For evidence relating to the absence of large-scale equine influenza outbreaks elsewhere in the world, see "Royal Veterinary College, London," *Canada Farmer*, April 30, 1873, 145; and "Contagious Diseases in Animals," *Canada Farmer*, July 30, 1873, 262.

4. My approach here is informed by Edmund Russell, *Evolutionary History: Uniting History and Biology to Understand Life on Earth* (Cambridge University Press, 2011).

5. This section draws heavily on David Swayne, *Animal Influenza*, 2nd ed. (Wiley Blackwell, 2017); and George Dehner, *Influenza: A Century of Science and Public Health Response* (University of Pittsburgh Press, 2012), 23–29.

6. Takeshi Noda, "Native Morphology of Influenza Virions," *Frontiers in Microbiology* 2 (2011), https://www.frontiersin.org/journals/microbiology/articles/10.3389/fmicb.2011.00269.

7. Quote from "The Influenza (Flu) Virus," in Michael W. Davidson, *Molecular Expressions: Cell Biology and Microscopy Structure and Function of Cells and Viruses*, last modified November 13, 2015, https://micro.magnet.fsu.edu/cells/viruses/influenzavirus.html. See also Suzanne Clancy, "Genetics of the Influenza Virus," *Nature Education* 1 (2008): 83.

8. Dan Dou et al., "Influenza A Virus Cell Entry, Replication, Virion Assembly and Movement," *Frontiers in Immunology* 9 (2018): article 1581.

9. See, e.g., Luis P. Villareal, "Are Viruses Alive?," *Scientific American*, December 2004, 100–105; Nigel Brown and David Bhella, "Are Viruses Alive," *Microbiology Today*, May 10, 2016, https://microbiologysociety.org/publication/past-issues/what-is-life/article/are-viruses-alive-what-is-life.html; and Eugene V. Koonin and Petro Starokadomskyy, "Are Viruses Alive? The Replicator Paradigm Sheds Decisive Light on an Old but Misguided Question," *Studies in the History and Philosophy of the Biological and Biomedical Sciences* 59 (2016): 125–34.

10. The hijacking metaphor is too ubiquitous to require citation; note, too, that influenza is rather unusual in its focus on cell nuclei.

11. Nicole M. Bouvier and Peter Palese, "The Biology of Influenza Viruses," *Vaccine* 26 (2008): D50–D52; Georgia K. Atkin-Smith et al., "The Induction and Consequences of Influenza A Virus-Induced Cell Death," *Cell Death and Disease* 9 (2018): 1002.

12. US Centers for Disease Control, "Antigenic Characterization," September 17, 2024, https://www.cdc.gov/flu/php/viruses/antigenic.html?CDC_AAref_Val=https://www.cdc.gov/flu/about/professionals/antigenic.htm.

13. Denison quoted in Laurel Oldach, "Slipping Past the Proofreader" (April 10, 2020), https://www.asbmb.org/asbmb-today/science/041020/slipping-past-the-proofreader.

14. On reassortment and pandemics, see Dehner, *Influenza*, 26; and Carl Zimmer, *Planet of Viruses*, 2nd ed. (University of Chicago Press, 2015), 23. On the Great Pandemic, see Jeffery K. Taubenberger, Johan V. Hultin, and David M. Morens, "Discovery and Characterization of the 1918 Pandemic Influenza Virus in Historical Context," *Antiviral Therapy* 12 (2007): 581–91.

15. Conrad E. Heidenreich and Robert W. C. Burgar, "Native Settlement to 1847," in *Special Places: The Changing Ecosystems of the Toronto Region*, ed. Betty I. Roots, Donald A. Chant, and Conrad E. Heidenreich (Royal Canadian Institute, 1999), 63. Kahkewaquonaby described his forebears as "exempt from sickness," explaining that "contagious disorders, were unknown to them before the landing of the white man." Peter Jones, *History*

of the Ojebway Indians: With Especial Reference to Their Conversion to Christianity; with a Brief Memoir of the Writer (London: A. W. Bennett, 1861), 141.

16. Heidenreich and Burgar, "Native Settlement to 1847," 67–71; Mississaugas of the New Credit First Nation, *The History of the Mississaugas of the New Credit First Nation* (Mississaugas of the New Credit First Nation, [2018]), n.p.; Jones, *History of the Ojebway Indians*, 111–14; Peter S. Schmalz, *The Ojibwa of Southern Ontario* (University of Toronto Press, 1991), chaps. 1–4; Michael John Witgen, *An Infinity of Nations: How the Native New World Shaped Early North America* (University of Pennsylvania Press, 2012), 44, 366. Jones explained that the Mississaugas comprised the Eagle tribe of the Ojibwe. Jones, *History of the Ojebway Indians*, 138.

17. Mississaugas of the New Credit First Nation, *History of the Mississaugas of the New Credit First Nation*, n.p.; Jones, *History of the Ojebway Indians*, 71; J. M. S. Careless, *Toronto to 1918: An Illustrated History* (James Lorimer & Company and National Museum of Man, 1984), 9.

18. The fort was also known as Fort Rouillé and Fort Portneuf; James H. Marsh, "Toronto Feature: Fort Rouillé," in *The Canadian Encyclopedia*, last modified July 2, 2015, https://www.thecanadianencyclopedia.ca/en/article/toronto-feature-fort-rouille.

19. On the Revolution as "civil war," see John Graves Simcoe, *Journal of the Observations of the Queen's Rangers from the End of the Year 1777, to the Conclusion of the Late American War* (Exeter, UK: Printed for the author, [1787]), 15; Wallace Brown, *The Good Americans: The Loyalists in the American Revolution* (William Morrow, 1969), 2, 225; and Maya Jasanoff, *Liberty's Exiles: American Loyalists in the Revolutionary World* (Penguin, 2012), 9.

20. Quoted in Wallace Brown, *Good Americans*, 199. See also Wallace Brown, *Good Americans*, 192, 226–27; and Jasanoff, *Liberty's Exiles*, 8. For more on Blacks as well as slavery in Canada, see Gerald M. Craig, *Upper Canada: The Formative Years, 1784–1841* (Oxford University Press, 1963), 28–31; Tiya Miles, *Dawn of Detroit: A Chronicle of Slavery and Freedom in the City of the Straits* (New Press, 2019), 105, 147; and Afua Cooper, "Acts of Resistance: Black Men and Women Engage Slavery in Upper Canada, 1793–1803," *Ontario History* 99 (2007): 5–17.

21. Nancy Shoemaker, "A Typology of Colonialism," *Perspectives on History* 53 (2015): https://www.historians.org/perspectives-article/a-typology-of-colonialism-october-2015/; Russell to Prescott, September 21, 1797, quoted in Gwen Reimer, "British-Canada's Land Purchases, 1783–1788: A Strategic Perspective," *Ontario History* 111 (2019): 55; John Johnson to W. Claus, October 19, 1787, quoted in Reimer, "British-Canada's Land Purchases, 1783–1788," 49; Russell to Prescott, January 21, 1798, quoted in Reimer, "British-Canada's Land Purchases, 1783–1788," 55. On these purchases, see also Alan Taylor, *The Divided Ground: Indians, Settlers, and the Northern Borderlands of the American Revolution* (Vintage, 2007), 343; and Robert J. Surtees, "Land Cessions, 1763–1830," in *Aboriginal Ontario: Historical Perspectives on the First Nations*, ed. Edward S. Rogers and Donald B. Smith (Dundurn Press, 1994), 107.

22. J. Ross Robertson, *The Diary of Mrs. John Graves Simcoe* [. . .] (William Briggs, 1911), 16–17.

23. J. Simcoe to Henry Dundas, April 28, 1792, in *The Correspondence of Lieut. Governor John Graves Simcoe with Allied Documents Relating to His Administration of the Government of Upper Canada*, vol. 4: 1795–1796, coll. and ed. E. A. Cruikshank (Champlain Society, 1926), 144.

24. E. Simcoe, entries for August 4, 1793, August 11, 1793, and October 25, 1793, and editor's footnotes in Robertson, *Diary of Mrs. John Graves Simcoe*, 180, 184, 109. See also Joseph Bouchette, *The British Dominions in North America* (London: Henry Colburn and Richard Bentley, 1831), 1:93.

25. Artem Blagodatski et al., "Avian Influenza in Wild Birds and Poultry: Dissemination Pathways, Monitoring Methods, and Virus Ecology," *Pathogens* 10, no. 5 (2021): 630, https://doi.org/10.3390/pathogens10050630.

26. E. Simcoe entry for August 4, 1793, in Robertson, *Diary of Mrs. John Graves Simcoe*, 180; Ali Raza, "Simcoe's Legacy: The Names of York Region Communities," *Newmarket (ON) Era*, April 24, 2018.

27. On concessions, see William Caniff, *History of the Settlement of Upper Canada (Ontario), with Special Reference to the Bay Quinté* (Toronto: Dudley & Burns, 1869), 165; and Lillian F. Gates, *Land Policies of Upper Canada* (University of Toronto Press, 1968), 19–23. Contemporaries understood the relative affordability of Upper Canada vis-à-vis American frontier regions; see, for instance, M. Smith, "Preface of the First Edition," in *Geographical View of the Province of Upper Canada* [. . .], 3rd ed. (Philadelphia: Thomas & Robert Desilver, 1813), n.p.

28. Taylor, *Divided Ground*, 18, 26, 29; Benjamin Mortimer journal entry, May 13, 1798, in Leslie R. Gray, ed., "From Bethlehem to Fairfield—1798," *Ontario History* 46 (1954): 60. On "four-fifths," see Wallace Brown, *Good Americans*, 197. The 1791 population figure is from Taylor, *Divided Ground*, 19–20; that for 1811 is from Bouchette, *British Dominions*, 1:108.

29. Among the many items in Simcoe's correspondence addressing the capital's location, see John Simcoe to the Duke of Portland, February 27, 1796, in *Correspondence of Lieut. Governor John Graves* [. . .], vol. 4: 1795–1796, coll. and ed. Cruikshank, 201.

30. J. Simcoe quoted in F. R. Berchem, *The Yonge Street Story 1793–1860: An Account from Letters, Diaries and Newspapers* (Natural Heritage / Natural History, 1977), 7. On this expedition, see Berchem, *Yonge Street Story*, 16–21.

31. Quotes from E. Simcoe, entry for October 25, 1793, in Mary Quayle Innis, ed., *Mrs. Simcoe's Diary* (1965; repr. Macmillan, 1983), 108–9; and Berchem, *Yonge Street Story*, 7.

32. J. Simcoe quoted in Berchem, *Yonge Street Story*, 9; E. Simcoe entry for February 18, 1796, in Innis, *Mrs. Simcoe's Diary*, 174; J. Simcoe to the Duke of Portland, February 27, 1796; "Canadian Railways XXVII: The Northern Railway," *Engineering*, November 21, 1879, 389. See also Berchem, *Yonge Street Story*, 22.

33. J. Simcoe to Duke of Portland, February 27, 1796; E. Simcoe quoted in Berchem, *Yonge Street Story*, 35–36. See also Berchem, *Yonge Street Story*, 30–31, 34–35, 53–56.

34. "Introduction," in Innis, *Mrs. Simcoe's Diary*, 21–24.

35. Quoted in Committee for the History of Markham Township, *Markham 1793–1900*, ed. Isabel Champion (Markham Historical Society, 1979), 93. See also William J. Cronon, *Changes in the Land: Colonists, Indians, and the Ecology of New England* (Hill & Wang, 1983); Brian Donahue, *The Great Meadow: Farmers and the Land in Colonial Concord* (Yale University Press, 2007); and Alan Taylor, "'Wasty Ways': Stories of American Settlement," *Environmental History* 3 (1998): 291–310.

36. E. Simcoe entry for January 19, 1794, in Innis, *Mrs. Simcoe's Diary*, 213–14.

37. Robert Leslie Jones, *The History of Agriculture in Ontario 1613–1880* (University of Toronto Press, 1946), quoted in J. David Wood, *Making Ontario: Agricultural Colonization and*

Landscape Re-Creation Before the Railway (McGill-Queen's University Press, 2000), 93; Anna Brownell Jameson, *Winter Studies and Summer Rambles in Canada* (London: Saunders and Otley, 1838), 1:96.

38. *Statistics of Canada*, vol. 4, *Censuses of Canada 1665 to 1871* (Ottawa: I. B. Taylor, 1876), 83, 128.

39. "Extracts from Diary of James Lesslie," June 19, 1832, in Edith G. Firth, ed., *The Town of York, 1815–1834: A Further Collection of Documents of early Toronto* (Champlain Society, 1966), 240; Strachan to Richard Whatley, September 24, 1832, in Firth, *Town of York, 1815–1834*, 253 (first quote); *Christian Guardian*, January 30, 1833, in Firth *Town of York, 1815–1834*, 255 (second quote); Wood, *Making Ontario*, 93 (third quote); *Report of the Commission Appointed by the Sanitary Board of the City Councils, to Visit Canada, for the Investigation of the Epidemic Cholera, Prevailing in Montreal and Quebec* (Philadelphia: Mifflin & Parry, 1832), 20 (fourth quote). The same outbreak struck New York on June 26, 1832; Charles Rosenberg, *The Cholera Years: The United States in 1832, 1849, and 1866* (University of Chicago Press, 1962), 25. On the 1832 influenza outbreak, see "Influenza," *American Journal of Medical Sciences* 18 (1832): 542.

40. David Boyle, ed., *Township of Scarboro, 1796–1896* (Toronto: William Briggs, 1896), 33, 271 (first quote and "last lynx"); Berchem, *Yonge Street Story*, 42 (quote on bounties). See also Wood, *Making Ontario*, 18–19, 158; and Janet Foster, *Working for Wildlife: The Beginning of Preservation in Canada*, 2nd ed. (University of Toronto Press, 1998), 10.

41. Wallace Brown, *Good Americans*, 210–11 ("pitchfork"); Karim M. Timo, "A Sorry Tale: Natives, Settlers, and the Salmon of Lake Ontario," *Historical Journal* 59 (2016): 1025 ("half-measures"). On efforts by Mississaugas to use the provincial government to conserve fishery resources in 1798, see Berchem, *Yonge Street Story*, 48.

42. Caniff, *History of the Settlement of Upper Canada*, 594; 1803 figures from Boyle, *Township of Scarboro*, 267.

43. Caniff, *History of the Settlement of Upper Canada*, 594; 1845 figures from Boyle, *Township of Scarboro*, 292.

44. On breed improvement in the United States and Britain, see, respectively, James Westfall Thompson, *A History of Livestock Raising in the United States, 1607–1860* (US Department of Agriculture, 1942); and Harriet Ritvo, *The Animal Estate: The English and Other Creatures in the Victorian Age* (Harvard University Press, 1987).

45. William Brown, *America: A Four Years' Residence in the United States and Canada* [. . .] (Leeds, UK: William Brown, 1849), 70, 77, 86.

46. William Brown, *America*, 96.

47. Boyle, *Township of Scarboro*, 75 ("thoroughbreds"); Committee for the History of Markham Township, *Markham*, 57–59 ("Merry Farmer"); William Brown, *America*, 77 ("everything you see and hear"). On cattle types, see William Brown, *America*, 84. The township's reputation for these draft horses endured; *History of Toronto and County of York, Ontario* [. . .](Toronto: C.B. Robinson, 1885), 1:111. On horse breeds popular among Canadian importers between the 1840s and 1870s, see Margaret E. Derry, *Horses in Society: A Story of Animal Breeding and Marketing, 1800–1920* (University of Toronto Press, 2006), chap. 3.

48. *Canadian Poultry Chronicle*, n.d., reprinted as "Fowls Don't Pay," *Canada Farmer*, n.s., July 15, 1872, 235–36 ("worthless"); "Our Poultry Retrospect, 1871," *Canadian Poultry Chronicle* 2 (1872): 97 ("red man of the forest"). See also "Ottawa Agricultural Exhibition—Poultry,"

Canadian Poultry Chronicle 1 (November 1870): 71; "Large Importation of Fowls," *Canadian Poultry Chronicle* 1 (October 1870): 55.

49. George P. Burnham, *The China Fowl: Shanghae, Cochin, and "Brahma"* (Melrose, MA: George F. Burnham, 1874), 47, 50 ("pictures"), 57 ("unequaled"). See also George P. Burnham, *The History of the Hen Fever, a Humorous Record* (Boston, New York, and Philadelphia: James French, J. C. Derby, and T. B. Peterson, 1855).

50. Quotes from Ontario Agricultural Commission (OAC), *Report of the Commissioners*, vol. 2: *Appendix B, Containing Returns Relating to the Soil, Climate, Topographical Features, Cultivable Area and Products of, and the Progress and Condition of Husbandry in the Province of Ontario* (Toronto: C. Blackett Robinson, 1881) (hereafter cited as OAC, *Report*), 654–55, 658, 664–67.

51. OAC, *Report*, 2:658–66.

52. Boyle, *Township of Scarboro*, 88.

53. Boyle, *Township of Scarboro*, 88 ("demand grew"). Other quotes from Boyle, *Township of Scarboro*, 88–90; and "Report of Home District Manufactures, 1828," quoted in *Town of York, 1815–1834*, 60. On Markham's factories producing "farm implements," carriages, and wagons, see OAC, *Report*, 2:650. In a column asking what proportion of farmers in their township employed such devices, the OAC's tables listed "the whole," "all, nearly," and "all of them" for Markham, Scarborough, and York, respectively. OAC, *Report*, 2:659.

54. Catharine Anne Wilson, "A Manly Art: Plowing, Plowing Matches, and Rural Masculinity in Ontario, 1800–1930," *Canadian Historical Review* 95 (2014): 170.

55. Foster, *Working for Wildlife*, 10 (quoted); Wood, *Making Ontario*, 19; "The Game Laws," TG, May 3, 1866.

56. Justice [pseud.], "The Game Laws," TG, February 28, 1871.

CHAPTER 2

1. Simon M. Firestone et al., "Influence of Meteorology on the Spread of Influenza," *PLoS ONE* 4 (2012): e5284.

2. Susan D. Jones, *Valuing Animals: Veterinarians and Their Patients in Modern America* (Johns Hopkins University Press, 2003), 29; James Law, "Influenza in Horses," in *Report of the Commissioner of Agriculture for 1872* (GPO, 1873).

3. A prime—and problematic—example is Sean Kheraj, "The Great Epizootic of 1872–73: Networks of Animal Disease in North American Urban Environments," *Environmental History* 23 (2018): 495–521.

4. Sarah R. B. King et al., "Behavior of Horses, Zebras, and Asses," in *Wild Equines: Ecology, Management, and Conservation*, ed. Jason I. Ransom and Petra Kaczensky (Johns Hopkins University Press, 2016), 23, 31 ("group living"); Wendy Williams, *The Horse: The Epic History of Our Noble Companion* (Scientific American / Farrar, Straus and Giroux, 2015), 26–32; Peter Mitchell, *The Donkey in Human History: An Archaeological Perspective* (Oxford University Press, 2018), 24–25.

5. Williams, *Horse*, 220 ("talk"); Kosuke Nakamura, Ayaka Takimoto-Inoese, and Toshikazu Hasegawa, "Cross-Modal Perception of Human Emotion in Domestic Horses (*Equus caballus*)," *Scientific Reports* 8 (2018): 8660 ("characteristic" and "call types"). On asses, see Petronella Vaarzon-Morel, "The Silence of the Donkeys: Sensorial Entanglements Between People and Animals at Willowra," *Australian Journal of Anthropology* 32

(2001): 119, 124–25; V. Sekhar et al., "Moffett's Muted Mules: The Science of Laryngology in the Art of War," *Journal of Laryngology and Otology* 132 (2018): 957; Mitchell, *Donkey in Human History*, 25–26.

6. King et al., "Behavior of Horses, Zebras, and Asses," 24; Marta De Santis et al., "Donkey Behaviour and Cognition: A Literature Review," *Applied Animal Behaviour Science* 244 (2021): 105485 (quote).

7. King et al., "Behavior of Horses, Zebras, and Asses," 27–32; De Santis et al., "Donkey Behaviour and Cognition."

8. "Horse Epidemic," *Toronto Mail*, October 5, 1872; "Horse Epidemic," TG, October 5, 1872; "Horse Epidemic," *Toronto Mail*, October 8, 1872. Boyd likewise asserted that "nearly every horse in the district was attacked." Special dispatch from Toronto, October 25, 1872, in "The Horse Disease," CT, October 28, 1872.

9. The novel influenza virus undoubtedly spread primarily through horse-to-horse transmission, but other flu-prone species may have played some role in the outbreak's initial stages.

10. Thomas McIlwraith, *Looking for Old Ontario* (University of Toronto Press, 1997), 50, 53, 58 (quoted), 267–68.

11. Robert Gourlay, *Statistical Account of Upper Canada: Compiled with a View to a Grand System of Emigration* (London: Simpkin & Marshall, 1822), 133, 459; John Goldie, entry for June 27, 1819, in John Goldie, *Diary of a Journey Through Upper Canada and Some of the New England States* (n.p.: Privately printed, n.d.), 12; Percy J. Robinson, "Yonge Street and the North West Company," *Canadian Historical Review* 24 (1943): 253–65; Edith G. Firth, introduction to *The Town of York, 1793–1815: A Collection of Documents of Early Toronto*, ed. Edith G. Firth (Champlain Society, 1962), lii; David Boyle, ed., *Township of Scarboro, 1796–1896* (Toronto: William Briggs, 1896), 115; F. R. Berchem, *The Yonge Street Story 1793–1860: An Account from Letters, Diaries and Newspapers* (Natural Heritage / Natural History, 1977), chap. 3; Edwin C. Guillet, *Pioneer Travel in Upper Canada* (1933; repr., University of Toronto Press, 1963), 142–43.

12. *Upper Canada Gazette*, August 25, 1825, in Berchem, *Yonge Street Story*, 110 ("Light"); Berchem, *Yonge Street Story*, 115 ("the traffic"); William Brown, *America*, 75–76 ("like").

13. Henry Scadding, "Toronto of Old: A Series of Collections and Recollections," *Canadian Journal of Science, Literature and History* 12 (February 1872): 256; Henry Scadding, "Yonge Street," TG, December 26, 1871.

14. "The Useful Horse," report dated Toronto, October 8, 1872, in *Daily Constitution* (Middletown, CT), October 9, 1872 ("interruption"); *Toronto Mail*, October 9, 1872 ("poor brutes"); *Buffalo Express*, n.d., quoted in "The Epizootic Disease Among Horses," *Watertown (NY) Times*, October 24, 1872 ("carriages").

15. *Toronto Mail*, October 22, 1872 ("probably"); "Is America to Be Horseless?," *Watertown (NY) Times*, November 15, 1872 ("an air").

16. *Ontario Workman* (Toronto), October 17, 1872 ("almost daily"); "Epidemic Among Horses," NYH, October 19, 1872 ("unable"); "The Markets," *Irish Canadian* (Toronto), October 19, 1872 ("scarce" and "supply"). On Angus, see *Toronto Mail*, October 10, 1872.

17. *Montreal Gazette*, October 17, 1872, reprinted in "The Canadian Horse Epidemic," *Wheeling (WV) Intelligencer*, October 23, 1872. The outbreak's arrival was placed at October 11 in "Latest from Montreal," TG, October 15, 1872. On snow, see "Télégraphie de toutes les parties du monde," *La Minerve* (Montreal), October 16, 1872.

18. "Canadian Horse Epidemic" ("effects"); "City Items" and "The Horse Epidemic," *Montreal Herald and Commercial*, October 17, 1872 (other quotes).

19. "The Horse Epidemic," *Montreal Herald and Commercial*, October 17, 1872; *Montreal Witness*, October 18, as quoted or paraphrased in "Canada," TG, October 22, 1872; "Revue commerciale pour la semaine finissant le 23 Octobre 1872," *Le Négociant Canadien* (Montreal), October 24, 1872; Margaret Heap, "La grève des charretiers à Montréal, 1864," *Revue d'Histoire de l'Amérique Française* 31 (1977): 371–95; and Sherry Olson, "The Urban Horse and the Shaping of Montreal, 1840–1914," in *Animal Metropolis: Histories of Human-Animal Relations in Urban Canada*, ed. Joanna Dean, Darcy Ingram, and Christabelle Sethna (University of Calgary Press, 2017), 58–66.

20. "The Horse Epidemic," *Montreal Herald and Commercial*, October 17, 1872 ("resolutely"); letter from J. T. Duncan, October 24, 1872, published as "The Horse Epidemic," *Ithaca Journal*, October 28, 1872 ("the disease").

21. *Montreal Witness*, October 18, 1872, as quoted or paraphrased in "Canada," TG, October 22, 1872. On timing of first fatality, see "Epidemic Among Horses," NYH, October 19, 1872.

22. *Montreal Witness*, quoted in "Canada," TG, October 22, 1872.

23. *Le Nouveau Monde*, n.d., quoted in "L'épizootie," *Le Journal des Trois-Rivières*, October 21, 1872.

24. "Notes locales," *Le Constitutionnel* (Trois-Rivières, PQ), October 21, 1872 ("no longer"); "L'épizootie," *Le Journal des Trois-Rivières*, October 21, 1872 ("few and far").

25. *Montreal Witness*, n.d., quoted in "Canada," TG, October 22, 1872.

26. William Somerville, "The Canada Horse Epidemic," *Buffalo Commercial*, October 15, 1872.

27. Somerville, "Canada Horse Epidemic."

28. "The Canadian Horse Plague," *Lexington (MO) Intelligencer*, October 30, 1872.

29. William Caniff, *History of the Settlement of Upper Canada (Ontario), with Special Reference to the Bay Quinté* (Toronto: Dudley & Burns, 1869), 568 (emphasis added); George S. Boutwell, *Reminiscences of Sixty Years in Public Affairs* (McClure, Phillips, & Co., 1902), 2:203.

30. Allan Nevins, *Hamilton Fish: The Inner History of the Grant Administration* (Dodd Mead, 1936), 490.

31. "Equine Epidemic," HC, October 24, 1872 ("to allow"); "The Prevailing Epizootic Among Horses," *Rochester Democrat Chronicle*, October 21, 1872 ("soon after"); *Rochester Democrat Chronicle*, October 21, 1872, in "The Epizootic and How to Treat It," NYH, October 22, 1872; "Evening Summary," *Montreal Witness*, October 22, 1872. For context, see Robert Craig Brown, "Canadian Opinion After Confederation, 1867–1914," in *Canada Views the United States* (University of Washington Press, 1967).

32. *Hamilton Times*, n.d., published as "'The Canadian Horse Disease,'" *Guelph (ON) Evening Mercury*, October 26, 1872.

33. "The Horse Disease," *Buffalo Commercial*, October 21, 1872 ("nine"); "The Horse Epidemic," *Buffalo Courier Express*, October 21, 1872 ("all branches"); "The City on Foot," *Buffalo Courier Express*, October 22, 1872 ("the disease"); "The Horse Disease," *Buffalo Courier Express*, October 23, 1872 ("to walk"); "The Horse Epidemic," *Buffalo Weekly Courier*, October 30, 1872 ("seventy-five").

34. *Syracuse Daily Journal*, October 22, 1872 ("noticed"); CT, October 30, 1872; and *Philadelphia Press*, October 29, 1872. On shipments, see Adoniram B. Judson, "Report on the

Origin and Progress of the Epizootic Among Horses in 1872, with a Table of Mortality in New York [. . .]," in Board of Health of the City of New York, *Third Annual Report of the Board of Health of the Health Department of the City of New York April 11, 1872 to April 30, 1873* (New York: D. Appleton & Co., 1873), 253–59. On US horse purchases from Canada, see "The Horse Market," *New England Farmer*, May 5, 1871, n.p.

35. "The Epizootic," CEP, October 30, 1872 ("follows"); Law, "Influenza in Horses," 235; "Epizootic," *Pittsburgh Gazette*, November 2, 1872.

36. "From Niagara Falls," *Buffalo Commercial*, October 21, 1872 ("every"); "The Prevailing Epizootic Among Horses," *Rochester Democrat and Chronicle*, October 21, 1872 ("sixty").

37. "Tribunings," *Medina (NY) Tribune*, November 7, 1872 ("met"); "News Summary," *Evening Gazette* (Port Jervis, NY), November 9, 1872 ("reigns supreme"). For context, see Susan Nance, *Entertaining Elephants: Animal Agency and the Business of the American Circus* (Johns Hopkins University Press, 2013).

38. Canadian canals, by contrast, were generally large enough to accommodate self-propelled vessels. Douglas McCalla, *Planting the Province: The Economic History of Upper Canada 1784–1870* (University of Toronto Press, 1993), 127. Not until 1874 were three proprietors "granted concessions" to operate steamboats on the Erie. Alvin F. Harlow, *Old Towpaths: The Story of the American Canal Era* (D. Appleton, 1926), 325.

39. "Miscellaneous News," *Buffalo Commercial*, October 26, 1872 ("Many boats"); "Epizootic," *Ithaca Journal*, October 28, 1872.

40. "The Horse Disease," BG, October 23, 1872.

41. "Commercial Effect of the Horse Distemper," MR (St. Louis), October 26, 1872 ("prevalence"); "By Telegraph," *Lewiston (ME) Sun-Journal*, October 29, 1872 ("forwarders"). On other canals, see, e.g., "The Epidemic Among Horses," *Lewis County Democrat* (Lowville, NY), November 6, 1872; and "The Epizootic in the Mines," *Iron Age*, November 28, 1872, 3.

42. "The Horse-Epidemic," *Niagara Falls (NY) Gazette*, October 16, 1872.

43. On quarantines, see, e.g., *Norfolk Virginian*, October 26, 1872; *Wilmington (DE) Journal*, November 27, 1872. On farmers, see "The Epizootic Plague," *Plattsburgh (NY) Sentinel*, November 8, 1872. On sanitary measures, see, e.g., *Ottawa (ON) Citizen*, October 21, 1872; "The Epizootic," *Meriden (CT) Republican*, October 24, 1872; "The Horse Epidemic," BS, October 30, 1872. On Prince Edward Island, see Adoniram B. Judson, "History and Course of the Epizoötic Among Horses upon the North American Continent," *Public Health Reports and Papers Presented at the Meetings of the American Public Health Association in the Year 1873* (New York and Cambridge, MA: Hurd and Houghton and the Riverside Press, 1875), 97.

44. Virologists emphasize the deposition of droplets and fomites—particles too large to behave as aerosols—in these dynamics; Gabriele A. Landolt and Thomas M. Chambers, "The Clinical Features, Pathobiology, and Epidemiology of Influenza Infections in Horses," in *Animal Influenza*, 2nd ed., ed. David E. Swayne (Wiley Blackwell, 2017), 513.

45. "The Epizootic," NYH, October 23, 1872 ("was creating"); "The Horse Disease," *New York Evening Post*, October 23, 1872 ("at once"); *Albany Express*, October 22, in "The Canadian Horse Disease," NYT, October 23, 1872 ("symptoms"); "The Horse Disease," *New York Evening Post*, October 23, 1872 ("alarming spread"); "The Epizootic," NYH, October 23, 1872 ("great public calamity"); "The Epizootic," NYH, October 23, 1872 ("no time").

46. "Horse Disease," *Galveston Tri-Weekly News*, October 23, 1872 ("many branches"); "Hippozymosis," BE, October 26, 1872 ("want of horses"); NYH, October 29, 1872, in "Incidents of the Horse Disease in New York and Boston," *Wyandot County Republican* (Upper Sandusky, OH), November 14, 1872 ("the epizoot").

47. "The Horse Epidemic in Boston," October 23, 1872, BET ("fifteen or twenty"); "The Disease in Boston," BG, October 24, 1872 ("so rapid"); "The Disease in Boston," BG, October 25, 1872 ("public misfortune"); "The Horse Epidemic," BET, October 24, 1872 ("two horses"); "Horse Epidemic," BET, October 26, 1872 ("almost complete"); "Local Intelligence: The Horse Plague," BG, October 28, 1872 ("In future years"); "The Scenes in Washington Street," BET, October 28, 1872 ("What the horse").

48. "The Horse Epidemic," *Detroit Free Press*, October 27, 1872.

49. "The Horse Epidemic," *Illustrated Journal of Agriculture* (St. Louis), November 1, 1872, 3.

50. Anne Norton Greene, *Horses at Work: Harnessing Power in Industrial America* (Harvard University Press, 2008), 167–70; Clay McShane, *Down the Asphalt Road: The Automobile and the American City* (Columbia University Press, 1994), 48–51.

51. PI, n.d., in "Epizootic Notes," *Pittsburgh Commercial*, October 28, 1872; "Doings of the Health Board," CE, October 30, 1872.

52. Quotes from Clay McShane and Joel A. Tarr, *Horse in the City: Living Machines in the Nineteenth Century* (Johns Hopkins University Press, 2007), 107–26; and Greene, *Horses at Work*, 170–77. See also "The Horse Disease," CT, October 31, 1872.

53. McShane and Tarr, *Horse in the City*, 103–7; McShane, *Down the Asphalt Road*, 52.

54. "The Position of the Horse in Modern Society," *The Nation*, October 31, 1872, 277–78.

55. "A City Without Means of Transit," NYH, October 30, 1872 ("enough unemployed"); CEP, November 5, 1872 ("Snow blockades"). For evidence that steamboat companies failed to respond to this opportunity, see "Out of the Traces," NYH, October 31, 1872. On steam railroads, see, e.g., "Jay" [pseud.], letter dated October 28, 1872, in "Letter from Boston," *Belfast (ME) Republican Journal*, October 31, 1872; and "Our Chevalric Sufferers," CEP, November 6, 1872.

56. "Epizootism," *Brooklyn Union*, October 30, 1872; "Steam Road Wagon," CEM, November 14, 1872; "The Unharnessed Horse," CEP, November 9, 1872. For more on dummies, see "Hipporhinorrhea," NYH, October 30, 1872; "Nambuat" [pseud.], November 12, 1872, in "Our American Letter," *Isle of Man Weekly Times* (Douglas, UK), December 28, 1872; "City Steam Cars," NYH, November 15, 1872; and Debra Brill, *History of the J. G. Brill Company* (University of Indiana Press, 2001), 15. On lifting such bans, see, e.g., "Hipporhinorrhea," NYH, October 30, 1872; "Our City Government," PI, November 1, 1872; "Hipporhinorrhea," CEP, November 2, 1872.

57. "The Horses in Baltimore to Have a Rest," NYH, November 3, 1872; "Local Matters," BS, November 7, 1872. On fifteen cents in Philadelphia, see "Plague Swept," PI, November 5, 1872. On twenty-five cents in Boston, see Browne [pseud.], letter dated October 29, 1872, in "Our Boston Letter," *Titusville (PA) Herald*, November 1, 1872.

58. "The Epidemic and Its Effect," *Buffalo Express*, n.d., in "The Horse Disease," *Titusville Herald*, October 24, 1872 ("radical change"); "The Epizootic," CEP, November 1, 1872 ("By pedestrianism"); "The Epizootic," *Summit County Beacon* (Akron, OH), November 20,

1872 ("People who"). On the difficulties faced by "the infirm," see "Hipporhinorrhea," NYH, October 30, 1872.

59. "'Quid Rides'?," *Raleigh News*, November 19, 1872; "Home Matters," *Troy (NY) Weekly Times*, November 2, 1872 ("large number"); Jay Bee [pseud.], "Epizooty," *Lebanon (PA) News*, November 19, 1872 ("Oh, epizoot"); "Jay" [pseud.], letter dated October 28, 1872, in "Letter from Boston," *Belfast (ME) Republican Journal*, October 31, 1872 ("singular trial").

60. On steam traction, see Anon., November 9, 1872, in "Letter from Washington," BS, November 9, 1872; Max [pseud.], n.d., in "Letter from Cincinnati," *Ottawa County News* (Port Clinton, OH), January 3, 1873; "Steam Power vs. Horse Power," BG, July 7, 1873.

61. "The Horse Epidemic," BET, October 24, 1872; "Household Marketing," BET, October 30, 1872; "The Extent of the Horse Epidemic," BET, October 26, 1872; "The Sick Horses," BG, October 30, 1872. On mail and police, see "The Horse Epidemic," BET, October 28, 1872; "The Police in a New Role," BET, October 30, 1872. See also "The Horse Disease," *Massachusetts Ploughman and New England Journal of Agriculture*, November 2, 1872, 32.

62. Anon. letter, November 5, 1872, in "From Chicago," *Topeka Commonwealth*, November 9, 1872 ("On every hand"); "Local Matters," BS, November 7, 1872; "Plague Swept," PI, November 5, 1872.

63. Undated letter quoted in "A Novel Team," *Muscatine (IA) Evening Journal*, November 15, 1872 ("steady Dutchmen"); "The Epizootic Catarrh—Again," *Richmond (VA) Dispatch*, November 13, 1872 ("loaded"); "Thirty Cents for Coal," *Pittsburgh Post*, November 16, 1872 ("stalwart"); "Lady Coal Haulers," *Pittsburgh Post*, November 16, 1872 ("several women").

64. "Pachydermatous Paragraphs," *Pittsburgh Weekly Gazette*, November 8, 1872 ("white stags"); "New York," BG, October 29, 1872 ("only solution"). On replacing horses with mules, see "The Afflicted Brutes," PI, November 2, 1872. On mules succumbing, see "Philadelphia and Its Suburbs," PI, November 7, 1872; "The Epizootic," NYH, November 8, 1872. On dogs, see "The Horse Epidemic," BS, November 4, 1872; "The Horse," CEP, November 8, 1872; "Letter from Portsmouth," *Cincinnati Inquirer*, December 4, 1872; "Fido," *Terre Haute Evening Gazette*, December 30, 1872. Ontario newspapers made no mention of oxen as replacements for horses stricken by the Great Horse Flu; when Québecois finally began introducing the bovines, they credited Americans as their inspiration. *Evenement*, n.d., in "Quebec," *La Minerve* (Montreal), November 2, 1872.

65. "The Horse Epidemic," *Buffalo Commercial*, October 26, 1872 ("primeval method"); "Fractional Currency," *The Chronicle* (Chicago), October 31, 1872, 279 ("multitude" and "bucolic"); "The Horse Disease," CT, October 29, 1872 ("sensation"); "Out of the Traces," NYH, October 31, 1872 ("each caravan").

66. Notice from B. G. Eastman, October 27, 1872, in "Equine Influenza," NYH, October 28, 1872; "Hipporhinorrhea," NYH, October 30, 1872.

67. "Out of the Traces"; "The Horse Epidemic," *Illustrated Journal of Agriculture* (St. Louis) 2, November 1, 1872, 3 ("sent"); "Lightning Flashes," *Salt Lake Herald-Republican*, November 19, 1872 ("carrying off").

68. "Horse Epidemic," BET, October 26, 1872; "Epizootic Incidents," *United States Club Advertiser*, November 21, 1872, 4; "Sidewalk Notes," *Nashville Republican Banner*, January 22, 1873.

69. "The Provoking Plague," CEP, November 5, 1872 ("demand for trained steers"); *New York Turf*, n.d., in *Canada Farmer*, November 15, 1872, 409 ("duly thankful"); "The

Epizootic," NYH, November 8, 1872 ("travelled"); "Our Equine Patients," CT, November 12, 1872. Price from "From Chicago," *Topeka Commonwealth*, November 9, 1872.

70. T. P. Wilson, "The Horse and Civilization," *Phrenological Journal* 56 (1873): 127; "The Horse Plague," BG, November 1, 1872. See also "Our Equine Patients"; *Pittsburgh Post*, November 30, 1872. On wooden paving, see Carl Abbott, "Plank Roads and Wood-Block Pavements," *Journal of Forest History* 25 (1981): 216–18.

71. "The Horse," CEP, November 8, 1872 ("curious crowds"); "A Week Without Horses," CT, November 10, 1872 ("a corps" and "steam-driven blasts"); R. [pseud.], December 2, 1872, in "Correspondence," BG, December 9, 1872. In addition to adapting to paved streets, oxen also had to adjust to drawing vehicles that had been built to equine rather than bovine specifications. "The Epizootic," *Petersburg (VA) Progress-Index*, November 9, 1872. For more on blacksmithing and oxen in other places, see P. P. Sibley to the *Boston Journal*, n.d., quoted in "Our Equine Patients"; "Our Patient Toilers," PI, November 6, 1872; and "Pachydermatous Paragraphs," *Pittsburgh Weekly Gazette*, November 8, 1872.

72. "Epizootic," *Tri-States Union* (Port Jervis, NY), November 16, 1872 ("get balky"); "Exit Episooty," PI, November 9, 1872 ("go into"); *Montgomery Advertiser*, December 5, 1872 ("run away").

73. "The Epizooty," *Nashville Union and American*, November 20, 1872.

74. C. [pseud.], November 7, 1872, in "Chicago," *Summit County Beacon* (Akron, OH), November 20, 1872 ("good number"); "The Provoking Plague," CEP, November 5, 1872 ("The number"); "The Chevalric Sufferer," CEP, November 6, 1872; "A Week Without Horses," CT, November 10, 1872 ("some fun"); Edwin Lee Brown, report of Illinois Humane Society for week ending November 16, 1872, in "The Horses," CT, November 17, 1872.

75. Quotes from "The Horses," CT, November 8, 1872. On commands, see "Week Without Horses." These same commands remain in use today throughout the world.

76. "Out of the Traces," NYH, October 31, 1872 ("the idea"); R. [pseud.], November 25, 1872, in "Correspondence," BG, December 2, 1872 ("interfered"). On oxen on canals, see "Brief Mentions," *Schenectady Reflector*, November 14, 1872.

77. "The Horses," CT, November 8, 1872; "Oxen in Favor," *Alton (IL) Telegraph*, December 13, 1872.

CHAPTER 3

1. All quotations in this and following paragraphs from Charley Bucephalus [pseud.], January 20, 1872, in "A Horse's Letter," trans. T. DeWitt Talmage, *Brooklyn Union*, February 6, 1872.

2. A[nna] Sewell, *Black Beauty, His Grooms and Companions: The "Uncle Tom's Cabin" of the Horse* (Boston: Lothrop Company, 1890). For context, see Adrienne E. Gavin, *Dark Horse: A Life of Anna Sewell* (Sutton, 2004); Gina M. Dorré, *Victorian Fiction and the Cult of the Horse* (Routledge, 2006).

3. Matthew Scully, *Dominion: The Power of Man, the Suffering of Animals, and the Call to Mercy* (St. Martin's, 2002).

4. "Our Dear Friend, the Horse," CT, October 26, 1872.

5. On the Paris Commune, see Gay L. Gullickson, *Unruly Women of Paris* (Cornell University Press, 1996); Patrick C. Jamieson, "Foreign Criticisms of the 1871 Paris Commune:

The Role of British and American Newspapers and Periodicals," *Intersections* 11 (2010): 113; and J. Michelle Coghlan, *Sensational Internationalism* (Edinburgh University Press, 2016).

6. "The New Horse Distemper," *New York Sun*, November 16, 1872 ("deeply depressed"); "Evanston," CT, December 6, 1872; "Death of a Valuable Horse," *Alexandria (VA) Gazette*, September 8, 1873. These burial honors hint at growing concerns about animal death and its theological implications; see, e.g., Joseph Hamilton, *Animal Futurity: A Plea for the Immortality of Brutes* (Belfast: C. Aitchison, 1877).

7. "Overworked and Overdosed," *Ottawa Citizen*, October 31, 1872; "Epizootic Brevities," MR, December 17, 1872; Mastodon [pseud.], December 6, 1872, in *New Bloomfield (PA) Times*, December 10, 1872; "Odds and Ends," *Portland (ME) Press Herald*, November 6, 1872. On abandoned horses, see "Philadelphia and Suburbs," PI, November 7, 1872.

8. "The Horse Disease," *Pittsburgh Post*, November 16, 1872; "Local Intelligence," *Wheeling Register*, November 22, 1872; *Galveston News*, December 17, 1872 ("stomach"); "Poisoning the Water," *Pittsburgh Post*, November 22, 1872.

9. "Removing Offal," BE, November 4, 1872; "Our Patient Toilers," PI, November 6, 1872 ("unwelcome thought"); "Malignant Epizootic," *Westminster (MD) Democratic Advocate*, November 23, 1872 ("bone yards" and "brisk business"); "General Intelligence," *Magnolia (MS) Gazette*, December 14, 1872; *Indianapolis Journal*, December 19, 1872; "'An Ill Wind That Blows Nobody Good,'" *Detroit Free Press*, November 24, 1872. Chicago leaders offered free disposal to that city's neediest residents after the price for hauling dead horses rose to five dollars; "The Horse," CEP, November 8, 1872.

10. *Scientific American*, n.d., in "What Becomes of a Dead Horse," *Western Rural*, February 18, 1871, 58.

11. "State News," *Bangor Whig and Courier*, December 11, 1872 ("valuable horse"); "Death and the Horse," CE, November 21, 1872 ("Fertilizing Company's stable"); "Diagnosis of the Horse Epidemic," *Leavenworth (KS) Commercial*, November 13, 1872 ("attached"). Another postmortem conducted by nonexperts, this one on Star, the same Virginia stallion whose mane was distributed to mourners as a keepsake, revealed that his "diaphragm was . . . inflamed and perforated like a seive [*sic*]." "Death of a Valuable Horse," *Alexandria (VA) Gazette*, September 8, 1873.

12. "The Horse Disease," *Buffalo Courier Express*, October 23, 1872.

13. J. Worth Estes, "Dropsy," in *The Cambridge World History of Human Disease*, ed. Kenneth F. Kiple (Cambridge University Press, 1993), 689–96.

14. "Local Matters," BS, November 7, 1872.

15. James Law, *Ithaca Journal*, n.d., in "The Epizootic," *Rochester Democrat and Chronicle*, October 28, 1872 ("epiglottic"); "The Epizootic," *Rochester Democrat and Chronicle*, October 28, 1872 ("present epizootic").

16. "Sanitary Measures," NYT, October 31, 1872 ("taken"); "Caution," *Lebanon (PA) News*, November 12, 1872; "Hippo-Malaria," NYH, October 29, 1872 ("prevent"). For early human cases, see "The Horse Epidemic," *Buffalo Courier Express*, October 25, 1872; "The Disease in Boston," PI, October 28, 1872; *Albany Express*, n.d., in "Shorts," *Saratogian* (Saratoga Springs, NY), October 28, 1872. Other authorities, meanwhile, raised the alarm about "the nearly simultaneous appearance of influenza and cholera." "The Noble Horse," *Reading Times*, November 1, 1872.

17. "Local Brevities," *Scranton Republican*, November 20, 1872; CT, November 19, 1872. On antelope, see "Curious Turn of the Epizootic," *Colorado Miner* (Georgetown), January

9, 1873; "Roundabout," *Leavenworth Commercial*, January 19, 1873; and *Kansas Democrat* (Oswego), February 7, 1873. On raccoons and opossums, see "Far South," *Wilmington (NC) Morning Star*, December 6, 1872; "News in Brief," *Memphis Avalanche*, December 12, 1872. On prairie chickens, see "State News," *Salt Lake Herald-Republican*, December 28, 1872. On zoo animals, see "The News of the Week," *Wilmington (OH) Journal*, November 21, 1872. On the rhino, see "News Summary," BE, November 19, 1872; "Live Topics About Town," *New York Sun*, November 19, 1872; ad for G. F. Bailey & Co., *New York Sun*, November 20, 1872.

18. *Galt (ON) Reporter*, n.d., in "Clippings," *Bowmanville (ON) Merchant*, November 29, 1872; *Luzerne Union* (Wilkes-Barre, PA), December 25, 1872. For other early reports of bovine cases, see "Cows Afflicted," *Ithaca Journal*, October 30, 1872; "Brief Local Items," BG, November 1, 1872.

19. "Epizootic," *Newmarket (ON) Era*, December 6, 1872; "Meeting of the Union Medical Association," *Saratogian* (NY), November 29, 1872. On the first mentioned case, see also *Catskill (NY) Recorder*, November 22, 1872; and "Poisoned by the Horse Distemper," *Port Jervis (NY) Evening Gazette*, November 23, 1872.

20. "Neighborhood News," *Cambridge City (IN) Tribune*, June 19, 1873 ("human epizootic"); "Local News," *Muscatine (IA) Weekly Journal*, December 13, 1872 ("coughing"); "Mere Mentions," *Sioux City Journal*, December 14, 1872 ("barking"); "The Human Epizootic or Influenza," *Georgia Weekly Telegraph, Journal and Messenger* (Macon), December 24, 1872 ("enlargement" through "or two"); "Illinois," CEP, January 18, 1873 ("painfully stiff"); "A New Disease," *Detroit Free Press*, January 23, 1873 ("sudden prostration"); Border [pseud.], "Orland Items," *Steuben (IN) Republican*, January 29, 1873 ("chills" to "back"); "The Horse Disease," *Carson City (NV) Appeal*, March 1, 1873 ("restlessness" through "sleeplessness"). For claims that epizootic preceded human cases, see, e.g., "The Epizootic," *Sedalia (MO) Democrat*, December 9, 1872; and *Pickens County Herald and West Alabamian* (Carrollton), January 29, 1873. For one exception, see "Got It," *Idaho World* (Idaho City), January 23, 1873. Claims of localized upswings include "News in Brief," *Memphis Avalanche*, November 29, 1872; "Brevities," *Pittsburgh Weekly Gazette*, December 6, 1872; "Local Intelligence," *Weston (WV) Democrat*, December 9, 1872.

21. "Brevities," *Port Huron (MI) Times Herald*, February 14, 1873; "California Locals," *Monongahela Valley Republican* (Monongahela, PA), December 26, 1872; "Epidemic Influenza," *Vermont Journal* (Windsor), March 1, 1873; "Sick of the Epizootic," *Wilmington (DE) News Journal*, December 23, 1872; *Georgetown (DE) Journal*, n.d., in "State Items," *Wilmington (DE) Commercial*, January 6, 1873; "Human Epizootic," *Lexington (MO) Intelligencer*, January 15, 1873. On the continuity of "epizootic," see Blind Pig and the Acorn, "Epizootic and Palpeetus of the Punk," February 21, 2018, https://blindpigandtheacorn.com/epizootic-and-palpeetus-of-the-punk/.

22. "Cut 'Em Shorts," *Minneapolis Star Tribune*, November 26, 1872; Charles Darwin, *The Descent of Man, and Selection in Relation to Sex* (New York: D. Appleton & Co., 1871), 1:11; "Citizens Suddenly and Singularly Affected," *Pioche (NV) Record*, February 1, 1873. One Illinois editor summed up his case for atmospheric causation; after asserting that "turkeys, chickens, geese, dogs, and even men, are having the epizo-otic, in this vicinity," he declared that the malady "is in the air." "Marseilles," *Ottawa (IL) Free Trader*, November 30, 1872. Contagionists, meanwhile, argued that species divides did little or nothing to prevent disease-causing agents from jumping from horses to humans, as when an Indiana paper quipped that "County Clerk Wallace is suffering fearfully with the epizootic,

contracted, as is supposed, from one of those fast nags that he drives so gracefully." "City Brevities," *Indianapolis Journal*, December 24, 1872 ("County Clerk")

23. Private letter from anon. to editor, October 28, 1872, in "The Epizootic in Montreal," *Burlington (VT) Free Press*, October 30, 1872. See also Everett B. Miller, "Private Veterinary Colleges in the United States, 1852–1927," *Journal of the American Veterinary Medical Association* 178 (1981): 584.

24. G. A. Hall, MS, "Epizootic Pathology and Homeopathic Treatment," *CEP*, November 23, 1872; "Veterinary Colleges," *Nebraska Advertiser* (Brownville, NE), January 9, 1873.

25. *CEP*, November 21, 1872; "The Horse Disease," *Scranton (PA) Republican*, October 30, 1872; "Dead and Dying," *CE*, November 20, 1872; "Just the Man for the Times," *Herkimer (NY) Democrat and Little Falls Gazette*, November 6, 1872. In Janesville, Wisconsin, Dr. J. B. Whiting, "an accomplished gentleman and one of the best physicians in the State," had likewise "examined quite a number of epizootic cases." "The Epizootic All Around Us," *Wisconsin State Journal* (Madison), November 20, 1872.

26. Hall, "Epizootic Pathology and Homeopathic Treatment."

27. Anonymous to Mayor of Rochester, October 24, 1872, in *Rochester Union*, n.d., in "New Cure for the Horse Distemper," *Oswego (NY) Palladium*, October 30, 1872; "The Horse Disease," *American Farmers Advocate* 1 (November 1872): 9; *Wilmington (DE) Journal*, November 27, 1872.

28. Letter dated October 25, 1872, in "The Horse Epidemic," *Times* (UK), November 6, 1872; *Rochester Democrat*, October 21, 1872. Mink's piece was subsequently republished, either in whole or in part, in "The Epizootic and How to Treat It," *NYH*, October 22, 1872; "The Epizootic Disease Among Horses," *Watertown (NY) Times*, October 24, 1872; "The Canada Horse Disease," *Troy (NY) Weekly Times*, October 25, 1872; "The Epizootic," *Malone (NY) Palladium*, October 30, 1872; "The Horse Disease," *Watertown (NY) Re-Union*, October 31, 1872; "The Horse Disease," *American Farmer and Rural Register* 1 (November 1872): 403; "The Horse Disease," *Moore's Rural New Yorker*, n.d., in "The Horse Disease," *American Farmers Advocate* 1 (November 1872): 9. Mink had previously published on influenza; e.g., E. Mink, "Influenza or Epizootic Catarrh," *American Farmer and School Visitor*, March 1, 1869, 69. A circular from General Roberts of the US Army and pointers from Robert Bonner, Irish-born publisher of the *New York Ledger* and perhaps the most famous trotting horse enthusiast on the continent, also made the rounds; see, e.g., "Hippozymosis," *BE*, October 26, 1872; "Epizootic Spreading," *Winchester (TN) Home Journal*, November 21, 1872; "Ep," *Bolivar (TN) Bulletin*, December 6, 1872; "Local," *Las Cruces (NM) Borderer*, December 7, 1872; "Hippozymosis," *BE*, October 26, 1872; "The Horse Disease," *American Farmers Advocate* 1 (November 1872): 9; "Gen. Roberts on the Horse Disease," *Salt Lake Herald-Republican*, January 19, 1873. "The newspapers," another correspondent concurred, "have had the disease as badly as the beasts themselves." "Jay" [pseud.], October 28, 1872, in "Letter from Boston," *Belfast (ME) Republican Journal*, October 31, 1872.

29. Ad, *CT*, November 10, 1872; ad in *Saratoga Springs (NY) Saratogian*, November 13, 1872; ad in *Troy (NY) Weekly Times*, November 30, 1872.

30. David P. Steensm and Robert A. Kyle, "Charles Fletcher, the Centaur Company, and Proprietary Medicine Revenue Stamps," *Mayo Clinic Proceedings* 92 (2017): e127; "The Horse Epidemic," *Wilmington (DE) Gazette*, October 29; "The Terrible Horse Disease," *Buffalo Weekly Courier*, October 30, 1872; "The Terrible Horse Disease," *The Independent* (New York), October 31, 1872; "The Terrible Horse Disease," *Chicago Inter Ocean*, November 6, 1872; "The Horse Epidemic," *The Independent* (New York), November 14, 1872.

31. *Berlin (WI) Courant*, n.d., in "Wisconsin Items," *Wisconsin State Journal* (Madison), November 26, 1872; *Boston Advertiser*, n.d., in "The Horse Disease," *Burlington (VT) Free Press*, November 4, 1872; CT, n.d., quoted in "A Run on Asafoetida," *Indianapolis News*, December 18, 1872. See also O. W. Gray, *Classified Business Directory—City of Chicago*, in *Gray's Atlas of the United States* (1873), 2–3.

32. "Round Abouts," *Nodaway Democrat* (Maryville, MO), December 26, 1872; "General News," *Seneca (KS) Courier-Tribune*, November 29, 1872 ("two hundred"); "The Epizootic," *Dunn County News* (Menominie, WI), December 7, 1872 ("some"); N. H. Paaren, letter to the editor, [November 8, 1872], in "Ready-Made Doctors," CEP, November 9, 1872.

33. Paaren, letter to the editor, [November 8, 1872].

34. "Influenza in Horses," *Canada Farmer*, January 1, 1868, 6; Smith quoted or paraphrased in "The Horse Epidemic," *Montreal Herald and Daily Commercial*, October 16, 1872.

35. "Épizotie [sic]," *La Minerve* (Montreal), October 19, 1872; "An Epizootic," *Bowmanville (ON) Merchant*, October 11, 1872.

36. W. T. Boyd, October 25, 1872, published in "The Horse Disease," CT, October 26, 1872; "The Horse Disease," *Ontario Workman*, October 24, 1872.

37. J. B. Johnson, "The Horse Disease," *Port Tobacco Times and Charles County Advertiser* (Port Tobacco, MD), November 22, 1872 ("bleeding"); W. Horne, "Epizootic," *Cultivator and Country Gentleman*, October 21, 1875, 667 ("very large"); J. S. McKenzie, "The Horse Disease," CT, October 26, 1872 ("reliance"); M. D. [pseud.], "Epizooty," *Bucyrus (OH) Telegraph-Forum*, November 30, 1872 ("no need"). This finding aligns with John Harley Warner, *The Therapeutic Perspective: Medical Practice, Knowledge, and Identity in America, 1820–1885* (Princeton University Press, 1997), 5, 125, 177, 209–19.

38. Letter from Cincinnati, December 2, in "Correspondence," BG, December 9, 1872; A. F. Cooper, *Manual of Veterinary Specific Homœopathy* (San Francisco: Cubery and Company, 1868), 4; F. A. Gunther, *New Manual of Homœopathic Veterinary Medicine, or, The Homœopathic Treatment of the Horse, the Ox, the Sheep, the Dog, and Other Domestic Animals*, 2nd American ed. (Otis Clapp, 1856), 19–23, 166; NYT, n.d., quoted in "The Epizootic," *Mineral Point (WI) Weekly Tribune*, November 7, 1872 ("less frequent"); Common Sense [pseud.], "The Horse Disease," *Troy (NY) Weekly Times*, November 9, 1872 (emphasis in original). The two most widely prescribed medicines for epizootic-afflicted equines by allopaths and homeopaths alike seem to have been aconite (a widely used, highly toxic analgesic made from wolfsbane and related plants) and belladonna (also known as poisonous nightshade, commonly used to treat pain and swelling).

39. "The Epizootic," CEP, November 1, 1872; letter from anon., November 17, 1872, in "Epizootic," *Nebraska State Journal* (Lincoln), November 22, 1872 (emphasis in original). For concurrence, see *Forest Republican* (Tionesta, PA), November 5, 1872; "The Horse Disease," *Reading (PA) Times*, November 7, 1872; "The Horse Disease," *West-Jersey Pioneer* (Bridgeton, NJ), November 8, 1872; "The Epihippic," *Raleigh News*, November 15, 1872; "The Horses," *Vergennes (VT) Enterprise and Vermonter*, November 15, 1872; "The Epizooty," *Point Pleasant (WV) Weekly Register*, December 5, 1872.

40. "Our Dear Friend, the Horse," CT, October 26, 1872.

41. "Lessons of the Horse Malady," ODA 5 (November 1872): 248 ("lessons"); "The Epizootic Disease," ODA 5 (December 1872): 256 ("awaken").

42. "Our Treatment of the Horse," HC, November 2, 1872.

43. "The Horse Disease," *New York Evening Post*, October 23, 1872; "From Chicago," *Topeka Commonwealth*, November 9, 1872.

44. "The Canadian Horse Disease," *Prairie Farmer* (Chicago), November 2, 1872; J. [pseud.], "Letter from Boston," dated October 28, 1872, in *Belfast (ME) Republican Journal*, October 31, 1872. The *Louisville Courier-Post's* New York correspondent described "the coughing and straining" of the sick animals he observed at several horsecar stables as "being most painful to look at." "A Horseless City," *Louisville (KY) Courier-Journal*, October 29, 1872.

45. "Dead and Dying," CE, November 20, 1872; "Epizooty Notes," *Saratogian* (Saratoga Springs, NY), November 16, 1872; *Fall River (MA) Evening News*, November 23, 1872 ("valuable young horse"); "Scarlatina Among Horses," CE, December 7, 1872 ("some of the cases"). See also "The Horse," *Memphis Appeal*, November 24, 1872. See also "Death of a Fine Horse," *Fort Scott (KS) Monitor*, March 2, 1873.

46. "Henry Bergh," *Scientific American*, March 24, 1888, 176; Lewis Gompertz, *Fragments in Defence of Animals, and Essays on Morals, Souls and Future State* [. . .] (W. Horsell, 1852), 174–75; Harriet Ritvo, *The Animal Estate: The English and Other Creatures in the Victorian Age* (Harvard University Press, 1987), 126–30. Some rural folks were also wise to the anticruelty movement; see, e.g., "Farmer's Club Read Our Paper," *ODA* 5 (December 1872): 260; and *Pottsville (PA) Miners Journal*, n.d., quoted in "Epizootic," *Sunbury (PA) American*, November 16, 1872.

47. "The Horse Disease," NYH, October 24, 1872 ("downright cruelty"); "Equine Influenza," NYH, October 28, 1872 ("rich"); "Hippo-Malaria," NYH, October 29, 1872 ("public feeling").

48. "A City Without Means of Transit," NYH, October 30, 1872 ("with an eye to their profits"); "Equine Influenza" ("the horses who are left").

49. "Equine Influenza."

50. "Horses in Town and Country," *New York Evening Post*, October 24, 1872.

51. "Hipporhinorrhea," NYH, October 30, 1872. That same day, Bergh justified his campaign to another transit president by asserting that "human and Divine law forbid the infliction of greater suffering on creatures already sick and diseased." "Out of the Traces," NYH, October 31, 1872.

52. "Henry Bergh on the Horse Disease," SFC, November 6, 1872.

53. "Stretched in the Straw," NYH, November 2, 1872 ("Mr. Bergh's"); "The Horse Disease," CT, October 31, 1872 ("sued"). On fatalities on the Third Avenue, see "The Epihippic Ending," NYH, November 3, 1872.

54. "Hipporhinorrhea," NYH, October 30, 1872; "Stretched in the Straw." For Bergh's response, see "The Sabbath of the Steeds," NYH, November 4, 1872.

55. "The Horse Disease," BG, October 26, 1872 ("daily bread"); "Hipporhinorrhea," NYH, October 30, 1872 ("owned by the poor"). On earning opportunities, see "A Horseless City," *Louisville Courier-Journal*, October 29, 1872.

56. "Tombs Police Court," NYH, October 29, 1872.

57. "Tombs Police Court" ("repent"); "Hipporhinorrhea," NYH, October 30, 1872 ("poor carter").

58. "The Horse Disease," MR (St. Louis), November 3, 1872.

59. "Overloading Cars," PI, November 19, 1872; "S.P.C.A.," PI, February 21, 1873. On humanitarians in other cities, see, e.g., James S. Branson to the editor, n.d., in "The Horse Disease," CT, October 31, 1872; "The Horse Disease," CEM, November 9, 1872; "The Epizootic Plague," *Plattsburgh (NY) Sentinel*, November 8, 1872 (on Washington, DC). In towns lacking SPCAs, municipal governments sometimes enacted regulations

empowering existing police forces to remove equines who displayed especially nasty signs of influenza from the streets. See, e.g., "Convalescent," *Pittsburgh Weekly Gazette*, November 15, 1872; "Local Briefs," *Raleigh News*, November 9, 1872; *Wilmington (NC) Journal*, November 27, 1872. Newspaper editors in many places implored readers to voluntarily withdraw their horses from labor. See *Republican Banner* (Nashville, TN), November 16, 1872; "The Epizooty," *Nashville Union and American*, November 22, 1872; and *Pottsville (PA) Miners Journal*, n.d., in "Epizootic," *Sunbury (PA) American*, November 16, 1872.

60. "The Hippo-Dropsy," NYH, November 18, 1872. The same account estimated that only 2 percent of horses overall developed dropsy. On the importance of rest in preventing dropsy, see "The Horse Disease," NYH, November 13, 1872; "The Horse," CEP, November 18, 1872. For evidence Americans were heeding the rest cure, see "The Horse Distemper," *Portland (ME) Press*, October 30, 1872; *Luzerne Union* (Wilkes-Barre, PA), November 20, 1872; "The Horse Epidemic," BS, November 5, 1872; and "The Noble Horse," CEM, November 7, 1872.

61. "The Metropolitan Horse-Railroad Versus Our Society," *ODA* 5 (December, 1872): 256–57.

CHAPTER 4

1. "Incidents of the Great Fire," *Youth's Companion*, December 5, 1872, 394.

2. Louisa May Alcott to Anna Alcott Pratt, [November 10, 1872], in *The Selected Letters of Louisa May Alcott*, ed. Joel Myerson and Daniel Shealy (Little, Brown, 1987), 170 ("so great"); C. A. Barton, *The Trial by Fire: A Sermon Preached in the West Church, Boston, Sunday, November 17, 1872* (Boston: Alfred Mudge & Son, 1872), 6 ("at twenty"); Carleton [pseud.], *The Story of the Great Fire, Boston, November 9–10, 1872* (Boston: Shepard and Gill, 1872), 22 ("visible"); H. E. Cole to Chief Signal Officer of the Army, November 13, 1872, reprinted in "The Boston Fire," *Army and Navy Journal* 10 (November 30, 1872), 247 ("flock"); William Burt testimony, *Report of the Commissioners Appointed to Investigate the Cause and Management of the Great Fire in Boston* (Boston: Rockwell & Churchill, 1873) (hereafter cited as RC), 393 ("so high"). For claims that the fire was visible fifty and sixty miles inland, see Russell H. Conwell, *History of the Great Fire in Boston November 9 and 10, 1872* (Boston: B. B. Russell, 1873), 81.

3. Carleton, *Story of the Great Fire*, 58 ("granite"); Sylvester Baxter, "A Reporter's Memories of Boston's Great Fire," *Boston Herald*, October 21, 1922; Alcott to Pratt, [November 10, 1872], in *Selected Letters of Louisa May Alcott*, 170.

4. John Damrell testimony, RC, 95; William Greenough testimony, RC, 307–9; Burt testimony, RC, 392–93; "Our Old Vets," BG, September 13, 1887. On subsequent explosions, see RC, xiv.

5. Quotes from "Ten Months After the Fire," BG, September 19, 1873; and "The Great Calamity! Vivid Pen Photographs," BG, November 12, 1872. On firefighters, see Austin Abbott, "Scenes at the Boston Fire," *Illustrated Christian Weekly*, November 30, 1872, 578; "Nearly 100 Fire Companies Fought the Great Boston Fire 30 Years Ago Today," BG, November 9, 1902; and "How the Great Boston Fire Was Fought," BG, November 10, 1912.

6. "The Boston Fire," *Harper's Weekly*, November 30, 1872, 934 (first and final quotes); "The Third Day," BG, November 13, 1872 ("so effectually").

7. Body counts varied. After the blaze's first anniversary, the *Globe* claimed that a dozen were killed and nineteen injured; "A Year's Progress," BG, November 11, 1873. Gas explosions and resulting fires killed an additional two. RC, xiv. Decades later, *Globe* articles

placed the body count at fourteen, including seven enrolled firemen and three volunteers and three veteran firefighters who were engaging in battling the blaze. See "How the Great Boston Fire Was Fought." On the number displaced, see "The Boston Fire," *Salt Lake Herald-Republican*, November 16, 1872. By the early 1870s, real estate development south of the Shawmut Peninsula had resulted in the construction of a neighborhood several miles away from downtown Boston that was already coming to be known as the South End. That area assumed the name that had previously applied to an older neighborhood south of Boston's core. As the place-name migrated, this former residential district lost its name. In the absence of an alternative, I refer to it simply as the "former South End."

8. "The Boston Fire," *Salt Lake Herald-Republican*, November 16, 1872. See also *RC*, iii, xiv; "Insurance Losses by the Boston Fire," *Independent*, February 6, 1873, 186; "The Boston Fire," *United States Club Advertiser*, December 5, 1872, 8; "The Ruins," *BG*, November 15, 1872. For comparisons to Chicago, see James M. Bugbee, "Fires and Fire Departments," *North American Review* 117 (July 1873): 131. For a listing of great nineteenth-century fires that shows the 1872 Boston blaze as exceeding any but the 1871 Chicago fire, see "Other Great Fires in the United States," *SFC*, July 15, 1874.

9. *CT*, November 13, 1872. See also "The Cause of the Boston Fire," *Sacramento Bee*, November 16, 1872. Historians have echoed this interpretation, with one prominent scholar lamenting that the blaze "burned unchecked[,] . . . all for a want of a few horses." Clay McShane, "Gelded Age Boston," *New England Quarterly* 74 (2001): 274.

10. My approach here meshes well with critical disaster studies; see Andy Horowitz and Jacob A. C. Remes, "Introducing Critical Disaster Studies," in *Critical Disaster Studies*, ed. Jacob A. C. Remes and Andy Horowitz (University of Pennsylvania Press, 2021), 1–5.

11. *Address Delivered by John S. Damrell, Before the Boston Veteran Firemen, February 2, 1886* (Boston: Babb & Stephen, 1886), 12 ("seeming indifference"); "Local Intelligence," *BG*, October 28, 1872 ("the well-being").

12. Cotton Mather, *Magnalia Christi Americana; Or, the Ecclesiastical History of New-England, from Its First Planting in the year 1620, unto the Year of Our Lord, 1698* (1702; repr., Hartford: Silas Andrus & Son, 1853), 1:92.

13. Arthur Wellington Brayley, *A Complete History of the Boston Fire Department* [. . .] (Boston: John P. Dale & Co., 1889), 29–33; William J. Novak, *The People's Welfare: Law and Regulation in Nineteenth-Century America* (University of North Carolina Press, 1996), chap. 2.

14. Caleb H. Snow, *A History of Boston, the Metropolis of Massachusetts, from Its Origin to the Present Period; with Some Account of the Environs*, 2nd ed. (Boston: Abel Bowen, 1828), 395–96; Gloria Austin and Mary Chris Foxworthy, *The Fire Horse: A Historic Look at Horses and Firefighting* (Equine Heritage Institute, 2018), 19–21. The most notorious incident of misrule by Boston firefighters was the Broad Street Riot of 1837.

15. Brayley, *Complete History of the Boston Fire Department*, 161, 200.

16. Charles Stearns quoted in "Fighting Fires," *BG*, May 3, 1886 ("to have"); Michael Rawson, *Eden on the Charles: The Making of Boston* (Harvard University Press, 2010), 117–18 ("over sixty").

17. "Old and New Engines," *BG*, February 23, 1890; "Early Fire Apparatus," *BG*, December 25, 1898; "Stories of Boston's Fire Department," *BG*, July 22, 1900; Paul C. Ditzel, *Fire Engines, Firefighters* (Rutledge, 1976), 102. Boston firemen "bitterly opposed" the engine, so it "was stored away and allowed to rust and go to pieces." F. E. Lowry, "The Development of the Electric Fire Alarm System," *American City* 5 (1911): 89.

18. Diane Tarmy Rudnick, "Boston and the Fire of 1872: The Stillborn Phoenix" (PhD diss., Boston University, 1971), 113–17; Brayley, *Complete History of the Boston Fire Department*, 233. This was but one instance of a broader, national process; Robert S. Holzman, "How Steam Blew the Rowdies Out of the Fire Departments," *American Heritage* 7, no. 1 (1955), available at https://www.americanheritage.com/how-steam-blew-rowdies-out-fire-departments?issue=61953; Ditzel, *Fire Engines, Firefighters*, chap. 12.

19. "The Fire Department Horses," *ODA* 5 (October 1872): 243 ("selected"); "Our Fire Interests," *BG*, July 9, 1873; H. C. Merwin, *Road, Track, and Stable: Chapters About Horses and Their Treatment* (Boston: Little, Brown, 1892), 34, 232, 245–46 (all other quotes). Some of these weights included attached hose carriages; none seem to have included firefighters who sometimes rode on engine carriages. Ditzel points out that "fire departments selected horses with greater care than they did firefighters." *Fire Engines, Firefighters*, 135.

20. All quotes from Merwin, *Road, Track, and Stable*, 237–39.

21. *Evening Post*, n.d., quoted in "Horses for Our Fire Department," *Phrenological Journal and Life Illustrated* 55 (November 1872): 337 ("so close"); "Fire Horses: What Constitutes a Model Animal for the Service," *Fire and Water* 32 (1902): 89 ("for hours"); "Grief Gives Up the Ghost," *BG*, September 9, 1890 ("He seemed"). Grief died at twenty-two, so he was probably on duty during the Great Fire eighteen years earlier.

22. "The Great Fire in Boston," *Illustrated Christian Weekly*, November 30, 1872, 577 ("the seat"); "The Sick Horses," *BG*, October 30, 1872 ("almost impossible").

23. "The Horse Disease," *BET*, October 31, 1872.

24. All quotes from "About Home," *BG*, October 26, 1872.

25. "About Home," *BG*, October 26, 1872 ("to seize"); *Address Delivered by Capt. John S. Damrell*, 12–13 ("visited all"). Damrell testified about this meeting and the orders that came from it in *RC*, 107–8. The chief also informed a Chicago fire captain "that oxen are being temporarily substituted for diseased horses in some instances," but sources from Boston fail to mention this recourse. "The Epizootic," *The Herald* (Chicago), November 1, 1872, 175.

26. *Address Delivered by Capt. John S. Damrell*, 13 ("drag ropes"); Damrell testimony, *RC*, 107 ("the different"); "Horse Epidemic," *BET*, October 26, 1873 ("to obtain," "Should the disease," "all good citizens"); "Local Intelligence: The Horse Plague," *BG*, October 28, 1872 ("to ensure"); "The Horse Epidemic," *BET*, October 28, 1872 ("the Fire-Department")

27. All quotes from *Address Delivered by Capt. John S. Damrell*, 13–14. Damrell claimed that only six horses remained well at this time, but the *Transcript* claimed that the epizootic had spread to all but three BFD horses. "The Horse Epidemic," *BET*, October 28, 1872.

28. "Local Intelligence," *BET*, November 2, 1872 ("Should the present"); "Brief Jottings," *BET*, November 5, 1872 ("nipped"). The "man-teams" merchants had previously hired to transport and advertise their wares at the outbreak's height were already "considered almost as things of the past." "The Horse Disease on the Wane," *BG*, November 5, 1872.

29. "The Horse Disease," *BET*, November 6, 1872 ("decided decline); "Epizootic," *Boston Advertiser*, n.d., in *Prairie Farmer* (Chicago), November 16, 1872 ("He is better").

30. "The Horse Epidemic and the Storm," *BET*, November 7, 1872 ("hundreds," "the owners," and "present weak"); and "Humanity," *BG*, November 8, 1872 ("to continue").

31. "Brief Jottings," *BET*, November 9, 1872 ("again lively"); T. S. Perry testimony, *RC*, 218 ("to investigate").

32. "Fire in Congress Street," BET, November 2, 1872; "Local Intelligence," BET, November 8, 1872; "The Fire on North Street," BET, November 6, 1872; "The Recent Fatal Accident to a Member of Engine Co. No. 6," BET, November 7, 1872.

33. Bugbee, "Fires and Fire Departments," 115.

34. Seman Klous testimony, RC, 79; Alexander K. Young testimony, RC, 1; *The Boston Directory, Embracing the City Record, a General Directory of the Citizens and Business Directory* (Boston: Sampson, Davenport, & Co., 1872), 210. The building occupied 83, 85, and 87 Summer Street.

35. Henry F. Bond, "Old Summer Street," *New England Magazine* 19 (1898): 350.

36. Enoch Cobb Wines, *A Trip to Boston: In a Series of Letters to the Editor of the United States Gazette* (Boston: Charles C. Little and James Brown, 1838), 208 ("decidedly"); and J. Elliot Cabot, "A Glimpse of Emerson's Boyhood," *Atlantic*, May 1887, 651 ("village-fashion").

37. Henry Piper testimony, RC, 63.

38. Frederick Hoffman testimony, RC, 70; Benjamin Farwell testimony, RC, 72; John Page testimony, RC, 359.

39. Bugbee, "Fires and Fire Departments," 115 ("practical electrician"); William F. Channing, *The American Fire-Alarm Telegraph: A Lecture Delivered Before the Smithsonian Institution, March, 1855* (Boston: Redding, 1855), 10 ("one of the ablest"), 7–9 ("the occurrence"). See also Joel A. Tarr, "The Municipal Telegraph Network: Origins of the Fire and Police Alarm Systems in American Cities," *Flux* 9 (1992): 16n15; "Boston's Fire Alarm 50 Years Old," BG, October 12, 1902; Lowry, "Development of the Electric Fire Alarm System," 88–89.

40. Channing, *American Fire-Alarm Telegraph*, 10 ("key-holders"); "Fires," *Insurance Monitor and Commercial Register* 2 (1854): 40 ("literal net-work"). On the number of boxes, see "J. F. Kennard, "Fire Alarm Telegraph: List of the Numbers and Localities of the Boxes," *New England Post Office Record*, March 14, 1868, 3; Theodore A. Glynn, "Progress in Fire Protection," *City Record* 14 (1922): 1195.

41. Kennard quoted in "Boston's Big Fire of 1872," BG, November 5, 1905. On gongs, see Bugbee, "Fires and Fire Departments," 115. Engineer John Regan, for instance, testified: "I have a fire-alarm telegraph in the room." Regan testimony, RC, 318.

42. "Fires," *Insurance Monitor and Commercial Register* 2 (1854): 40.

43. Bugbee, "Fires and Fire Departments," 115 ("the electric current"); "The Fire Department Horses," *ODA* 5 (October 1872): 243 ("fourteen"); and Merwin, *Road, Track, and Stable*, 235–36 ("Often"). See also "Improvement in Horse Stalls for Steam Fire Engine House," *Patent Rights Gazette* 5 (December 1872): 10.

44. RC, iii. On the timeline, see RC, iv; Stearns quoted in "Boston's Big Fire of 1872." See also Charles Andrew Bodge testimony, RC, 293–96; Julius F. Gage testimony, RC, 297–98.

45. James Powers testimony, RC, 262–63 ("as sudden"). For similar accounts, see RC, iii; John S. Holmes testimony, RC, 215; Daniel Marden testimony, RC, 26; Charles Pratt testimony, RC, 66; Regan testimony, RC, 318; "How the Great Boston Fire Was Fought," BG, November 10, 1912.

46. Olin Paine testimony, RC, 228–30 ("light"); William Halsall testimony, RC, 63–65 ("cracking" and "saturated"); Alonzo Pratt testimony, RC, 68 ("The instant"). At precisely the same time, attorney John S. Holmes, who had begun to run over to the scene of the fire after seeing its flames, "saw, in the basement story, what at first looked like a large globe of fire." Holmes testimony, RC, 215.

47. Damrell testimony, RC, 84 ("not as fully"); Damrell quoted by Stearns in "Boston's Big Fire of 1872" ("pretty"). Damrell's timing is based on RC, iii; Damrell testimony, RC, 85, 113; and Regan testimony, RC, 323.

48. Damrell testimony, RC, 113 ("on fire"), 84–85 ("flying"); and L. E. Shaw testimony, RC, 191 ("a very far"). Alderman Samuel Little had much the same reaction; he later recalled that "when I got to the scene of the fire . . . I saw that Boston was in for a serious blaze and there was no discovering the extent of the probable damage." "Boston's Fire Alarm 50 Years Old," BG, November 5, 1905. Shaw estimated that it took him seven and a half minutes to reach the fire after he heard the alarm given at 7:24. Stephanie Schorow places Damrell's home at 60 Temple Street; Stephanie Schorow, *The Great Boston Fire: The Inferno That Nearly Incinerated the City* (Globe Pequot, 2022), 49.

49. See RC, iv; Damrell testimony, RC, 13; and "How the Great Boston Fire Was Fought," BG, November 10, 1912.

50. Nathan Brown testimony, RC, 31–32, 39 ("our hose-carriage"); Holmes testimony, RC, 215–16 ("attempting"); Marden testimony, RC, 26 ("inside of"); Joseph Pierce testimony, RC, 42 ("what I"). Older downtown stations like Engine 4's, Pierce explained, lacked the automatic, telegraph-operated doors of their newer counterparts in outlying parts of Boston; RC, 44.

51. George Upton testimony, RC, 355–56.

52. Bugbee, "Fires and Fire Departments," 119 ("old portion"); Damrell testimony, RC, 104–5 ("constantly").

53. Lawrence Curtis testimony, RC, 462–65.

54. Clarence Dorr testimony, RC, 15 ("The water"). On failed attempt to climb stairs, see Brown testimony, RC, 36; Burt testimony, RC, 386.

55. J. M. Crafts testimony, RC, 458–59.

56. Damrell testimony, RC, 103.

57. Glynn, "Progress in Fire Protection," 1195; Bugbee, "Fires and Fire Departments," 120; William Woolley testimony, RC, 167.

58. Phineas Allen testimony, RC, 196–97; Woolley testimony, RC, 166; David Chamberlain testimony, RC, 225.

59. RC, viii ("for larger mains"); Damrell testimony, RC, 116–17 ("every one"). See also Daniel H. Johnson testimony, RC, 474, 476.

60. Damrell testimony, RC, 116; John Cooligan testimony, RC, 205.

61. Burt testimony, RC, 385.

62. Quotes from William Russell testimony, RC, 462. See also George Gardner testimony, RC, 269; Charles A. R. Dimon testimony, RC, 324; Burt testimony, RC, 385.

63. Regan testimony, RC, 323.

64. Damrell testimony, RC, 108. See also Regan testimony, RC, 323.

65. Wooley testimony, RC, 151.

66. Daniel Lord testimony, RC, 477–78.

67. RC, vii.

68. Damrell testimony, RC, 115. Assistant engineer L. E. Shaw corroborated the chief's assessment; Shaw testimony, RC, 194–95. On forty-two streams, see Glynn, "Progress in Fire Protection," 1196.

69. Woolley testimony, RC, 166.

70. William Delano testimony, RC, 340.

71. "The 'Mansard' Roof," *Youth's Companion* 45 (December 12, 1872): 402 ("beauty of effect"); "The Mansard Roof," *Circular*, February 22, 1869, 391 ("attic story"); "The 'Mansard' Roof," *Colman's Rural World*, May 15, 1869, 316 ("equal to").

72. A. C. Martin testimony, RC, 22.

73. *Chicago Chronicle*, n.d., quoted in "The Mansard Roof," *Baltimore Underwriter* 6 (September 1870), 81 ("gorgeous tinder box"); Chamberlain testimony, RC, 226.

74. Gardner testimony, RC, 273 ("thirty"); Henry Bigelow testimony, RC, 143 ("When one"); Chamberlain testimony, RC, 224 ("so uncontrollable," emphasis added).

75. "Sixty-Five Acres Burned Over 40 Years Ago in Boston's Worst Conflagration," BG, November 9, 1912 ("assumed such"); Burt testimony, RC, 385 ("beyond"). Harvard President Charles W. Elliot presented a much more critical recollection of this same moment; Elliot testimony, RC, 372, 379.

76. Quotes from Woolley testimony, RG, 155–56; Damrell testimony, RC, 104, 106.

77. Powers testimony, BG, 285–88 ("very clamorous"); Regan testimony, BG, 321–22 ("there was"); Burt testimony, RC, 398 ("counted"). On boxes, see Dexter R. Dearing testimony, RC, 126; William T. Cheswell testimony, RC, 131; Bigelow testimony, RC, 144; Delano testimony, RC, 341; and Joseph Dunbar testimony, RC, 176. On use of a human-powered wagon to fetch coal, see Powers testimony, RC, 288.

78. Woolley testimony, RC, 155; Bigelow testimony, RC, 144; Burt testimony, RC, 398.

79. Damrell testimony, RC, 121 ("Your horses"). On Engine 7, see RC, 109.

80. Alcott to Pratt, [November 10, 1872], in *Selected Letters of Louisa May Alcott*, 170. See also Brown testimony, RC, 36; Burt testimony, RC, 389; James Quinn testimony, RC, 74; Damrell testimony, RC, 112.

81. Robert C. Nichols testimony, RC, 350 ("to allow"). On the Common, see also Damrell testimony, RC, 92; Burt testimony, RC, 388–89; *Boston Advertiser*, n.d., in "The Great Boston Fire," *Green-Mountain Freemen* (Montpelier, VT), November 13, 1872.

82. "Another Account," NYT, November 10, 1872 ("the horse distemper"); "The Great Fire in Boston," *Illustrated Christian Weekly*, November 30, 1872, 577 ("reputed").

83. "Another Account."

84. Damrell testimony, RC, 90–93.

85. Damrell testimony, RC, 90–93, 97–98. See also RC, xiv–xviii.

86. Damrell testimony, RC, 117. On brigades saving structures, see Pratt testimony, RC, 66–67.

87. Entry for November 10, 1872, in Emily Marshall Eliot Morison Journals, vol. 3, Boston Athenaeum, Boston, MA. Morison would become the mother of famous historian Samuel Eliot Morison.

88. Alcott to Pratt, [November 10, 1872], in *Selected Letters of Louisa May Alcott*, 171; Schorow, *Great Boston Fire*, 9; Dearing testimony, RC, 127.

89. "Great Fire in Boston," *Illustrated Christian Weekly*, November 30, 1872, 577.

90. F. E. Frothingham, *The Boston Fire, November 9th and 10th, 1872. Its History, Together with the Losses in Detail of Both Real and Personal Estate* [. . .] (Boston: Lee & Shepard, 1873), 16. On losses, see "Ten Months After the Fire," BG, September 19, 1873; "A Year's Progress," BG, November 11, 1873; "Insurance Losses by the Boston Fire," *Independent*, February 6, 1873, 186; "The Boston Fire," *United States Club Advertiser*, December 5, 1872, 8; William Claflin, Francis A. Perry, and Jacob Sleeper, "Boston University and the Great Fire," *College Courant*, December 21, 1872, 255–56; "Fire-Proof Buildings," *Boston Medical and Surgical*

Journal (December 26, 1872), 458–59; Rudnick, "Boston and the Fire of 1872," 193–94; Carleton, *Story of the Great Fire*, 28.

91. Carleton, *Story of the Great Fire*, 28 ("the accumulation"); "The Burnt District," BET, November 29, 1872 ("carting away"); "Brief Jottings," BET, November 20, 1872 ("horse distemper"). On job losses, see Frothingham, *Boston Fire*, 15; and Rudnick, "Boston and the Fire of 1872," 206–7. On relief, see Rudnick, "Boston and the Fire of 1872," 201. On early stages of reconstruction, see "The Third Day," BG, November 13, 1872; and W. H. Fay and S. A. Choate, "Laborers in Boston," BET, December 2, 1872.

92. *Harper's Weekly*, November 30, 1872, 934 ("historic relics"); HC, November 12, 1872 ("Nothing"); quotes on Abbotts from "Two More Bodies Found," BET, November 25, 1872; and "'The Burnt District,'" BET, November 29, 1872. Neither of the dead Abbotts were current members of the Charlestown Fire Department.

93. Quotes from "The Epizootic," *Memphis Public Ledger*, November 19, 1872; "Miscellaneous," NOR, November 22, 1872. For human-powered pullers' successes elsewhere, see, e.g., "The Horse Disease," *McArthur (OH) Enquirer*, November 20, 1872; and John Morrow, "Volunteers!," *Nashville Republican Banner*, November 20, 1872.

94. The deployment of engines from all six downtown companies might have checked the fire at the Klous Building. Schorow, *Great Boston Fire*, 166.

95. "The Newly Built District," BET, November 8, 1873.

96. Quotes from Christine Meisner Rosen, *The Limits of Power: Great Fires and the Process of City Growth in America* (Cambridge University Press, 1986), 246, 245. On the May 1873 fire, see Rosen, *Limits of Power*, 210; Schorow, *Great Boston Fire*, 144–45; Rudnick, "Boston and the Fire of 1872," chap. 11. On the BFD's composition, see Glynn, "Progress in Fire Protection," 1195. Over the previous decades, the department had periodically sold its "worn-out fire horses . . . at auction to the highest bidder." By 1907, however, the BFD began sending its superannuated equines to a pioneering workhorse refuge, Red Hill Farm, the pet project of Boston socialite Harriet G. Bird. "'Red Acre Farm'—A Rest Cure for Horses," NYT, January 6, 1907. Despite the commission's call for Boston to invest in self-propelling fire engines, the BFD did not retire its last firehorse until 1925.

CHAPTER 5

1. Excelsior [pseud.], December 28, 1872, in "From the South," CE, January 2, 1873 ("could not"); *St. Paul Pioneer*, November 27, 1872, reprinted in "The Epizoot in St. Paul," *Minneapolis Star Tribune*, November 28, 1872 ("a vast"); "The Epizootic," *Tensas Gazette* (St. Joseph, LA), December 7, 1872 ("no longer").

2. Frere [pseud.], letter dated December 6, 1872, published as "Louisiana," BG, December 14, 1872 ("Nothing"); M.A.Y. [pseud.], December 11, 1872, in "Correspondence," *Hutchinson (KS) News*, December 19, 1872 ("very curious").

3. "Phoenixiana," *Columbia (SC) Phoenix*, December 7, 1872 ("No horse"); "The Horse Plague Spreading," *Hagerstown (MD) Herald and Torch Light*, November 27, 1872; *Oswego (NY) Palladium*, November 20, 1872 ("destined").

4. W. E. B. Du Bois, *Black Reconstruction in America 1860–1880* (1935; repr., Free Press, 1992), 585. As this chapter shows, I do not subscribe to Du Bois's Beardian interpretation of the economics of war and Reconstruction. Statistics from Abraham Gibson, "War Horses: Equine Perspectives on the Confederacy," in *Animal Histories of the Civil War*

Era, ed. Earl J. Hess (Louisiana State University Press, 2022), 94; and Kathryn Olivarius, *Necropolis: Disease, Power, and Capitalism in the Cotton Kingdom* (Harvard University Press, 2022), 236. Mortality rate from Drew Gilpin Faust, *This Republic of Suffering: Death and the American Civil War* (Knopf, 2008), 266. A Senate report tallied up "southern war losses in property (exclusive of slave property) at $1.1 billion," while two economists later placed the "final aggregate estimate of the cost of the war at $6.6 billion"—truly massive sums. Jeremy Atack and Peter Passell, *A New Economic View of American History from Colonial Times to 1940*, 2nd ed. (W. W. Norton, 1994), 361–62.

5. Michael W. Fitzgerald, *Splendid Failure: Postwar Reconstruction in the American South* (Ivan R. Dee, 2007), 172–73. On livestock levels, see Atack and Passell, *New Economic View of American History*, 373, 380–81. As of 1870, populations of mules, horses, milk cows, swine, and working oxen stood at 75, 71, 68, 65, and 60 percent of 1860 levels, respectively; Eugene M. Lerner, "Southern Output and Agricultural Income, 1860–1880," *Agricultural History* 33 (1956): 117–18. On the roots of these Republican policies as well as their ideological foundations, see Heather Cox Richardson, *The Greatest Nation on Earth: Republican Economic Policies During the Civil War* (Harvard University Press, 1997); and Mark W. Summers, *Railroads, Reconstruction, and the Gospel of Prosperity: Aid Under the Radical Republicans* (Princeton University Press, 1984). For more on economic growth as the sine qua non in containing intra- and intersectional tensions (but with an emphasis on national policy rather than market dynamics), see Richard Franklin Bensel, *Yankee Leviathan: The Origins of Central State Authority in America 1859–1877* (Cambridge University Press, 1991).

6. *Ogdensburg (NY) Journal*, November 19, 1872; "Local Brevities," *Reading (PA) Times*, November 18, 1872; "Epizootics," *Davenport (IA) Morning Democrat*, November 27, 1872; "The Epizoot," *Minneapolis Star Tribune*, November 27, 1872; "Neighborhood News," *Hickman (KY) Courier*, December 21, 1872; "Injury to the Manufacturing Interests," *Summit County Beacon* (Akron, OH), November 20, 1872; "Local Affairs," *Cecil Whig* (Elkton, MD), November 23, 1872; "Shut Down," *Wheeling Register*, November 23, 1872; *Plattsburgh (NY) Sentinel*, November 29, 1872; "Work Resumed," *Wheeling Register*, December 9, 1872.

7. "The Horse Plague," *Appleton (WI) Post*, November 21, 1872 ("lumbermen"); *Oshkosh Northwester*, November 21, 1872, in "The Epizootic in Wisconsin," *Wisconsin State Journal* (Madison), November 23, 1872 ("great consternation"). On horses in logging, see Jason L. Newton, *Cutover Capitalism: The Industrialization of the Northern Forest* (University of West Virginia Press, 2024), chaps. 3–4. On logging rhythms, see William J. Cronon, *Nature's Metropolis: Chicago and the Great West* (W. W. Norton, 1991), chap. 4.

8. *Bangor Whig*, n.d., in *BG*, February 1, 1873; and William A. Thayer, January 3, 1873, in "From the Pineries," *Muscatine (IA) Weekly Journal*, January 17, 1873. On delays, see also "November Blasts," *Appleton (WI) Crescent*, November 23, 1872; "Reed Village," *Detroit Free Press*, November 30, 1872; "Muskegon," *Chicago Inter Ocean*, December 8, 1872; Waukan [pseud.], letter dated "December 1872," *New England Farmer*, December 28, 1872; D. [pseud.], January 20, 1873, in "Cherry Tree Chips," *Pittsburgh Weekly Gazette*, January 29, 1873. For corroboration on losses, see "Marinette," *Green Bay Weekly Gazette*, January 18, 1873; "Chisago County," *Minneapolis Star Tribune*, January 19, 1873; "Charles W. Morrill," *Newport (VT) Express and Standard*, February 18, 1873. Although the ongoing recovery of flu-stricken horses in February and March enabled lumberjacks to make up for some of these losses, the overall harvest for 1872–73 still fell far short of projections. *Eau Claire (WI) Weekly Free Press*, April 3, 1873.

9. "The Epizooty," *Nashville Union and American*, November 19, 1872; "The Epizootic," *Indianapolis Journal*, November 30, 1872. See also "The Epizooty," *Nashville Union and American*, November 22, 1872; *Louisiana Journal*, n.d., in *La Grange (MO) Democrat*, December 26, 1872; and "Epizootic," *Valley Virginian* (Staunton), November 21, 1872.

10. "City and Vicinity," *Carbondale (PA) Leader*, November 23, 1872 ("becoming general"); "How Did They Get It?," *Norfolk Virginian*, November 30, 1872 ("one of the toughest"); "Marseilles," *Ottawa (IL) Free Trader*, November 30, 1872 ("four hundred feet"); "Streator," CT, December 23, 1872 ("hacking coughs"). See also "The Horse Disease," *Sunbury (PA) American*, November 23, 1872; Saltus Mohegan [pseud.], November 29, 1872, in "A Flying Trip to the Ohio," *Nashville Union and American*, December 1, 1872; and "City and Neighborhood," *Terre Haute Evening Gazette*, December 13, 1872. Outside Akron, Ohio, mine mules housed on the surface fell ill first; "The Epizootic," *Summit County Beacon* (Akron, OH), November 20, 1872.

11. "The Price of Coal," *Wheeling Register*, November 21, 1872. On layoffs, see, e.g., "The Monthly Coal Sale," *Iron Age*, November 28, 1872, 3.

12. For evidence on disrupted harvests, see, e.g., "The Horse Disease," CT, November 18, 1872. On oxen, see Henry [pseud.], December 21, 1872, *Knoxville Chronicle*, December 25, 1872; "Kingsville," *Ashtabula (OH) Weekly Telegraph*, December 14, 1872; "The Noble Horse," *Des Moines Register*, January 3, 1873.

13. Robert Lamb Byron, *The Mule in Southern Agriculture* (University of California Press, 1963), 18 ("before winter"); "From Georgia," *Interior Journal* (Sanford, KY), December 13, 1872 ("excitement"); "The Horse Malady," *Nashville Union and American*, December 10, 1872 ("sixty head"). For advertisements, see, e.g., ad for "FORTY KENTUCKY MULES, which I want to sell quick!," posted by R. W. Owen, who claimed "they have all had the Epizootic, and are now ready for work, so that persons buying from me need lose no time." *Livingston (AL) Journal*, January 17, 1873. For a human version of such immunocapital, see Olivarius, *Necropolis*. On intraregional trade in horses and mules, see also Thomas D. Clark, "The Trade Between Kentucky and the Cotton Kingdom in Livestock, Hemp and Slaves from 1840 to 1860" (MA thesis, University of Kentucky, 1929), 34–42; Ulrich Bonnell Phillips, *Life and Labor in the Old South* (Little, Brown, 1963), 144. On average value, see "The Horse Population," BE, November 8, 1872.

14. "The Epizootic Catarrh—Again," *Richmond (VA) Dispatch*, November 13, 1872 ("haul a hogshead"); "Letter from Petersburg," *Richmond (VA) News Leader*, November 9, 1872.

15. "Industrial Department," NOTP, December 7, 1872. Louisiana sugar production for 1872 was 108,520 hogsheads; the next year, only 89,498 hogsheads were produced. These were far and away the smallest harvests of any year after 1870. Eugene V. Smalley, "Sugar-Making in Louisiana," *Century Illustrated Monthly Magazine* 35 (1887): 103. By the early 1870s, most mills were steam-powered, though some still used mules.

16. "Cotton Financing," *Federal Reserve Bulletin*, May 1923, 567.

17. John Peabody, 1883, quoted in Gavin Wright, *The Political Economy of the Cotton South: Households, Markets, and Wealth in the Nineteenth Century* (W. W. Norton, 1978), 173 ("The people"); "Cotton—No. 11," *Atlanta Constitution*, November 17, 1872 ("burned up" through "blue"); *Memphis Public Ledger*, November 20, 1872. Statistics from John Hope Franklin, *Reconstruction After the Civil War* (1961; repr., University of Chicago Press, 2013), 175; Ewen Bro's, "Cotton: Cotton Trade of the United States" (n.p.: n.p., ca. 1884). W. E. B. Du Bois underestimated the volatility of cotton agriculture when he noted that "by 1870,

the Cotton Kingdom was reëstablished": That year's harvest would not be equaled until 1875–76. *Black Reconstruction in America*, 587.

18. *Charlotte Observer*, n.d., in "State News," *Wilmington (NC) Journal*, November 29, 1872; "The Small Pox in Harnett," *Raleigh News*, November 23, 1872; "Horse Talk About Town," *NOR*, November 25, 1872 ("nearby plantations"). On oxen, see also *Wilmington (NC) Journal*, November 28, 1872; and "Financial and Commercial," *Memphis Avalanche*, November 20, 1872.

19. "Financial and Commercial," *Memphis Avalanche*, November 20, 1872; Frederick Law Olmsted, *Journeys and Explorations in the Cotton Kingdom* (London: S. Low, Son & Co., 1861), 2:366.

20. "Cotton," *Memphis Appeal*, November 26, 1872; "Stricken Savannah," *Charleston (SC) News*, November 21, 1872. See also "Hoisting by Steam," *Wilmington (NC) Morning Star*, November 20, 1872.

21. "Horse Talk About Town," *NOR*, November 30, 1872 ("joint committees"); "Plans for Moving Freight," *NOR*, December 1, 1872 ("abandoned"); "The Jackson Railroad All Over Town," *NOR*, December 1, 1872 ("fifteen hundred" and "expense of receiving"); "The Epizootic," *NOTP*, November 29, 1872 ("up-town cotton presses"); "The City," *NOTP*, December 1, 1872 ("Cotton languishes"); "Horse Gossip and Stock Items," *Turf, Field and Farm*, December 6, 1872, 358 ("but a meagre"). Savannah took similar precautions; "Midnight Dispatches," *Atlanta Constitution*, November 21, 1872.

22. "The Equine Influenza," *Memphis Appeal*, November 27, 1872; Frere [pseud.], letter dated December 6, 1872, published as "Louisiana," *BG*, December 14, 1872.

23. "Industrial Department," *NOTP*, December 7, 1872 ("Truly"); Frere [pseud.], letter dated December 6, 1872.

24. "The Cotton Trade," *The Guardian* (London, UK), January 13, 1873 ("unprecedently" and "telegraphed planters"); "News in Brief," *Memphis Avalanche*, December 16, 1872 ("such an extent"); "Epizootic," *Nashville Union and American*, November 24, 1872 ("afraid"); "Cotton," *Atlanta Constitution*, December 15, 1872 ("interior towns"); "The Freight Blockade," *NOR*, December 29, 1872.

25. "1872–3," *Nashville Union and American*, September 2, 1873; "Atlanta," *Atlanta Herald*, September 14, 1873.

26. "The Epizootic," *Plymouth (IN) Weekly Republican*, November 14, 1872.

27. "Epizootic Items," *Sedalia (MO) Democrat*, December 7, 1872 ("Frightful reports"); "The Horse Disease," *Nashville Tennessean*, November 21, 1872.

28. "The Epizootic Catarrh," *Richmond (VA) Dispatch*, November 13, 1872; "Fancy Prices," *Nashville Union and American*, November 24, 1872; Digby [pseud.], November 18, 1872, in "Letter from Cumberland," *York (PA) Democratic Press*, November 22, 1872 ("to trudge").

29. "Hipporhinorrhea," *Atlanta Constitution*, November 20, 1872; "The Equine Epidemic," *Atlanta Weekly Constitution*, November 26, 1872; "Epizooty," *Janesville Gazette*, November 18, 1872. On merchants' longer-running critiques, see Erwin H. Ackerknecht, "Anticontagionism Between 1821 and 1867," *Bulletin of the History of Medicine* 22 (1948): 562–93.

30. "The Horse Market," *Charleston Courier*, November 26, 1872. On local quarantines, see "The Epizootic," *NOTP*, November 13, 1872; "The Horse Disease," *NOTP*, November 15, 1872; "The Horse Malady," *NOR*, November 16, 1872; "The Horse Market," *Charleston Courier*, November 26, 1872; "Alabama Items," *Columbus (GA) Ledger-Enquirer*, November 22, 1872; "Notice," *Nashville Union and American*, November 22, 1872.

31. Lithograph [pseud.], "From Lynchburg," *Highland News* (Hillsboro, OH), December 19, 1872; "The Horse Disease," *Nashville Republican Banner*, November 23, 1872.

32. "The Horse Disease," *Chicago Inter Ocean*, November 4, 1872; Nicolas Barreyre, *Gold and Freedom: The Political Economy of Reconstruction*, trans. Arthur Goldhammer (University of Virginia Press, 2015), 73. See also "Review of the Market for the Week Ending Friday Morning, April 18th, 1873," *Commercial Herald and Market Review* (San Francisco), April 18, 1873.

33. N. [pseud.], December 2, 1872, in "Letter from New Orleans," *Montgomery Advertiser*, December 4, 1872 ("number six"); "Financial and Commercial," *Memphis Avalanche*, November 23, 1872; "Pittsburgh Markets," *Pittsburgh Weekly Gazette*, November 28, 1872. For corroboration, see "Financial and Commercial," *Memphis Avalanche*, November 27, 1872; "The Father of Waters," NYH, December 30, 1872.

34. 1870 US Agricultural Census. Between 43,700 and 87,400 of these fatalities occurred in states west of Indiana and south of Virginia. Given the US GDP in 2023 of $29.184 trillion, an analogous loss today would involve $29 to $58 billion.

35. "Horse Gossip and Stock Items," *Turf, Field and Farm*, December 20, 1872, 390–91; "Local Brevities," *Andrew County Republican* (Savannah, MO), March 7, 1873; *Louisville Courier-Journal*, January 6, 1873, reprinted in "Mortality Among the Jacks," *Columbia (SC) Phoenix*, January 17, 1873; "Report of the Department of Agriculture for April," *St. Alban's (VT) Messenger*, May 22, 1873. For other accounts of heavy fatalities among donkeys, see "Why Is It?," *Crawford Mirror* (Steelville, MO), January 17, 1873; "Fatal Epizootic," *Sedalia (MO) Democrat*, January 20, 1873; "Remedy for the Epizootic," *Lexington (MO) Intelligencer*, January 22, 1873; "Fatality Among Jacks," *Gadsden (AL) Times-News*, January 23, 1873; "Indiana News," *Cambridge City (IN) Tribune*, January 23, 1873. On recent science, see, e.g., Megan M. Ahearne et al., "Disease Progression, Pathologic, and Virologic Findings of an Equine Influenza Outbreak in Rescue Donkeys," *Journal of Veterinary Internal Medicine* 36 (2022): 2230–37. Although these figures supposedly pertained to donkeys and mules, there is no clear-cut evidence to suggest that the latter actually perished at higher rates than horses.

36. "Effects of the Epizootic," *Buffalo Commercial*, April 14, 1873; Grit [pseud.], May 13, 1873, in "Carrollton, Ills.," MR, May 14, 1873; "A Disagreeable Inheritance by Spring Colts," *Sioux City Journal*, May 21, 1873; *Tionesta (PA) Forest Republican*, June 11, 1873. For similar reports pertaining to other areas, see "The Northwest," CEP, May 14, 1873; "News Items," *Alton (IL) Telegraph*, June 13, 1873; "The Epizootic Again," *Decatur (IL) Weekly Republican*, June 19, 1873; "Maury County Farmers's [*sic*] Club," *Columbia (TN) Herald and Mail*, July 4, 1873.

37. *Denver News*, n.d., in *Laramie (WY) Sentinel*, January 18, 1873 ("all the colts"); Fleur Whitlock et al, "A Review on Equine Influenza from a Human Influenza Perspective," *Viruses* 14 (2022): article 1312, n.p. See also Juliana Gonzalez-Obando et al. "Equine Influenza Virus: An Old Known Enemy in the Americas," *Vaccines* 10 (2022): article 1718.

38. "Ithaca Farmers' Club," *Ithaca Journal*, November 18, 1872 ("most marked"); "The Epizooty," *Wheeling Register*, December 3, 1872 ("leaves the animals"). See also "Local," *Wilmington (NC) Journal*, January 3, 1873. For a contrary view, see "The Horse Disease," *Urbana (OH) Citizen and Gazette*, December 26, 1872.

39. *West Chester (PA) Record*, n.d., in "Another Horse Disease," *Wilmington (DE) News Journal*, April 8, 1873; "City Department," *Decatur (IL) Republican*, April 19, 1873; "Baltimore and Yorktown Turnpike Road Company," BS, October 21, 1873; *Troy Times*, n.d., in "The Equine Epidemic," *Pittsburgh Commercial*, October 25, 1872 ("sometimes"). For similar accounts, see "Our Fire Department," CT, April 27, 1873.

40. "Around Town," *Columbia (TN) Herald and Mail*, February 7, 1873 ("lost one"); "The Epizootic Returned," *Harrisburg (PA) Telegraph*, April 23, 1873 ("lost two"). Fatality rates from CEM, December 11, 1872. In October, prior to the Great Horse Flu's arrival, the average daily death rate was seven. "Convalescing Chargers," CEP, November 13, 1872. For other examples, see *Warrenton Gazette*, n.d., in *Raleigh Sentinel*, June 2, 1873; "Caroline County," *Wilmington (DE) Commercial*, April 5, 1873; "The Epizooty," *Sunbury (PA) Gazette*, February 7, 1873.

41. "Ithaca Farmers' Club," *Ithaca Journal*, November 18, 1872 (emphasis added); "The Canadian Horse Disease," *Prairie Farmer* (Chicago), November 2, 1872 (emphasis added). These depictions anticipate Mark Honigsbaum, *A History of the Great Influenza Pandemics: Death, Panic and Hysteria, 1830–1920* (I. B. Tauris, 2014), 2.

42. *Charlotte Observer*, n.d., in "North Carolina News," *Yorkville (SC) Enquirer*, March 6, 1873; "Alabama News," *Eufaula (AL) Weekly Times*, February 6, 1873. See also, e.g., "State News," *Miami Republican* (Paola, KS), December 21, 1872; and "Epizootic," *Salt Lake Herald-Republican*, April 26, 1873.

43. "The Horse Distemper," *Sunbury (PA) Gazette*, November 15, 1872; "Epizootic," *Nashville Banner Republican*, November 17, 1872; "The Horse Disease," *Jackson (TN) Whig and Tribune*, November 23, 1872; "The Horse Plague," *Quad-City Times* (Davenport, IA), November 16, 1872; "The Horse Disease," *St. Joseph (MO) Gazette*, December 11, 1872.

44. "Epizootic in St. Louis," MR (St. Louis), December 4, 1872; "News of the Day in Brief," *St. Joseph (MO) Gazette*, January 3, 1873. See also O. Nyx [pseud.], "From Shelbina," *Shelby County Herald* (Shelbyville, MO), December 11, 1872; "The Epizootic," MR (St. Louis), December 6, 1872; "Wellington Items," *Lexington (MO) Intelligencer*, December 18, 1872; *Louisiana Sugar-Bowl* (New Iberia), December 19, 1872; Jim [pseud.], December 30, 1872; in "Sherman, Tex.," *Kansas City (MO) Times*, January 9, 1873.

45. "La enfermedad de los caballos," *Juan Palomo*, December 15, 1872, 397 ("first"); "Menestra semanal," *Juan Palomo*, December 15, 1872, 393 ("All the horses"); CT, December 26, 1872 ("lighter" to "very great"); *Indianapolis News*, December 30, 1872 ("a malignant type"). See also "Cronica general," *Diario de la Marina* (Havana), January 3, 1873 ("In many cases"); *Panama Star and Herald* (Panama City, Panama), January 18, 1873. See also *El Mercurio* (Mexico City), February 5, 1873. For concurrence on the outbreak's spread to *ganado vacuno* (bovine cattle), see "Telegramas," *La Cronica* (Los Angeles), January 11, 1873; and *Panama Star and Herald* (Panama City, Panama), January 18, 1873. See also *El Mercurio* (Mexico City), February 5, 1873.

46. *Highland Weekly News* (Hillsboro, OH), February 6, 1873 ("universal traveler"); *Highland Weekly News* (Hillsboro, OH), January 9, 1873 ("pine apples").

47. Holbrook [pseud.], December 12, 1872, in "From Beloit," *Western Home* (Lawrence, KS), December 19, 1872 ("Westward"). See also *Galveston News*, November 5, 1872; and *Osage Mission (KS) Transcript*, November 22, 1872.

CHAPTER 6

1. Untitled and "Beautiful Picture," PH (Auburn, CA), March 1, 1873; David Scobey, "Looking West from the Empire City: National Landscape and Visual Culture in Gilded Age New York," in *New York: Art and Cultural Capital of the Gilded Age*, ed. Margaret R. Laster and Chelsea Bruner (Routledge, 2019), 19. Rosalyn R. LaPier notes that "the Blackfeet do

not have an official orthography." Rosalyn R. LaPier, *Invisible Reality: Storytellers, Storytakers, and the Supernatural World of the Blackfeet* (University of Nebraska Press, 2017), xvi–xvii. This chapter uses spellings from the Blackfoot Language Resources and Digital Dictionary (https://blackfoot.algonquianlanguages.ca) unless otherwise noted.

2. All citations from the PH from "Beautiful Picture." On this technique, see "How Chromos Are Made," *New York World*, n.d., in *York (PA) Democratic Press*, November 29, 1872.

3. "What the Western Press Says About Our 'American Progress,'" *Crofutt's Western World*, April 1873, 56 (quoted). On Crofutt, see Jennifer Raab, "Panoramic Vision, Telegraphic Language: Selling the American West, 1869–1884," *Journal of American Studies* 47 (2013): 495–520.

4. "Beautiful Picture"; "Explanation and Response," *Crofutt's Western World*, March 1873, 40. The magazine also had a San Francisco office, but Crofutt and Gast were both based in New York in late 1872 and early 1873.

5. [Myron Angel], *History of Placer County, California, with Illustrations and Biographical Sketches of Its Prominent Men and Pioneers* (Oakland, CA: Thompson & West, 1882), 140, 177; and *Sacramento Union*, n.d., 1857. Walkup was long remembered as "The Father of Placer County." [Angel], *History of Placer County*, 174; Norman McLeod, "Joseph Walkup," *Auburn (CA) Journal*, October 14, 1984, 44–45. See also *Hutchings' California Magazine* 2 (March 1858): 387–88; and "Death of Ex-Lieutenant-Governor Walkup," *Sacramento Union*, October 16, 1873.

6. [Angel], *History of Placer County*, 174–78, 205–6, 240, 365. On settler-Indigenous conflicts in the area, see [Angel], *History of Placer County*, 68–72; and Benjamin Madley, *American Genocide: The United States and the California Indian Catastrophe, 1846–1873* (Yale University Press, 2016), chap. 3. Neither of these works mentions Walkup as a perpetrator of anti-Indigenous violence, but accounts of anti-Native violence in California often elided settlers' identities.

7. [Angel], *History of Placer County*, 140; and *Sacramento Union*, n.d., 1857.

8. "Beautiful Picture." Helpful works on this image include Scobey, "Looking West from the Empire City"; Raab, "Panoramic Vision, Telegraphic Language"; Valerie J. Fifer, *American Progress: The Growth of the Transport, Tourists, and Information Industries in the Nineteenth-Century West* (Globe Pequot, 1988); and Samantha Rothenberg, "Beyond *American Progress*: The Legacy of John Gast" (MA thesis, Sotheby's Institute of Art, 2012). Most interpreters of *American Progress* have neglected to note its relationship to an engraving Crofutt had commissioned more than a year earlier, J. Beard's *Progress*. See *Crofutt's Western World*, November 1871, 1.

9. Walkup addressed individual aspects of the picture in nearly the same order as Crofutt; "Description of Our Oil Chromo Entitled AMERICAN PROGRESS!," *Crofutt's Western World*, February 1873, 32 (emphasis in original).

10. "Description of Our Oil Chromo."

11. "Description of Our Oil Chromo"; "Description of Our Premium Oil Chromo, Entitled 'American Progress,'" *Crofutt's Western World*, June 1873, 7; "Beautiful Picture."

12. *Osage Mission (KS) Transcript*, November 22, 1872. See also *Kansas Chief* (Troy), December 19, 1872.

13. "The Horse Epidemic," *Salt Lake Herald-Republican*, January 9, 1873; *Virginia City (NV) Enterprise*, February 1, 1873, reprinted in "Swiftness of the Epizootic," *Sacramento Union*, February 3, 1873.

14. On Cheyenne, see "By Telegraph," *Cheyenne Leader*, January 13, 1873. On Salt Lake, see "It Has Arrived," *Deseret News*, January 15, 1873. On railway status, see *Maps Showing the Atlantic & Pacific and Leased Lines* (New York: G. W. and C. B. Colton and Co., 1873).

15. "Mails, Epizootic, &c.," *Las Cruces Borderer*, February 15, 1873; *Santa Fe Weekly New Mexican*, February 11, 1873; Veterinary [pseud.], February 2, 1873, in "Mails, Epizootic, &c.," *Las Cruces Borderer*, February 15, 1873; *Santa Fe New Mexican*, February 20, 1873. On claims that between 180 and 200 burros had died in and around Taos, compared to just "three horses and one mule," see Influenza [pseud.], February 12, 1873, in "The Epizootic in Taos," *Santa Fe New Mexican*, February 20, 1873.

16. "The Lesson of the Epizootic," *SFEB*, May 22, 1873.

17. Peter Mitchell, *Horse Nations: The Worldwide Impact of the Horse on Indigenous Societies Post-1492* (Oxford University Press, 2015).

18. *Cheyenne Leader*, January 13, 1873; "Items," *Helena Weekly Herald*, January 30, 1873; US Commissioner of Indian Affairs, *Annual Report of the Commissioner of Indian Affairs to the Secretary of the Interior for 1873* (GPO, 1874) (hereafter cited as ARCIA), 3. For accounts of the Modoc War that mention epizootic among army horses but say nothing about Native-owned horses, see, e.g., "Skirmish at Colonel Mason's Camp," *Sacramento Union*, April 16, 1873; "The Modoc War," *Sacramento Union*, April 19, 1873; *Puget Sound Dispatch* (Seattle, WA), April 24, 1873. Yavapai is pronounced like "YAH-vuh-pie." Dilzhę́'é is pronounced similarly to "dill-ZHAY-ay."

19. Undated item from *Denver News*, in *Laramie Sentinel*, January 18, 1873 ("all," etc.). On housing as a factor in equine influenza, see "Videx" [pseud.], "Veterinary Department: Equine Epidemic Influenza—The Physiology and Pathology of the Disease," *Turf, Field and Farm*, January 17, 1873, 38–39.

20. Mooney quoted in Russell Thornton, *American Indian Holocaust and Survival: A Population History Since 1492* (University of Oklahoma Press, 1987), 107. On California, see Benjamin Madley, "Understanding Genocide in California Under United States Rule, 1846–1873," *Western Historical Quarterly* 47 (2016): 449. Pekka Hämäläinen and Richard White claim that Comanche and Western Sioux populations rose through the 1840s and '50s, respectively. Pekka Hämäläinen, *Comanche Empire* (Yale University Press, 2008), 347–48; Richard White, "The Winning of the West: The Expansion of the Western Sioux in the Eighteenth and Nineteenth Centuries," *Journal of American History* 65 (1978): 329–30. For two useful discussions of epidemics in Indian Country, see David S. Jones, "Virgin Soils Revisited," *William & Mary Quarterly* 60 (2003): 703–42; and Tai S. Edwards and Paul Kelton, "Germs, Genocides, and America's Indigenous Peoples," *Journal of American History* 107 (2020): 52–76. On the Civil War in Indian Country, see Ned Blackhawk, *The Rediscovery of America: Native Peoples and the Unmaking of US History* (Yale University Press, 2023), chap. 9.

21. Population figures from Thornton, *American Indian Holocaust and Survival*, 133; John Douglas Belshaw, *Canadian History: Post-Confederation* (BCcampus, 2016), https://opentextbc.ca/postconfederation/. Historian Maurice Crandall, a member of the Yavapai-Apache Nation, refers to this as "our time of terror." Crandall, "When the City Comes to the Indian: Yavapai-Apache Exodus and Return to Urban Indian Homelands, 1870s–1920s," in *Indian Cities: Histories of Indigenous Urbanization*, ed. Kent Blansett, Cathleen D. Cahill, and Andrew Needham (University of Oklahoma Press, 2022), 141. On storied lands and "place-making" among Western Apaches, see Keith H. Basso, *Wisdom Sits*

in Places: Landscape and Language Among the Western Apache (University of New Mexico Press, 1996).

22. My terminology here borrows from Thornton, *American Indian Holocaust and Survival*. John C. Ewers posited that Indigenous horse holdings stabilized after the early 1800s; see *The Horse in Blackfoot Indian Culture: With Comparative Material from Other Western Tribes*, Smithsonian Institution Bureau of American Ethnology Bulletin 159 (1955; repr., Smithsonian Institution Press, 1969), 23.

23. Entry for May 21, 1862, in Lewis Henry Morgan, "Journal of an Expedition to the Rocky Mountains by the Missouri River in May, June, and July, 1862," in *Lewis Henry Morgan: The Indian Journals*, ed. Leslie A. White (University of Michigan Press, 1959), 143–44. Although Blackbird died in the smallpox epidemic of 1800–1801, such burial practices remained common into the late 1800s; see W. E. Walsh, "A Reexamination of the Historic Indian Burial from Yellowhouse Canyon, Texas," *Plains Anthropologist* 42 (1997): 243; Richard White, *Roots of Dependency: Subsistence, Environment, and Social Change Among the Choctaws, Pawnees, and Navajos* (University of Nebraska Press, 1983), 105; and Robert Neighbors to Henry Schoolcraft, "The Na-U-Ni, or Comanches of Texas: Their Traits and Beliefs, Their Divisions and Intertribal Relations," n.d., in Winfrey H. Dormian, *Texas Indian Papers, 1846–1859: Edited from the Original Manuscript Copies in the Texas State Archives* (Texas State Library, 1960), 357. On horses as food, see Dormian, *Texas Indian Papers, 1846–1859*, 356; Thomas G. Andrews, *Coyote Valley: Deep History in the High Rockies* (Harvard University Press, 2015), 72; D. O. Kennedy (Ochankugahe), *Recollections of an Assiniboine Chief* (McClelland and Stewart, 1972), 57–60. On sales to outsiders, see Dan Flores, "Bringing Home All the Pretty Horses: The Horse Trade in the Early American West, 1785–1825," *Montana: The Magazine of Western History* 58 (2008): 3–21, 94–96; Alexander Morris, *The Treaties of Canada with the Indians of Manitoba and the Northwest* (Toronto: Willing & Williamson, 1880), 9; and Report from Constantine Scollen to Alexander Morris, September 8, 1876, in Morris, *Treaties of Canada*, 248. For an example of the US Army killing Native horses, see Kathleen DuVal, *Native Nations: A Millennium in North America* (Random House, 2024), 498–99. On intertribal warfare, see, e.g., figure 154 ("Summer 1873") in James Mooney, *Calendar History of the Kiowa Indians, Seventeenth Annual Report of the Bureau of American Ethnology 1895–1896* (GPO, 1898), 337; and Janet C. Berlo, ed., *Plains Indian Drawings 1865–1935: Pages from a Visual History* (Harry N. Abrams, 1996), 106, 108, 110, 132. Droughts, blizzards, and other climatic and meteorological vicissitudes may also have taken a toll; see, e.g., drawings for winter 1865–66 in the Dakota and Corbusier Winter Counts found in Garrick Mallery, "Pictographs of the North American Indians—A Preliminary Paper," in *Fourth Annual Report of the Bureau of Ethnology to the Director of the Smithsonian Museum* (GPO, 1886), 124, 144.

24. Ryan Hall, "Negotiating Sovereignty: US and Canadian Colonialisms on the Northwest Plains," in *Remaking North American Sovereignty: State Transformation in the 1860s*, ed. Jewel L. Spangler and Frank Towers (Fordham University Press, 2020), 132–52.

25. *Report of the Indian Branch of the Department of the Secretary of State for the Provinces* (Ottawa: I. B. Taylor, 1872), 19–24; *Report of the Indian Branch of the Department of the Minister of the Interior, For the Year Ended 30th June, 1873* (Ottawa: I. B. Taylor, 1874), 5; Morris, *Treaties of Canada*, 287–88; Sarah Carter, *Lost Harvests: Prairie Indian Reserve Farmers and Government Policy* (McGill-Queen's University Press, 1990); and C. Joseph Genetin-Pilawa, *The Crooked Paths to Allotment: The Fight over Federal Indian Policy After the Civil War* (University of North Carolina Press, 2012).

26. On reduced raiding along the US-Mexico borderlands, see Hämäläinen, *Comanche Empire*, conclusion; Brian DeLay, *War of a Thousand Deserts* (Yale University Press, 2008), epilogue; Lance R. Blyth, *Chiracahua and Janos: Communities of Violence in the Southwestern Borderlands, 1680–1880* (University of Nebraska Press, 2012), chap. 6; and Karl Jacoby, *Shadows at Dawn: An Apache Massacre and the Violence of History* (Penguin, 2009). For mentions of raids in 1872–73, see ARCIA 1873, 6, 42, 153, 167, 201, 219, 231, 248.

27. ARCIA 1873, 221 ("plenty"); ARCIA 1873, 234 ("In former times"); "Extract of a Despatch, W. J. Christie, Chief Factor at Edmonton House to Lieut. Governor Archibald," April 13, 1871, in *Report of the Indian Branch of the Department of the Secretary of State for the Provinces*, 33 ("the visible"); Sweet Grass, quoted in "Messages from the Creek Chiefs of the Plains, Saskatchewan, to Gov Archibald," n.d., in *Report of the Indian Branch of the Department of the Secretary of State for the Provinces*, 33–34 ("the Chief").

28. All quotes here and below from Walkup from *PH*, March 1, 1873. I have chosen to alternate this leader's Piikani and English names to balance respect for the name by which he knew himself with the imperative of honoring the many hundreds of his descendants who continue to use the English translation of his name as their family name. On Heavy Runner's Piikani name, see Adolf Hungry-Wolf, *The Blackfoot Papers*, vol. 4, *Biographies* (Good Medicine Cultural Foundation, 2006), 1115. Although Calf Tail called this a "mixed camp," Issokui-omachkan led the Worm band. Hungry-Wolf, *Blackfoot Papers*, 4:1018. On the Piikani name for the Marias River, see Nora Mabie, "A Story of Genocide, Survival and Resilience: Blackfeet Nation Remembers Baker Massacre," *Great Falls Tribune*, January 16, 2020. The best book-length studies are Andrew Graybill, *The Red and the White: A Family Saga of the American West* (Liveright, 2013); and Paul R. Wylie, *Blood on the Marias: The Baker Massacre* (University of Oklahoma Press, 2016). Also useful are Blanca Tovías, "Diplomacy and Contestation Before and After the 1870 Massacre of Amskapi Pikuni," *Ethnohistory* 60 (2013): 269–93; and Rodger C. Henderson, "The Piikuni and the US Army's Piegan Expedition: Competing Narratives of the 1870 Massacre on the Marias River," *Montana: The Magazine of Western History* 68 (2018): 48–70, 93–96. For published Blackfoot narratives, see James White Calf, "My Memories of the Baker Massacre," in Hungry-Wolf, *Blackfoot Papers*, vol. 1, *Pikunni History and Culture* (Good Medicine Cultural Foundation, 2006), 52; and Ramona Big Head, "'Strike Them Hard!': The Baker Massacre Play" (MEd thesis, University of Lethbridge, 2009). Baker and others repeatedly invoked the figure of 173 dead but changed their story over time about how many women, children, and other noncombatants this figure included; see Wylie, *Blood on the Marias*, chap. 9. On Sheridan's role, see Paul A. Hutton, "Phil Sheridan's Pyrrhic Victory: The Piegan Massacre, Army Politics, and the Transfer Debate," *Montana: The Magazine of Western History* 32 (1982): 32–43.

29. Angel quotes from [Angel], *History of Placer County*, 176. On 1864 meeting, see "Proceedings of the County Central Committee," *PH*, April 16, 1864.

30. Philip Henry Sheridan, *Personal Memoirs of P. H. Sheridan, General, United States Army* (New York: C. L. Webster & Co., 1888), 1:3–7; US Grant to Philip Sheridan, August 26, 1864, in Sheridan, *Personal Memoirs of P. H. Sheridan*, 1:486–87; and Scott C. Patchan, *Shenandoah Summer: The 1864 Valley Campaign* (University of Nebraska Press, 2007).

31. See "Another Chance," *PH*, October 31, 1868; and "Telegraphic Summary," *PH*, November 11, 1871. For a detailed discussion, see Carl Smith, *Urban Disorder and the Shape of Belief: The Great Chicago Fire, the Haymarket Bomb, and the Model Town of Pullman*, 2nd ed. (1995; University of Chicago Press, 2007), 77–80. No indictment was issued.

32. "Letter from Roseville," PH, May 10, 1872; "To Governor Booth," PH, March 8, 1873; and "The Heathen Chinee," PH, June 7, 1873.

33. "Sudden Demise," *Placer Argus* (Auburn, CA), October 18, 1873. Foucault was especially fond of this inversion of Clausewitz's famous formulation. Mark Kelly, "Carl von Clausewitz," in *The Cambridge Foucault Lexicon*, ed. Leonard Lawlor and John Nale (Cambridge University Press, 2014), 693–94.

34. *Cincinnati Enquirer*, quoted in Wylie, *Blood on the Marias*, 234; "Just Retribution," *Fayetteville (TN) Observer*, January 4, 1872. This smallpox narrative unfolded as part of a broader push by Democratic newspapers to impugn Grant's Indian policies by identifying Sheridan with the Marias Massacre; see, e.g., "Over the Plains," *Memphis Appeal*, June 15, 1872; "The Indian Problem," *Buffalo Weekly Courier*, July 3, 1872.

35. "The Small-Pox," PH, January 20, 1872.

36. Bear Head affidavit, January 18, 1915, Heavy Runner Records, 1914–1921, MF 53, Montana Historical Society, Helena (hereafter cited as Heavy Runner Records); Mrs. Frank Monroe affidavit, January 18, 1916, and H.[orace] J. Clarke affidavit, November 9, 1920, Heavy Runner Records. See also Buffalo Trail Woman affidavit, January 16, 1916, Heavy Runner Records. Good Bear Woman's affidavit mentioned that soldiers set lodges on fire but made no mention of robes. January 16, 1916, Heavy Runner Records. For other evidence of soldiers destroying robes, see Joseph Kipp affidavits, February 8, 1913, and December 29, 1914, Heavy Runner Records. For concurring evidence, see Henry Myers to Franklin Lane, January 11, 1916, Heavy Runner Records.

37. Wylie, *Blood on the Marias*, chap. 11 (quote from 233).

38. Smallpox first appeared in the French countryside in 1869 and reached Paris in 1870. Donald R. Hopkins, *The Greatest Killer: Smallpox in History, with a New Introduction* (1983; repr., University of Chicago Press, 2002), 89–93; Matthew Smallman-Raynor and Andrew D. Cliff, "The Geographical Transmission of Smallpox in the Franco-Prussian War: Prisoner of War Camps and Their Impact upon Epidemic Diffusion Processes in the Civil Settlement System of Prussia, 1870–71," *Medical History* 46 (2002): 241–64. On this epidemic in North America, see Robert Higgs, "Cycles and Trends of Mortality in 18 Large American Cities, 1871–1900," *Explorations in Economic History* 16 (1979): 399; "The Small Pox in Harnett," *Raleigh News*, November 23, 1872; "Ledger Lines," *Memphis Public Ledger*, December 17, 1872; "It Has Arrived," *Deseret News*, January 15, 1873.

39. "Smallpox and the Administration," *Memphis Appeal*, October 28, 1872.

40. James Law, "Influenza in Horses," in *Report of the Commissioner of Agriculture for the Year 1872* (GPO, 1872), 218; and Adoniram B. Judson, "History and Course of the Epizoötic Among Horses upon the North American Continent," *Public Health Reports and Papers Presented at the Meetings of the American Public Health Association in the Year 1873* (New York and Cambridge, MA: Hurd and Houghton and the Riverside Press, 1875), 88–109.

41. "Origin of the Epizootic," *Helena Weekly Herald*, February 13, 1873. Walkup may have read of this article in "Where the Epizootic Came From," SF *Examiner*, February 25, 1873.

42. Henry Myers to Franklin Lane, January 11, 1916, Heavy Runner Records ("reimburse"); other quotes from Bear Head, Clarke, and Kipp affidavits, as well as William Upham, Emma Miller, and Dick Kipp to Commissioner of Indian Affairs (CIA), March 16, 1914, Heavy Runner Records. Factual disagreements in the affidavits gathered by Heavy Runner's heirs and disparities between their recollections and official US Army reports filed in 1870 gave Secretary of the Interior Franklin Lane a pretext for ignoring the heirs'

cause. Franklin Lane to Henry Ashurst, January 24, 1916, and April 25, 1917, Heavy Runner Records.

43. Quotes from Wylie, *Blood on the Marias*, 230–32.

44. Wylie, *Blood on the Marias*, chaps. 9–11; Henderson, "Piikuni and the US Army's Piegan Expedition."

CHAPTER 7

1. Stephen H. Haber, *Industry and Underdevelopment: The Industrialization of Mexico, 1890–1940* (Stanford University Press, 1989), 13–15.

2. Gustavo Ruiz y Sandoval, *La epizootia de los años de 1872 y 1873 en el Continente America, presentado como tesis de concurso, para la oposicion a la Plaza de Catedratico de 40. Año de Veterario* (Mexico: n.p., 1874), 10–11; "Foreign," *Frank Leslie's Illustrated Newspaper*, April 12, 1873, 71 ("many regiments").

3. "Mas sobre la epizootia," *El Eco de Ambos Mundos* (Mexico City), April 15, 1873; "Zacatecas," *El Correo del Comercio*, April 18, 1873; "Tamaulipas," *El Eco de Ambos Mundos* (Mexico City), April 30, 1873; "La epizootia," *La Iberia* (Mexico City), August 1, 1873; "Sonora," *La Iberia* (Mexico City), December 3, 1873; David M. Pletcher, "The Building of the Mexican Railway," *Hispanic American Historical Review* 30 (1950): 26–27; John H. Coatsworth, "Obstacles to Economic Growth in Nineteenth-Century Mexico," *American Historical Review* 83 (1978): 91–92.

4. "Epizootia y hidrofobia," *El Siglo Diez y Nueve* (Mexico City), March 20, 1873 (quoted); "Mexico," *NYH*, March 27, 1873; "Epizootia," *El Correo del Comercio* (Mexico City), March 22, 1873; "La epizootia," *La Voz de México*, March 22, 1873.

5. Ruiz y Sandoval, *La epizootia*, 14–17; José Maria Lugo, "Estudio de la epizotia [*sic*]," *Gaceta Medica* 8 (1873): 160.

6. Ruiz y Sandoval, *La epizootia*, 14 ("in contact"); José V. del Collado, letter of March 7, 1873, in "Epizootia," *La Iberia* (Mexico City), March 13, 1873 ("all the horses"); "Gacetilla-La epizootia," *El Siglo Diez y Nueve* (Mexico City), March 10, 1873 ("fear that the epidemic"); I. Alvarado, March 16, 1873, in "La epizootia," *El Cultivador*, May 1, 1873, 159–62; "La epizootia," *Eco de Ambos Mundos* (Mexico City), March 11, 1873; letters from District Governor and M. A. Mercado, March 12 and 13, 1873, Expediente 25, Caja 1, Seres-HV [Higiene veterinaria, Secretaria-HP [Higiene publica], Fondo-SP [Salud publica], Archivo Historico/Centro de la Documentacion Institucional de la Secretario de la Salud, Mexico City; "La epizootia en Veracruz," *El Eco de Ambos Mundos* (Mexico City), March 29, 1873; *El Siglo Diez y Nueve* (Mexico City) April 14, 1873.

7. "La epizootia," *El Monitor Republicano* (Mexico City), March 16, 1873 ("an effective remedy"); "Curacion de la epizootia," *El Siglo Diez y Nueve* (Mexico City), March 18, 1873 ("four hundred and fifty-seven"); "Ciencias," *El Pajaro* (Mexico City), March 20, 1873; "Mejico," *Estrella de Panamá* (Panama City), June 10, 1873.

8. "Remedio eficaz," *El Padres Cobos* (Mexico City), March 16, 1873 ("news"); "La epizootia," *El Correo del Comercio*, March 13, 1873 ("serious disturbances"); "Charla de los Domingos," *El Monitor Republicano* (Mexico City), March 23, 1873 ("extremely sad"). See also "La epizootia," *El Correo del Comercio*, March 14, 1873; "Revista de la semana," *El Eco de Ambos Mundos* (Mexico City), March 23, 1873; "Ecos de Tacubaya," *El Monitor Republicano* (Mexico City), March 29, 1873; "Ferrocarril de Tacubaya," *La Voz de México* (Mexico City), April 1, 1873; "La epizootia," *La Orquesta* (Mexico City), April 4, 1873.

9. "Moneda y comestibles," *El Correo del Comercio* (Mexico City), March 28, 1873 ("basic necessities"); "Varias noticias," *La Iberia* (Mexico City), April 9, 1873 ("succumbed in greater proportions"); Ruiz y Sandoval, *La epizootia*, 15 ("was noted"); "Varias noticias," *La Iberia* (Mexico City), March 25, 1873 ("prices of various items"); "Consecuencias de la epizootia," *Bandera de Juarez* (Mexico City), April 9, 1873 ("very scarce"). Statistics on San Luis Potosí from "La epizootia," *La Reconstrucción* (Mexico City), May 14, 1873. The same source also mentioned the death of one hundred "foals [*potros*]," but since this term could apply to any species of equine, I have excluded it from these figures. On the stickiness of prices, see "Varias noticias," *La Iberia* (Mexico City), May 8, 1873; and "Consecuencias de la epizootia," *El Monitor Republicano* (Mexico City), May 9, 1873.

10. "La epizootia," *El Siglo Diez y Nueve* (Mexico City), March 18, 1873 ("pestiferous miasmas"); "Muladares," *El Monitor Republicano* (Mexico City), March 23, 1873 ("full of the cadavers"); "Epizootia," *El Siglo Diez y Nueve* (Mexico City), March 24, 1873 ("the prevailing epizootic"); "La epizootia," *La Voz de México* (Mexico City), March 26, 1873 ("to prevent"); "Boletin del 'Monitor,'" *El Monitor Republicano* (Mexico City), April 3, 1873 ("complain[ed]"). On incineration, see "La epizootia," *El Monitor Republicano* (Mexico City), April 2, 1873. On the lack of municipal funds, see "Falta de fondos," *La Voz de México* (Mexico City), March 27, 1873; and "La epizootia," *El Monitor Republicano* (Mexico City), April 2, 1873. On reports of influenza among humans, see Ruiz y Sandoval, *La epizootia*, 20–21.

11. Ruiz y Sandoval, *La epizootia*, 11–12. The Sierra Mixtec was much more heavily populated before the disease, violence, and displacement of Spanish conquest.

12. Maurice Crandall, "When the City Comes to the Indian: Yavapai-Apache Exodus and Return to Urban Indian Homelands, 1870s–1920s," in *Indian Cities: Histories of Indigenous Urbanization*, ed. Kent Blansett, Cathleen D. Cahill, and Andrew Needham (University of Oklahoma Press, 2022), 140; Timothy Braatz, *Surviving Conquest: A History of the Yavapai Peoples* (University of Nebraska Press, 2003), 25. Crandall is quoting here from Daniel J. Herman, *Rim Country Exodus: A Story of Conquest, Renewal, and Race in the Making* (University of Arizona Press, 2012), 27. Tribal elders say that "all Yavapai come from Sedona first. But in time they spread around." Mike Harrison and John Williams, *Oral History of the Yavapai*, ed. Sigrid Khera and Carolina C. Butler (Acacia, 2012), 168. For Yavapai and Dilzhę́'é perspectives, see Mike Burns (Hoomothya), *All My People Were Killed: The Memoir of Mike Burns (Hoomothya), a Captive Indian* (Sharlot Hall Museum, 2010); Maurice Crandall, "Yava-Who? Yavapai History and (Mis)Representation in Arizona's Indigenous Landscape," *Journal of Arizona History* 61 (2020): 487–510; and Maurice Crandall, "Captive Cousins: Hoomothya, Wassaja, and a Lifetime of Unwellness," *Western Historical Quarterly* 54 (2023): 117–36. All Yavapai and Dilzhę́'é terms from Yavapai-Apache Nation, *Wipukpa-Tolkapaya Yavapai Dictionary Online* (2026), https://dictionary.yavapailanguage.org/; and Yavapai-Apache Nation, *Dilzhe'e Apache Dictionary Online* (2026), https://dilzhee.western-apache.org/.

13. Braatz, *Surviving Conquest*, 29–33 ("Families"); Inyo-kutavêre ("Vanishedpursue"), "In the Desert with Hipahipa," ed. A. L. Kroeber, in *Surviving Through the Days: Translations of Native California Stories and Songs: A California Indian Reader*, ed. Herbert W. Luthin (University of California Press, 2002), 448 ("We have taken").

14. Crandall, "Captive Cousins," 119–20 ("our traditional enemies"); John C. Cremony, "The Apache Race," *Overland Monthly* 1 (1868), in Peter Cozzens, *Eyewitnesses to the Indian Wars, 1865–1890*, vol. 1: *The Struggle for Apacheria* (Stackpole Books, 2001), 13 ("horses captured by them"); L. Y. Loring, "Report on [the] Coyotero Apaches," n.d., in Cozzens,

Eyewitnesses to the Indian Wars, 1:187, 191 ("esteemed as a delicacy"). See also Harrison and Williams, *Oral History of the Yavapai*, 215; Braatz, *Surviving Conquest*, 64–68.

15. Harrison and Williams, *Oral History of the Yavapai*, 132.

16. Braatz, *Surviving Conquest*, 70–72; Natale Zappia, "Revolutions in the Grass: Energy and Food Systems in Continental North America, 1763–1848," *Environmental History* 21 (2016): 43.

17. "Come at Last," AM (Prescott), March 8, 1873; Thaddeus Harlan Stanton, "Itinerary of a Journey to and through Arizona in the Winter of 1871–72," Rare Page Manuscripts, Huntington Library, San Marino, CA, page 95 ("about one thousand people"); entry for March 11, 1873, in *The Diaries of John Gregory Bourke*, vol. 1: *November 20, 1872–July 28, 1876*, ed. Charles M. Robinson (University of North Texas Press, 2003), 71 ("has broken out"); *Puget Sound Dispatch* (Seattle), March 27, 1873 ("to an alarming extent"). On the outbreak's initial arrival, see "The Direct Eastern Mail," *Arizona Citizen* (Tucson), March 1, 1873. Crook famously beefed with Philip Sheridan; George Crook, *General George Crook: His Autobiography*, ed. Martin F. Schmitt (1946; repr., University of Oklahoma Press, 1960), 134n7.

18. Cremony, "Apache Race," 13; "Description of Our Oil Chromo Entitled AMERICAN PROGRESS!," *Crofutt's Western World*, February 1873, 32. For a military historian's take on these events, see Paul Andrew Hutton, *The Apache Wars: The Hunt for Geronimo, the Apache Kid, and the Captive Boy Who Started the Longest War in American History* (Crown, 2016), chaps. 11, 13.

19. "General Howard's Mission," *Army and Navy Journal*, April 27, 1872, in Cozzens, *Eyewitnesses to the Indian Wars*, 1:114; Sylvester Mowry, NYH, May 14, 1871, in Cozzens, *Eyewitnesses to the Indian Wars*, 1:68. See also Charles B. Genung, "Indians and Indigo," *Los Angeles Mining Review* (1909–11), in Cozzens, *Eyewitnesses to the Indian Wars*, 1:71; John G. Bourke, "Crook's Campaign in '72," *Chicago Inter Ocean*, July 5, 1883, in Cozzens, *Eyewitnesses to the Indian Wars*, 1:141.

20. Entry for December 11 and 21, 1872, in Bourke, *Diaries*, 1:34, 42. See also Dan L. Thrapp, *Al Sieber: Chief of Scouts* (1964; repr., University of Oklahoma Press, 1995), 108. In the following weeks, Crook supplemented these five columns with troops from other posts.

21. "General Crook," from the *Denver News*, April 23, 1873, in SFC, May 11, 1873. See also Crook, *General George Crook*, 160–62.

22. John G. Bourke, *On the Border with Crook* (New York: Charles Scribner's Sons, 1891), 150 ("made pack-trains") and ("as nearly perfect"), 138. On the units involved, see US Adjutant General, *Chronological List of Actions, &c., with Indians, from January 1, 1866, to January, 1891* (GPO, 1891), in *Indian Battles and Skirmishes on the American Frontier, 1790–1898*, ed. Joseph P. Peters (Argonaut Press, 1966), 30–31. One military source later listed several of Crook's packers; most bore Anglo names, with the exception of "Chileno John" and "Manuel Lopez." H. W. Daly, *Manual of Pack Transportation* (GPO, 1917), 17. Bourke remarked on the death of another packer, "the sick Mexican Presiliano Mongo." Entries for March 22 and 24, 1873, in Bourke, *Diaries*, 1:75–77.

23. Bourke, *On the Border with Crook*, 150, 154; Emmett M. Essin III, "Mules, Packs, and Packtrains," *Southwestern Historical Quarterly* 74 (1970): 54–55. Each train also had a bell mare and fourteen saddle mules.

24. "Peace Prospect Brighter," *Arizona Weekly Citizen* (Tucson), April 5, 1873 ("suffering much"); *Juniata Sentinel* (Mifflintown, PA), March 19, 1873 ("Indian ponies"); Bourke, *On the Border with Crook*, 208 ("crippling the resources"). See also Crandall, "Captive Cousins," 120.

25. Bourke, *On the Border with Crook*, 208–9.

26. George Crook, "General Orders No. 14," April 9, 1873, quoted in Dan L. Thrapp, *Conquest of Apacheria* (University of Oklahoma Press, 1967), 143. For Bourke's claim of five hundred killed, which may have been a serious undercount, see entry for April 7, 1873, in Bourke, *Diaries*, 1:82.

27. Crook, *General George Crook*, 179.

28. Escheteplan quoted in Crook, *General George Crook*, 179; Bourke, *On the Border with Crook*, 200 ("San Carlos agency"). Bourke was referring specifically to the Skeleton Cave Massacre, but a broader sense of trauma permeates written and oral histories from Hoomothya (Mike Burns), Mike Harrison, John Williams, and other Yavapai and Dilzhę́'é people.

29. Headquarters, Military Division of the Pacific, "General Orders No. 10," November 21, 1871, Arizona Superintendency, Letters Received, 1863–1880, Microfilm Publication M234: Letters Received by the Office of Indian Affairs, 1824–1881, National Archives and Records Administration (hereafter cited as Arizona Superintendency, Letters Received), reel 9.

30. See, for example, M. Soule to H. Bendell, November 17, 1872, and A. H. Nickerson to Commander, Camp Apache, November 5, 1872, both in Arizona Superintendency, Letters Received, reel 5. Crook and Bourke each placed the total number of such auxiliaries at 200 to 250, but Bourke added that his number was "exclusive of any operating from [Fort] McDowell or Prescott." Crook, *General George Crook*, xii, 175; entry for December 21, 1872, in Bourke, *Diaries*, 1:42. On scout leaders, see Michael Lynn Tate, "Apache Scouts, Police, and Judges as Agents of Acculturation, 1865–1920" (PhD diss., University of Toledo, 1974), 56–57; and Thrapp, *Al Sieber*.

31. Figures based on Gregory F. Michno, ed., *Encyclopedia of Indian Wars: Western Battles and Skirmishes, 1850–1890* (Mountain Press, 2003), 259–61. US officers rarely identified their victims by nation or band; any identifications they offered, moreover, remain unreliable.

32. Thrapp, *Conquest of Apacheria*, 134–35.

33. Crook, *General George Crook*, 177–78. On band name, see Greenville Goodwin, *The Social Organization of the Western Apache* (1942; repr., University of Arizona Press, 1969), chap. 1.

34. Crook, *General George Crook*, 177–78.

35. Crook, *General George Crook*, 177–78; *Buffalo Commercial*, April 7, 1873. For lower figures, see AM (Prescott), March 28, 1873, quoted in "The Arizona Apaches," SFC, April 7, 1873. Later dispatches raised the body count to forty-one and forty-seven. "Indian News," AM (Prescott), April 5, 1873; "The Modoc War," CT, April 18, 1873. Retrospective sources, though, claimed that twenty-three were killed and ten captured. Michno, *Encyclopedia of Indian Wars*, 264.

36. Eschetlepan quoted in Bourke, *On the Border with Crook*, 213. See also AM, March 28, 1873, quoted in "The Arizona Apaches," SFC, April 7, 1873.

37. AM, March 28, 1873, quoted in "Gen. Crook's Operations," CT, April 21, 1873. See also "The Apache Troubles Subsiding," *New York Tribune*, May 1, 1873; "Indian Policy Epitomized," *Arizona Weekly Citizen* (Tucson), May 24, 1873.

38. Burns (Hoomothya), *All My People Were Killed*, 95, 106–7, 113–16; William H. Corbusier, *Soldier, Surgeon, Scholar: The Memoirs of William Henry Corbusier, 1844–1930*, ed. Robert Wooster (University of Oklahoma Press, 2003), 83–84; William H. Corbusier, "Del-Cha, or Wa-Po-Wa-Ta, Big Rump, and Yavapai, Tulkepa and Walapai Apache Geographic

Names in Arizona," p. 1, typescript in William Henry Corbusier Indian Language Vocabularies, HM 63703, Huntington Library, San Marino, CA. Elsewhere, Corbusier placed those "collected" at Rio Verde in May 1873 at "about 2000." Untitled photostat in Corbusier Indian Language Vocabularies, HM 63694, Huntington Library, 105.

39. Bourke, *On the Border with Crook*, 213.

40. Harrison and Williams, *Oral History of the Yavapai*, 144; Braatz, *Surviving Conquest*, 146. On the daily practice of calling roll, see Nickerson to Commanding Officer, November 5, 1872, and A. G. Buttoner to H. Bendell, April 28, 1873, Records of the Arizona Superintendency, 1863–1873, Microfilm Publication M734, Records of the Bureau of Indian Affairs, RG 75, National Archives and Records Administration, reel 7.

41. Braatz, *Surviving Conquest*, chaps. 3, 4; William Corbusier, manuscript copy made in 1928 of undated manuscript authored by Corbusier and held by the Bureau of American Ethnology, Corbusier Indian Language Vocabularies, p. 105.

42. In August 1873, for instance, Verde Agent Josephus Williams reported that "Apache Tontos numbering over nine hundred left reservation last night supposed induced to leave by renegade Apaches from Camp Apache." Joseph Williams to Commissioner of Indian Affairs, August 12, 1873, Arizona Superintendency, Letters Received, reel 9. "Most" returned within a few weeks. Williams to Commissioner of Indian Affairs (CIA), August 28, 1873, Arizona Superintendency, Letters Received, reel 9. On earlier escapees, see T. M. K. Smith to Assistant Adjutant General, Department of Arizona, May 1, 1872, and Philip Dwyer to Captain A. H. Nickerson, May 12, 1872, Arizona Superintendency, Letters Received, reel 5; Herman, *Rim Country Exodus*, 82–85.

43. "The Indians," CT, July 19, 1873; "The Indians," *Detroit Free Press*, July 22, 1873; "A Brush with the Apaches," *Rochester Democrat and Chronicle*, August 18, 1873; William H. Corbusier, "The Apache-Yumas and Apache-Mojaves," *American Antiquarian and Oriental Journal* 8 (1886): 276–78; "Indian Affairs," *New York Tribune*, November 11, 1873; Albert H. Schroeder, *A Study of Yavapai History* (1959), in *Yavapai Indians* (Garland, 1974), 287. This list of atrocities is undoubtedly incomplete; in his table for 1872, for instance, Schroeder omitted any mention of the Skeleton Cave Massacre.

44. Corbusier, "Apache-Yumas and Apache-Mojaves," 276–78; Corbusier, *Soldier, Surgeon, Scholar*, 73. A former army colleague who served with Corbusier in Arizona told a mutual acquaintance in 1928 that he had refrained from using the physician's name in a story he published on the Grand Offensive "because of the one gruesome thing of his boiling the flesh off the heads of the specimen skulls he purposed shipping to the Smithsonian Institution." George O. Eaton to Charles King, September 14, 1928, Charles King Papers, HM 63684, Huntington Library. In 1879 Corbusier was credited with contributing "the complete skeletons . . . of seven Sioux" he had "exhumed" while stationed on the Plains. "Anthropology," *American Naturalist* 13 (1879): 48.

45. Corbusier quoted in "Veteran of Valley's Early History Visits," July 11, 1921, clipping from unidentified newspaper from Jerome, AZ, in box 1, folder 11, Mike Burns (Hoomothya) Papers, SHM MS-8, Sharlot Hall Library and Archives, Prescott, AZ; Burns (Hoomothya), *All My People Were Killed*, 115. Agent Josephus Williams claimed that "at present about 70 or 80 per cent. of the Indians" at the Rio Verde Reserve were "sick from Malarial Fever and Scurvey [*sic*]." Williams to Commissioner of Indian Affairs, September 20, 1873, Arizona Superintendency, Letters Received, reel 9. See also Williams to CIA, November

26, 1873, Arizona Superintendency, Letters Received, reel 9. On earlier routes of malaria transmission to Indigenous populations in Arizona, see Heidi Roberts and Richard V. N. Ahlstrom, "Malaria, Microbes, and Mechanisms of Change," *Kiva* 63 (1997): 117–35.

46. Corbusier, "Apache-Yumas and Apache-Mojaves," 277–78; Corbusier, *Soldier, Surgeon, Scholar*, 73–74.

CHAPTER 8

1. Quotes from "Local Brevities," SFAC, April 14, 1873; and "An Official Tribute to General Canby's Memory," SFAC, April 15, 1873. For coverage of Crook's campaigns, see "The Modoc War," CT, April 18, 1873; and "Peace in Arizona," SFC, April 18, 1873. Human population figure from Henry G. Langley, *The San Francisco Directory for the Year Commencing March, 1873* [. . .] (San Francisco: Henry G. Langley, 1873), n.p. ("Prefatory" section). In 1869–70, the city assessor supposedly recorded 9,000 horses, 180 mules, and 5 asses; in 1874–75, these numbers had fallen to 7,068, 16, and 0, respectively, bucking the national trend of equine population growth (intervening reports provide no equine population figures). *San Francisco Municipal Reports for the Fiscal Year 1869–70, Ending June 30, 1870* (San Francisco: Cosmopolitan, 1870), 84 and *San Francisco Municipal Reports for the Fiscal Year 1874–5, Ending June 30, 1875* (San Francisco: Spaulding & Barto, 1875), 110.

2. "Brief Mention," SFEB, July 31, 1873.

3. William Simpson, *Meeting the Sun: A Journey All Round the World, Through Egypt, China, Japan and California, Including an Account of the Marriage Ceremonies of the Emperor of China* (Boston: Estes & Lauriat, 1877), 351.

4. US Const. amend. XIV, sec. 1. The body of the 1866 act largely pertained to "citizens," but section 2 referred to "inhabitants," and the terms "person" and "persons" appear throughout; Civil Rights Acts of 1866, 14 Stat. 27–30. Also relevant was the Burlingame-Seward Treaty of 1868; *Text of the Treaty Between China and the United States, Generally Known as the "Burlingame Treaty"* (n.p.: n.p., n.d.), article VI, 6. See also the Civil Rights or Enforcement Act of 1870, 16 Stat. 140.

5. This approach builds on Beth Lew-Williams's exemplary deployment of "transscalar" analysis in *The Chinese Must Go: Violence, Exclusion, and the Making of the Alien in America* (Harvard University Press, 2018).

6. "The Horse Disease," SFC, April 18, 1873 ("a good many"); "San Francisco News," *Marysville (CA) Appeal*, April 19, 1873 ("over a thousand"); "The Epizootic," SFC, April 22, 1873 ("rapidity"); "The Epizootic," SFC, April 25, 1873 ("alarming"). Three-quarters estimate from "Epizootic," SFEB, April 26, 1873. The disease had already struck animals in Oakland on April 12; "The Epizootic," SFC, April 16, 1873.

7. "The Epizootic," SFC, April 25, 1873 ("great suffering"); "Review of the Market for the Week Ending Friday Morning, May 2d, 1873," *SF Commercial Herald and Market Review*, May 2, 1873 ("lessened cargoes"); "The Epizootic," SFC, April 25, 1873 ("newspaper carriers").

8. "The Epizooty," *SF Examiner*, April 26, 1873 ("a large number"); "California Items," *Two Republics* (Mexico City), June 7, 1873 ("The spread"). See also "The Epizooty," *SF Examiner*, April 26, 1873. Another account, by contrast, claimed that the CP had fired twenty men. "Epizootic," SFEB, April 26, 1873. In addition to several dozen laundry and sprinkling wagons, San Franciscans registered 211 "Coaches, Omnibuses, Hacks and

Coupees," 464 "Double Wagons and Trucks" (all of which boasted two axles), 1,392 "Grocery, Milk, Bakery and Market Wagons" (a group composed largely or entirely or two-axle vehicles), and 2,361 "Single Wagons, Trucks, Drays and Carts" (which probably had a single axle). License Collector's Report, in San Francisco Board of Supervisors, *San Francisco Municipal Reports for the Fiscal Year 1872–73, Ending June 30th, Ending June 30th, 1873* (San Francisco: Spaulding & Barto, 1873), 238.

9. "Auction Sale of Paintings," *SFC*, April 24, 1873 (quoted). On ads, see *SFEB*, April 18, 1873. By April 26, bran had increased from $19 to $35 a ton, while carrot prices increased from 75 cents per hundredweight to $2.50 or $3.00. "The Epizooty," *SFC*, April 26, 1873. Intriguingly, one local magazine claimed that the epizootic's effects included "raising the price of bran, Chinese carrots and vegetables in general." "What Thistleton's Jolly Giant Saw and Heard About the Streets," *Thistleton's Jolly Giant (The Critic)*, May 3, 1873. Although carrots originated in Central Asia and have been grown in China for millennia, they had become a fixture in Europe and the Americas long before the 1870s. This reference to "Chinese carrots," then, hints that Chinese American farmers may have contributed significantly to San Francisco's supply.

10. "The Epizootic," *SF Examiner*, April 24, 1873 ("$15"); "Epizootic," *SFEB*, April 26, 1873 ("rates"); "The Epizooty," *SF Examiner*, April 26, 1873 ("as high as"); "The Epizooty," *SFC*, April 27, 1873 ("large prices"); "The Horse Disease," *SFAC*, April 26, 1873 ("nine"); "Epizootic," *SFEB*, April 26, 1873 ("more [arrests]"). On farmers' recognition of the risks their profit-seeking entailed, see, e.g., "The Horse Disease," *SFC*, April 23, 1873. On the SFSPCA, see Andrew Robichaud, *Animal City: The Domestication of America* (Harvard University Press, 2019), chap. 4. More broadly, see Jessica Wang, *Mad Dogs and Other New Yorkers: Rabies, Medicine, and Society in an American Metropolis, 1840–1920* (Johns Hopkins University Press, 2019).

11. "The Epizooty," *SF Examiner*, April 26, 1873 ("first ox team"); Henry G. Langley, *The San Francisco Directory for the Year Commencing March, 1872 [. . .]* (San Francisco: Henry G. Langley, 1872), 622 ("importers"); "The Equine-Noctial," *SFC*, May 1, 1873 ("several yoke"); "The Epizooty," *SFC*, April 27, 1873 ("tender memories").

12. "Epizootic," *SFEB*, April 26, 1873; "The Epizooty," *SF Examiner*, April 28, 1873.

13. "The Epizootic," *SF Examiner*, April 24, 1873.

14. "Epizootic in California," *Harrisburg (PA) Telegraph*, April 25, 1873 ("hire"); "The Value of Horse Flesh," *Sacramento Bee*, April 25, 1873 ("Unable"). On behavior-based laws, see Beth Lew-Williams, *John Doe Chinaman: Race and Law in the American West* (Harvard University Press, 2025).

15. Samuel Wells Williams to Rev. W. F. Williams, March 26, 1849, in *The Life and Letters of Samuel Wells Williams, LL.D., Missionary, Diplomatist, Sinologue* (New York: G. P. Putnam's Sons, 1889), 169–70. Other claims here and below draw on Yong Chen, *Chinese San Francisco, 1850–1943: A Trans-Pacific Community* (Stanford University Press, 2000), 35–36; and Mae Ngai, *The Chinese Question: The Gold Rushes and Global Politics* (W. W. Norton, 2021), 19–21. Roughly forty Chinese arrived before this English-sponsored ship landed. Ngai, *Chinese Question*, 325n5.

16. Shi-Shan Henry Tsai, *China and the Overseas Chinese in the United States, 1868–1911* (University of Arkansas Press, 1984), 14; Chen, *Chinese San Francisco*, chap. 1; Kil Young Zo, *Chinese Emigration into the United States, 1850–1880* (1971; repr., Arno Press, 1978), chap. 3;

June Mei, "Socioeconomic Origins of Emigration: Guangdong to California, 1850–1882," *Modern China* 5 (1979): 468–69.

17. *Taishan xianxhi* (Local gazetteer of Taishan County), quoted in Tsai, *China and the Overseas Chinese in the United States*, 14. See also Mei, "Socioeconomic Origins of Emigration," 469–74, which offers a slightly terser translation.

18. Pyan Ling, "Causes of Chinese Immigration," *Annals of American Academy of the Political and Social Science* 39 (1912): 80. Throughout this paragraph, I state figures in rough terms because extant sets of statistics on Chinese immigration to the United States conflict. Statistics throughout this paragraph draw from tables 1 and 2 of Tsai, *China and the Overseas Chinese in the United States*, 19, 22. For more on the politics of population estimates for Chinese San Franciscans in the 1870s, see Chen, *Chinese San Francisco*, 51–54. On diaspora, see Wang Ling-chi and Wang Gungwu, eds., *The Chinese Diaspora: Selected Essays*, vol. 1 (Times Academic Press, 1998); and Adam McKeown, "Conceptualizing Chinese Diasporas, 1842 to 1949," *Journal of Asian Studies* 58 (1999): 306–37. For an example of a returned migrant inspiring others, see Thomas W. Chinn, *Bridging the Pacific: San Francisco Chinatown and Its People* (Chinese Historical Society of America, 1989), 71–72.

19. See Charles J. McClain Jr., "The Chinese Struggle for Civil Rights in Nineteenth Century America: The First Phase, 1850–1870," in *Chinese Immigrants and American Law*, ed. Charles McClain (Garland, 1994), 167–76. Return migration exceeded 40 percent during this period. Tsai, *China and the Overseas Chinese in the United States*, 22, table 2; Chen, *Chinese San Francisco*, 40, 50. Chinese emigration to San Francisco cratered in 1871 but picked up in 1872. On the arrival of 1,258 Chinese to San Francisco concurrent with the epizootic's invasion, see "Review of the Market for the Week Ending Friday Morning, April 18th, 1873," *SF Commercial Herald and Market Review*, April 18, 1873.

20. Chen, *Chinese San Francisco*, 48.

21. Chen, *Chinese San Francisco*, 55, 57, 68; Catherine Lee, "'Where the Danger Lies': Race, Gender, and Chinese and Japanese Exclusion in the United States, 1870–1924," *Sociological Forum* 25 (2010): 255. Women comprised just 7.2 percent of the overall Chinese American population in the US in 1870; Sucheng Chan, "The Exclusion of Chinese Women, 1870–1943," in McClain, *Chinese Immigrants and American Law*, 2.

22. Zo, *Chinese Emigration*, 111 ("had no"); Tsai, *China and the Overseas Chinese in the United States*, 17 ("do not"). See also Mei, "Socioeconomic Origins," 481; and Chen, *Chinese San Francisco*, 68.

23. Mary Roberts Coolidge, *Chinese Immigration* (Henry Holt and Company, 1909), 411; Chen, *Chinese San Francisco*, 71. Loomis noted, "There are but few Chinamen in California not connected with one of the six companies." Augustus Loomis, "The Chinese Companies," *Overland Monthly* 1 (1868): 225.

24. Chen, *Chinese San Francisco*, 71; Ngai, *Chinese Question*, 38; L. Eve Armentrout-Ma, "Urban Chinese at the Sinitic Frontier: Social Organizations in United States' Chinatown, 1849–1898," *Modern Asian Studies* 17 (1983): 107–35; Him Mark Lai, "Historical Development of the Chinese Consolidated Benevolent Association/Huiguan System," *Chinese America: History and Perspectives* (1987): 16; and Hao Zou, "Tracing Their Transpacific Tradition: A Reconstruction of the Organization and Functional Characteristics of the Nineteenth-Century San Francisco Huiguan," *Chinese America: History and Perspectives* (2019), n.p. For more on huiguan in China, see Bryna Goodman, *Native Place, City, and*

Nation: Regional Networks and Identities in Shanghai, 1853–1937 (University of California Press, 1995); and Richard Belsky, *Localities at the Center: Native Place, Space, and Power in Late Imperial Beijing* (Harvard University Asia Center, 2005). Zou notes that "immigrants had no choice, but automatically became huiguan members." "Tracing Their Transpacific Tradition," n.p.

25. Loomis, "Chinese Companies," 223 ("help[ing] them") and 225 ("Congress"). See also Chen, *Chinese San Francisco*, 72; Ngai, *Chinese Question*, 50–53; Zo, *Chinese Emigration*, 57; Chinn, *Bridging the Pacific*, chap. 1. Loomis alleged that members of the Sze Yup Company paid "fifty cents to the 'lawyer's fund,' which is the same in all the companies." "Chinese Companies," 224–25. As Lai notes, the companies coordinated political action as early as 1853; Lai, "Historical Development of the Chinese Consolidated Benevolent Association/ Huiguan System," 24–27.

26. David Abeel, *Journal of a Residence in China, and the Neighboring Countries, from 1829 to 1833* (New York: Leavitt, Lord & Co., 1834), 67; B. E. Lloyd, *Lights and Shades in San Francisco* (San Francisco: A. L. Bancroft, 1876), 245.

27. "The Basket Ordinance," SFAC, January 10, 1871 (quoted). On this upswing, see Henry George, "The Chinese in California," *New York Tribune*, May 1, 1869; "The Yellow-Skinned Horde," SFC, July 9, 1870; and "The Asiatic Locusts," SFC, July 16, 1870. In November 1870, supervisor Flaherty "introduced an amendatory clause to an ordinance, ordaining, among other things, that 'no person shall carry a basket or baskets upon any sidewalk, suspended from or attached to poles across or upon the shoulders, and no person shall carry upon any sidewalk, so as to be offensive to pedestrians, any rubbish, garbage, or filth.'" "Board of Supervisors," SFC, November 29, 1870. The supervisors enacted the ordinance that December. "The Basket Ordinance," SFAC, February 5, 1871. On the relative tranquility of the 1860s, see McClain, "Chinese Struggle for Civil Rights in Nineteenth Century America," 187. California's legislature refused to ratify the Fourteenth Amendment, largely because many lawmakers understood that the amendment would make it harder to discriminate against Chinese Americans.

28. "The Basket Ordinance," SFAC, January 14, 1871.

29. "The Basket Ordinance," SFAC, January 14, 1871. See also "Police Court Record," SFC, January 14, 1871; and "The Basket Ordinance," SFAC, February 5, 1871.

30. Quote from Charles J. McClain, *In Search of Equality: The Chinese Struggle Against Discrimination in Nineteenth-Century America* (University of California Press), 47. See also Todd Stevens, "Brokers Between Worlds: Chinese Merchants and Legal Culture in the Pacific Northwest, 1852–1925" (PhD diss., Princeton University, 2003).

31. "Police Court Record," SFC, January 14, 1871. On Porter, see One Voter Project, JoinCalifornia: Election History for the State of California (2005–2024), at www.joincalifornia.com/candidate/7793. Porter went on to represent Alameda County in the California State Senate until his death in 1878, when he was replaced by an ardently anti-Chinese opponent. Theodore H. Hittell, *History of California*, vol. 4 (San Francisco: N. J. Stone, 1898), 610.

32. "Police Court Record," SFC, January 14, 1871; "The Basket Ordinance," SFAC, February 4, 1871; "The Basket Ordinance," SFAC, February 5, 1871; McClain, *In Search of Equality*, 46–47; Lucile Eaves, *A History of California Labor Legislation, with an Introductory Sketch of the San Francisco Labor Movement* (University of California Press, 1910), 140. Sawyer based his decision on the supervisors' failure to specify that baskets constituted a nuisance. "The Police Court Record," SFC, January 19, 1871.

33. San Francisco Police recorded sixty arrests for violations of the Basket Ordinance in the year ending June 30, 1872; "Crime," SFAC, August 13, 1872. Enforcement of the ordinance resumed by summer 1873; "Local Brevities," SFAC, August 21, 1873; "Arrests for August," SFAC, September 1, 1873. Other cities copied the ordinance: see, e.g., "Board of City Trustees," *Sacramento Union*, November 9, 1875; "The Basket Ordinance," *San Jose Herald*, April 14, 1885. The city's building trades remained lily-white for decades to come; Michael Kazin, *Barons of Labor: The San Francisco Building Trades and Union Power in the Progressive Era* (University of Illinois Press, 1987).

34. "The Epizootic," SFC, April 25, 1873 ("some"); *Victoria (BC) Colonist*, May 2, 1873 ("entered").

35. "The Epizooty," SFC, April 27, 1873 ("thick and fast"); "A Novel Team," *SF Examiner*, April 26, 1873. On non-Chinese pullers, see, e.g., "The Epizootic," SFC, April 25, 1873, which described "vegetable and milk wagons" as "being drawn in the city by men." On Terwilliger's location, see *San Francisco Directory for the Year Commencing March, 1873*, 594.

36. "Novel Team"; "The Epizootic," SFAC, April 27, 1873. On "likely," see Walter Johnson, *Soul by Soul: Life Inside the Antebellum Slave Market* (Harvard University Press, 1999), 72–73.

37. "Novel Team"; "The Epizootic," SFAC, April 27, 1873; "The Epizooty," SFC, April 27, 1873.

38. "The Epizootic," SFAC, April 27, 1873; "Novel Team."

39. Robert G. Lee, *Orientals: Asian Americans in Popular Culture* (Temple University Press, 1999), 38–39 ("mice and rats"); Claire Jean Kim, *Dangerous Crossings: Race, Species, and Nature in a Multicultural Age* (Cambridge University Press, 2015), 53 ("menacing"). On bees, see Gordon H. Chang, *Ghosts of Gold Mountain: The Epic Story of the Chinese Who Built the Transcontinental Railroad* (Houghton Mifflin Harcourt, 2019), 104; Lisa Yun, *The Coolie Speaks: Chinese Indentured Laborers and African Slaves in Cuba* (Temple University Press), 230. On sheep, see Daniel Cleveland report, quoted in Chang, *Ghosts of Gold Mountain*, 53. On Chinese as "human leeches, sucking the life-blood of the country," see Hubert Howe Bancroft, *History of California*, vol. 7: 1860–1890, in *The Works of Hubert Howe Bancroft*, vol. 24 (San Francisco: History Company, 1890), 338. On Chinese as dogs, cattle, pigs, vermin, and even horses, see Kim, *Dangerous Crossings*, 54–57. The Chinese themselves, however, sometimes described those caught up in the transnational trade in unfree laborers as "pigs." See Elmer Sandmeyer, *The Anti-Chinese Movement in California* (University of Illinois Press, 1939), 27; Peter Kwong and Dušanka Dušana Miščevič, *Chinese America: The Untold Story of America's Oldest New Community* (New Press, 2005), 36; Moon-Ho Jung, *Coolies and Cane: Race, Labor, and Sugar in the Age of Emancipation* (Johns Hopkins University Press, 2006), 22; Yun, *Coolie Speaks*, 84, 121.

40. "Monkey, Chinaman, and Pig," *Thistleton's Jolly Giant (The Critic)*, February 21, 1874, 6; "Chinese Abomination," *Thistleton's Jolly Giant (The Critic)*, August 1873, 2.

41. Kim, *Dangerous Crossings*, 24, 53 ("never"); "The Epizootic," SFAC, April 27, 1873.

42. "Novel Team."

43. "The Epizooty," SFC, April 27, 1873.

44. "Team of Chinamen," *Idaho World* (Idaho City, ID), May 8, 1873; *Dakota Republican* (Vermillion, SD), May 29, 1873. See also "Pacific Coasters," *Albany (OR) States Rights Democrat*, May 2, 1873; "News Items," *Grass Valley (CA) Morning Union*, April 29, 1873; and *Puget Sound Dispatch* (Seattle, WA), May 3, 1873. Here I follow Ngai, *Chinese Question*, chap. 3.

45. "Brief Mention," SFEB, July 31, 1873 (emphasis mine).

46. Despite the biographical details mentioned by the *Bulletin*, the contractor's identity remains elusive. An 1873 city directory listed three companies doing business on Sacramento Street under the family name Quong. Quong Chung Lung & Co. and Quong Hing & Co., two firms of "merchants" doing business at 712 and 719 Sacramento Street, and Quong Song, which sold "provisions" from 751 Sacramento. Langley, *San Francisco Directory for the Year Commencing March, 1873*, 506, 581. Quong Hing & Co., Quong Son & Co., and several other firms are also listed as doing business on Sacramento Street in Wells Fargo Express Company, *Directory of Principal Chinese Business Firms in San Francisco* (n.p.: n.p., 1882), 36–42. An earlier version of the same directory included fewer listings for businesses starting with Quong on Sacramento Street, but still too many to identify Ah Quong. Wells Fargo Express Company, *Directory of Chinese Business Houses* (n.p.: n.p., 1878). In an 1878 newspaper ad, Stivers described himself as a "lumber inspector" and noted that he offered "Storage for Lumber and all kinds of Merchandise," though by that time he had moved his offices to South Beach. SFAC, February 10, 1878.

"Ah" was usually a diminutive rather than a first name, but other sources document at least two men named "Ah Quong." One had been "murdered in broad daylight in the streets of Sacramento" several weeks earlier. A second Ah Quong—a prominent railroad labor contractor with long-standing ties to the Central Pacific—operated out of Reno rather than San Francisco. Charles Crocker, "C.P.R.R. Pay Roll, No. 332 for the Month of November 1866, Egbert & Co. 'China' P Roll," November 1866, series 4, box 23, MS 79, Central Pacific Railroad Collection, California State Railroad Museum Library and Archives, http://purl.stanford.edu/nx173vn8674; American Federation of Labor, *Meat vs. Rice: Some Reasons for Chinese Exclusion* [. . .] (GPO, 1902), 6; John Jung, "Chinese Labor Contractors," *Chinese American History by Chance* (blog), March 24, 2014, https://chineseamericanhistorian.blogspot.com/2014/03/chinese-labor-contractors.html.

47. Although Congress would ultimately pass laws restricting Chinese immigration starting in 1875, state lawmakers continued to perceive immigration as well within their purview prior to the US Supreme Court's 1876 decision in the Passenger Cases. Lucy Salyer, *Laws Harsh as Tigers: Chinese Immigrants and the Shaping of Modern Immigration Law* (University of North Carolina Press, 1995), 5.

48. Abeel, *Journal of a Residence in China*, 67 ("one class"); W. F. Mayers, "Bibliographical: The Record of Marvels; or Tales of the Genii," *Notes and Queries on China and Japan* 1 (1867): 25 ("chair coolies"); William Speer, *The Oldest and the Newest Empire: China and the United States* (Cincinnati: National Publishing Company, 1870), 473n1. The "hired runners" who carried silver from Hong Kong remittance firms to the family members of Chinese emigrant miners in California and Australia were sometimes referred to via a term that translated as "horses patrolling the city." Ngai, *Chinese Question*, 55. On the Turkic root قول (*qul*), see *Oxford English Dictionary*, "coolie (n.)," last modified September 2025, https://www.oed.com/dictionary/coolie_n?tab=factsheet#8314631. As was well understood in the late 1800s, "coolie" also drew on a second and distinct etymology. One Briton explained in the late 1860s that it was "a purely Tamil word. It means *hire*, or *wages*; and by Europeans has been applied to the *native labourers*, who work for hire." G. P., "The Word Coolie," *Notes and Queries About China and Japan* 1 (1867): 77. Other respondents to the same query, however, pointed to other etymological lineages; R. S. G., "The Word Coolie," *Notes and Queries About China and Japan* 1 (1867): 77; and E. C. Bowra, "Etymology of the Word 'Coolie,'" *Notes and Queries About China and Japan* 1 (1867): 77. Later that same year,

another authority who was conversant in Tamil from time spent in Madras noted that "in Tamil 'coolie' means *hire*, but *Cooliekara* signifies and is applied to those who earn their livelihood by outdoor work in carrying burdens." This author went on to propose that this term's ending had disappeared when Indian laborers were introduced to Mauritius: "Thus to 'become a coolie' was considered to surrender one's self unconditionally to the will of the *Saheeb*." This writer concluded by claiming that "the indiscriminate application of the term 'coolie' in China to the domestics, chair and burden-carriers, compradore's bill-collectors, and emigrants, would appear to an Indian observer as much a puzzler as the misnomer *Amah*." J., "The Term 'Coolie,'" *Notes and Queries on China and Japan* 1 (1867): 94. The esteemed Chinese linguist Herbert Giles noted this dual etymology for "coolie," the meaning of which he summarized as "the menial of the east." Giles traced one etymology to "*Kholees* or *Kolis*, the Hindee name of a degenerate race of Rajpoots in Guzerat," and the second to "a Tamil word *Kûli*, meaning wages," adding that "the Chinese write the word in various ways without reference to its meaning." Herbert A. Giles, "Coolie," in *A Glossary of Reference on Subjects Connected with the Far East* (Hong Kong: Lane, Crawford, 1878), 31.

49. Vijay Prashad, *Everybody Was Kung Fu Fighting: Afro-Asian Connections and the Myth of Cultural Purity* (Beacon, 2001), 71. "The familiar use of *Cooly* has extended," a leading Anglo-Indian dictionary noted, "to the Straits Settlements, Java, and China, as well as to all tropical and subtropical colonies, whether English or foreign." *Hobson-Jobson: The Anglo-Indian Dictionary*, "Cooly," ed. Henry Yule and A. C. Burnell (1886; repr., Wordsworth, 1996), 250. This sense of "coolie" seems to have first entered English in the early seventeenth century; see, e.g., William Bruton, *Newes from the East-Indies* [. . .] (London: I. Okes, 1638), 6. On the persistence of this usage in California, see Coolidge, *Chinese Immigration*, 41.

50. "Men as Horses," *Belleville (KS) Weekly Telescope*, June 13, 1878; David Strand, *Rickshaw Beijing: City People and Politics in the 1920s* (1989; repr., University of California Press, 1993), 23–24; James Francis Warren, *Rickshaw Coolie: A People's History of Singapore, 1880–1940* (Singapore University Press, 2003), 14, 51–54.

51. E. T. C. Werner, *Autumn Leaves: A Sheaf of Papers, Sociological and Sinological, Philosophical and Metaphysical with an Autobiographical Note* (Kelly & Walsh, 1928), 167 ("rapidly supplanted" and "threw"); and *Millard's Review*, November 8, 1919, in Strand, *Rickshaw Beijing*, 25–26. See also Warren, *Rickshaw Coolie*, 15.

52. Quoted in Strand, *Rickshaw Beijing*, 34.

53. Lau She, *Rickshaw Boy: The Novel Lo-T'o Hsiang Tzu*, trans. Jean M. James (University of Hawai'i Press, 1979), 233.

54. Tim Wright, "Shanghai Imperialists Versus Rickshaw Racketeers: The Defeat of the 1934 Rickshaw Reforms," *Modern China* 17 (1991): 77.

55. Quoted in Chi Ming Fung, *Reluctant Heroes: Rickshaw Pullers in Hong Kong and Canton, 1874–1954* (Hong Kong University Press, 2005), 90. Strand notes that "rickshaw men carried out the first strikes in Japanese and Korean labor history." *Rickshaw Beijing*, 61. The plight of rickshaw coolies prompted reform as well as revolution; see Wright, "Shanghai Imperialists Versus Rickshaw Racketeers," 76–111. On 1940s bans, see Edward J. M. Rhoads, "Cycles of Cathay: A History of the Bicycle in China," *Transfers* 2 (2012): 104. Cycle rickshaws, which were present in Singapore by 1929, reached China in the 1930s and remained legal under both Nationalist and Communist regimes.

56. "How John Chinaman Goes for Property in Frisco," *Thistleton's Jolly Giant (The Critic)*, May 3, 1873, 6.

57. "Pagan Ordinances," SFAC, May 27, 1873.

58. Charles McClain and Laurene Wu McClain, "A Chinese Contribution to American Law: *Yick Wo Versus Hopkins*," *Chinese America: History and Perspectives* (2003): 141. Reverand Abeel perceptively noted that queues, once a "mark of subjugation," had since "become an ornament and a mark of proud distinction." Abeel, *Journal of a Residence in China*, 93. On the ordinance, see Eaves, *History of California Labor Legislation*, 144–45; Lee, *Orientals*, 39–40; "Pagan Ordinances," SFAC, May 27, 1873. Taking matters a step further, *Thistleton's Jolly Giant* hopefully noted that requiring "each Chinaman and Chinawoman to have their tails cut off close to their scalps before they are allowed to land on our barbarian shore" would "stop their coming on the coast, and save" California from becoming "a Celestial Kingdom." "How John Chinaman Goes for Property in Frisco," 6. See also "Our Illustrations," *Thistleton's Jolly Giant (The Critic)*, June 8, 1873.

59. Goodwin's original language would have based license fees on the number of male and "male minor" employees a laundry engaged; Supervisor Kenny amended Goodwin's ordinance to base fees on horse ownership instead. "Pagan Ordinances," SFAC, May 27, 1873. See also Eaves, *History of California Labor Legislation*, 144–45.

60. "Pagan Ordinances," SFAC, June 3, 1873.

61. "Pagan Orders," SFAC, June 24, 1873. Curiously enough, the city made little effort to enforce the Laundry Ordinance until February 1874. "War on the Washmen," SFAC, February 7, 1874. See also McClain and McClain, "Chinese Contribution to American Law," 140–48; Eaves, *History of California Labor Legislation*, 144–45. A similar measure, which also used horse ownership as a foil for race, was enacted by the board in 1876. "Board of Supervisors," SFAC, March 7, 1876. It met the same fate; "The Laundrymen's License," SFAC, May 3, 1876.

CHAPTER 9

1. *Minneapolis Star Tribune*, May 4, 1873. In December 1873, Honolulu's *Pacific Advertiser* remarked that "a disease had appeared among horses in town, thought to resemble the epizootic that prevailed so extensively in the United States," with "numbers of dray and carriage horses . . . sick with colds and fever," but this is the only indication I can find that the Great Horse Flu hit Hawai'i. "Epizootic Among Horses," *Pacific Advertiser* (Honolulu), December 6, 1873.

2. "The Epizootic," *Lake County Bee* (Lakeport, CA), May 3, 1873; "Pacific Coasters," *States Rights Democrat* (Albany, OR), May 2, 1873; "Epizootic," *Statesman Journal* (Salem, OR), May 15, 1873; *Corvallis Gazette-Times*, May 17, 1873; "Pacific Coast Brevities," SFEB, May 28, 1873; "Home and Abroad," *Albany (OR) Democrat*, May 30, 1873; "Cheering Prospects in Washington County," *Portland Morning Oregonian*, June 2, 1873; "First Case," *Salem Oregon Statesman*, July 8, 1873.

3. "Washington Territory," *Victoria (BC) Colonist*, June 3, 1873; "Here and There," *Mound City (KS) Border Sentinel*, June 20, 1873; "British Columbia," *Portland Morning Oregonian*, September 13, 1873; "Epizootic," *Washington Standard* (Olympia), September 20, 1873; "By Telegraph and Mail," *North American and United States Gazette* (Philadelphia), October 2, 1873 ("all the horses"). The outbreak also struck Ochoco Valley, Oregon, during June,

"having a big run . . . but doesn't seem to hurt much." J. H. Douthit, June 11, 1873, in "Ochoco," *Albany (OR) Register*, June 20, 1873. On Cariboo Country, see *Portland Oregonian*, September 28, 1873; "British Columbian Jolts," *SF Examiner*, October 6, 1873.

4. "State News," *Statesman Journal* (Salem, OR), May 27, 1873; "Far West Points," *Fort Scott (KS) Monitor*, July 2, 1873; Pierce Eaton, May 20, 1873, in "Upper Lake Letter," *Lake County Bee* (Lakeport, CA), May 24, 1873; "Items," *Helena Weekly Herald*, October 23, 1873 ("get enough"). On influenza in bovines, see *Sacramento Record*, n.d., in "Coast Items," *Petaluma Evening Argus*, May 5, 1873. On dogs, see "Brief Mention," *SFEB*, May 12, 1873; *Weekly Trinity Journal* (Weaverville, CA), May 17, 1873. On turkeys, see "Pacific Coast Items," *Stockton (CA) Evening Herald*, May 16, 1873; "Pacific Coast Brevities," *San Francisco Commercial*, June 5, 1873; "Evening Echoes," *Wilmington (DE) New Journal*, June 4, 1873; "Hog Disease," *Petaluma Evening Argus*, June 14, 1873.

5. Gustavo Ruiz y Sandoval, *La epizootia de los años de 1872 y 1873 en el Continente America, presentado como tesis de concurso, para la oposicion a la plaza de Catedratico de 40. Año de Veterario* (Mexico: n.p., 1874), 11–12; Adoniram B. Judson, "History and Course of the Epizoötic Among Horses upon the North American Continent," *Public Health Reports and Papers Present at the Meetings of the American Public Health Association in the Year 1873* (New York and Cambridge, MA: Hurd and Houghton and the Riverside Press, 1875), 107. Elsewhere, Judson claimed that the Great Horse Flu reached Guatemala in July and San Salvador in August. A. B. Judson, "Report on the Origin and Progress of the Epizoötic Among Horses in 1872, with a Table of Mortality in New York," in New York Department of Health, *Third Annual Report of the Board of Health of the Health Department of the City of New York* (New York: D. Appleton & Co., 1873), 251.

6. Ruiz y Sandoval, *La epizootia*, 12.

7. "Morrow County," *Bucyrus (OH) Telegraph-Forum*, January 28, 1873; Optic [pseud.], February 24, 1873, in *Cedar Falls Gazette*, February 28, 1873; *Shippensburg (PA) News*, April 5, 1873 ("The fact"). Sources often employed the term "relapse" in reference to the first instance, e.g., "The Epizootic Still Around," *Monmouth Democrat* (Freehold, NJ), January 9, 1873. For examples of the second category, see "Chester Briefs," *Montpelier (VT) Argus and Patriot*, January 16, 1873; "Delphos Column," *Solomon Valley Pioneer* (Lindsey, KS), March 1, 1873; *Jasper (IN) Weekly Courier*, April 4, 1873; *La Crosse Republican*, n.d., in "Wisconsin Items," *Wisconsin State Journal*, April 17, 1873; *Marengo (IL) Beacon/Republican-News*, April 19, 1873; *Lebanon (PA) Courier*, n.d., in "State News," *Pittsburgh Commercial*, May 13, 1873; "Items of News," *Westminster (MD) Democratic Advocate*, June 7, 1873; "Collinsville," *HC*, June 10, 1873. For other accounts of second infections, see *Greensburg (PA) Tribune and Herald*, n.d., in *Pittsburgh Weekly Gazette*, November 27, 1873. Reports such as this are consistent with influenza—or at least agnostic on the malady in question. In other instances, though, purported "second cases" undoubtedly involved another disorder; e.g., "bilious pneumonia accompanied by inflammation of the bowels" in "Massachusetts," *BET*, January 14, 1873; and cerebro-spinal meningitis in "More Sick Horses," *Vermont Journal* (Windsor), February 1, 1873. For more ambiguous reports, see, e.g., *Reading (PA) Eagle*, n.d., in *Stroudsburg (PA) Jeffersonian*, July 24, 1873.

8. "Michigan," *Chicago Weekly Post*, June 12, 1873; *Wood County Reporter*, n.d., in "State News," *Watertown (WI) News*, February 5, 1873; *Muscatine (IA) Weekly Journal*, April 4, 1873; *NOTP*, June 1, 1873; "The Week," *Newport (VT) Express and Standard*, June 3, 1873; *Minneapolis Star Tribune*, June 4, 1873.

9. "Epizootic," *Indianapolis Journal*, June 13, 1873; "Local Department," *Kansas Tribune* (Lawrence), October 23, 1873.

10. Statistics Canada, *Census of Agriculture, Ontario, 1871–1911* (Borealis, 2016), https://borealisdata.ca/dataset.xhtml?persistentId=hdl:10864/11150. No comparable figures seem to be available for Mexico or Cuba. "Horses, Mules, and Asses on Farms," US Bureau of the Census, *Census Bulletin No. 103* (Washington, DC), August 19, 1891, 6–7, tables 2 and 3.

11. "Cruelty," *Buffalo Morning Express*, March 4, 1873.

12. "Retrospect," *Reading (PA) Times*, January 15, 1873.

13. All material on this event here and below comes from "Lecture by Henry Bergh," *Buffalo Commercial*, November 26, 1873.

14. On the controversies that surrounded Descartes's "doctrine of animal automatism," see Peter Harrison, "Descartes on Animals," *Philosophical Quarterly* 42 (1992): 219–27; Deborah J. Brown, "Animal Souls and Beast Machines: Descartes's Mechanical Biology," in *Animals: A History*, ed. Peter Adamson and G. Fay Edwards (Oxford University Press, 2018), 187–210.

15. Quote from Darcy Ingram, "Beastly Measures: Animal Welfare, Civil Society, and State Policy in Victorian Canada," *Journal of Canadian Studies* 47 (2013): 23. See also Bernard Oreste Unti, "The Quality of Mercy: Organized Animal Protection in the United States 1866–1930" (PhD diss., American University, 2002); Diane L. Beers, *For the Prevention of Cruelty: The History and Legacy of Animal Rights Activism in the United States* (Swallow Press / Ohio University Press, 2006); Reinaldo Funes Monzote, "Animal Labor and Protection in Cuba: Changes in Relationships with Animals in the Nineteenth Century," in *Centering Animals in Latin American History*, ed. Martha Few and Zeb Tortorici (Duke University Press, 2013), 209–42; Janet M. Davis, *The Gospel of Kindness: Animal Welfare and the Making of Modern America* (Oxford University Press, 2016); and Ernest Freeburg, *A Traitor to His Species: Henry Bergh and the Birth of the Animal Rights Movement* (Basic Books, 2020), chap. 7.

16. *Louisville Courier-Journal*, n.d., quoted in "Steam Railroads," *Salt Lake Herald-Republican*, February 7, 1873; *Louisville Commercial*, February 12, 1873, in "Steam Power on Street Cars," *American Artisan and Illustrated Journal of Popular Science*, March 15, 1873, 178; "Rapid Transit in the City," CEM, February 10, 1873.

17. "City Hall," NOTP, January 24, 1873.

18. Statistics from "Horse Production Falling," US Department of Agriculture, *Yearbook of Agriculture, 1926* (GPO, 1927), 437–38; Grant Macewan, "Horse," last edited March 22, 2015, *The Canadian Encyclopedia*, https://www.thecanadianencyclopedia.ca/en/article/horse#; Larry Sawers, "The Mule, the South, and Economic Progress," *Social Science History* 28 (2004): 667. It is worth noting that the Mexican Revolution may well have caused equine populations there to plummet during the 1910s. Presumably Mexican equine populations peaked either in the first decade of the 1900s, or perhaps later, after donkeys, horses, and mules made good their losses. On street transit more generally, see Brian Cudahy, *Cash, Tokens, and Transfers: A History of Urban Mass Transit in North America* (Fordham University Press, 1990).

19. "The City," NOTP, December 27, 1872.

20. Alfred W. Crosby, *America's Forgotten Pandemic: The Influenza of 1918*, 2nd ed. (New York, 2003); Nancy K. Bristow, *The American Pandemic: The Lost Worlds of the 1918 Influenza*

Epidemic (New York, 2012), 7–8. On fatalities, see World Population Review, "Spanish Flu Deaths by Country 2026," https://worldpopulationreview.com/country-rankings/spanish-flu-deaths-by-country; Enrique Beldarraín Chaple, Bélgica Cabrera, and Ileana Armenteros Vera, "La Gripe de 1918 en Cuba," *Revista Cubana de Salud Pública* 45 (2019): 8.

21. A. Liautard, "Influenza, or 'Pink-Eye' in Horses," *American Agriculturist*, n.d., in *Lane (KS) Advance*, December 23, 1881; "The Same Diseases but Different Names," *Wilkes-Barre Sunday Leader*, January 3, 1897.

22. *St. Louis Globe-Democrat*, n.d., in "Worse Than the Strike," *BE*, August 25, 1900; "Epizootics Halted Business in 1872," *Indianapolis Star*, May 19, 1907.

23. *Pittsburgh Dispatch*, n.d., in "The Epizooty," *St. Louis Globe-Democrat*, October 9, 1875; "The Horse Disease," *HC*, October 4, 1880. The view that influenza had "recurred each spring to a more or less extent," as one Buffalo veterinary surgeon put it, also lent continuing relevance to the Great Horse Flu; Dr. Hutchins quoted in "Grip Among Horses," *Buffalo Courier*, April 8, 1891.

24. "The Disease at Boston," *CE*, December 19, 1889; "Be Ready to Sneeze," *Two Republics* (Mexico City), December 28, 1889. For evidence that equines also suffered flu-like outbreaks around the same time, see "The Epizootic Again," *Atlanta Constitution*, May 1, 1891.

25. "Automatic Carriages," *Knoxville Journal and Tribune*, July 10, 1895; F. J. McCafferty, *BG*, n.d., quoted in "New Horse Disease," *Independence (KS) Daily*, July 18, 1901; "The Equine Plague," *BET*, July 1, 1901.

26. "'Horse Influenza' Crippled Street Cars," *HC*, October 8, 1918. Interestingly, the *Courant* recalled that "gangs of colored men were pressed into service to draw the cars through the streets of New York." I have not found contemporary accounts documenting this contingency, though it seems plausible and even likely.

27. "Must Be Avoided," *Greenfield (IN) Reporter*, November 19, 1918; "Turf and Diamond," *CE*, November 24, 1918.

28. "Horse 'Flu' Resembles Human Ailment," *Glasgow (MT) Courier*, November 22, 1918; George A. Soper, "Influenza in Horses and in Man," *New York Medical Journal* 109 (1919): 720; "Live Farm Works for Tennesseeans," *The Parisian* (Paris, TN), December 6, 1918.

29. Soper, "Influenza in Horses and in Man," 720; J. W. Rainey, "The Army Veterinary Service," *Journal of the US Cavalry Association*, April 1, 1918, 475; C. E. Gapen, "When Dobbin Gets the 'Flu,'" *Country Gentleman*, December 21, 1918, 5; Yousuke Maeda and Masa-aki Oikawa, "Patterns of Rectal Temperature and Shipping Fever Incidence in Horses Transported over Long-Distances [sic]," *Frontiers in Veterinary Science* 6 (February 2019): article 27; Kara M. Lascola and Lindsey Boone, "Overview of Respiratory Diseases of Horses," rev. July 2023, in *Merck Veterinary Manual*, https://www.merckvetmanual.com/respiratory-system/respiratory-diseases-of-horses/overview-of-respiratory-diseases-of-horses. Horses also suffer from asthma and allergies.

30. *New York Tribune*, n.d., in "Epizootic and Influenza," *Spokane Spokesman-Review*, January 23, 1919 (also reprinted in "Animals Immune from Influenza," *Victoria (BC) Colonist*, May 2, 1919). On the successful search for the responsible variant, see Gina Kolata, *Flu: The Story of the Great Influenza Pandemic of 1918 and the Search for the Virus That Caused It* (Farrar, Straus and Giroux, 1999); and Pete Davies, *The Devil's Flu: The World's Deadliest Influenza Epidemic and the Scientific Hunt for the Virus That Caused It* (Henry Holt & Co., 2000). On H1N1

in other-than-human creatures, see, e.g., Mark D. Schrenzel et al., "Pandemic (H1N1) 2009 Virus in 3 Wildlife Species, San Diego, California, USA," *Emerging Infectious Diseases* 17 (2011): 747–49.

31. For an excellent overview, see David L. Suarez, "Influenza A Virus," *Animal Influenza*, 2nd ed., ed. David E. Swayne (Ames, IA, 2017), 3–30.

32. Martha I. Nelson and Michael Worobey, "Origins of the 1918 Pandemic: Revisiting the Swine 'Mixing Vessel' Hypothesis," *American Journal of Epidemiology* 12 (2018): 2501.

33. Nelson and Worobey, "Origins of the 1918 Pandemic," 2501. Note that the hypothesis of other-than-human animals as "mixing vessels" remains controversial; Suarez, "Influenza A Virus," 7. On 2009 H1N1, see Charles R. Bartolotti, ed., *The H1N1 Influenza Pandemic of 2009* (Nova Science, 2010); F. Dawood et al., "Estimated Global Mortality Associated with the First 12 Months of 2009 Pandemic Influenza A H1N1 Virus Circulation: A Modelling Study," *Lancet Infection* 12 (2012): 687–95; Theresa MacPhail, *The Viral Network: A Pathography of the H1N1 Influenza Pandemic* (Cornell University Press, 2014).

34. W. I. Beveridge, "Unravelling the Ecology of Influenza A Virus," *History and Philosophy of the Life Sciences* 15 (1993): 23–24. For an accessible account of twentieth-century influenza research from a leading virologist, see Robert G. Webster, *Flu Hunter: Unlocking the Secrets of a Virus* (Otago University Press, 2018).

35. "The 'Pink-Eye,'" *Kansas City (MO) Times*, September 28, 1881. The literature on these broader transformations is immense. See, for instance, John S. Haller Jr., *American Medicine in Transition, 1840–1910* (University of Illinois Press, 1981); John Harley Warner, *The Therapeutic Perspective: Medical Practice, Knowledge, and Identity in America, 1820–1885* (Harvard University Press, 1986); and Owen Whooley, *Knowledge in the Time of Cholera: The Struggle over American Medicine in the Nineteenth Century* (University of Chicago Press, 2013).

36. Judson, "History and Course of the Epizoötic," 106–7.

37. Judson, "History and Course of the Epizoötic," 109 ("apparently sudden"), 89 ("darkness"); "Morbid Anatomy of the Epizootic," MR, January 2, 1873; and Ruiz y Sandoval, *La epizootia*, 18 ("too little").

38. Eric Foner, *Reconstruction: 1863–1877* (Harper & Row, 1988), chap. 11.

39. George Templeton Strong, entries for September 18 and 20, 1873, *The Diary of George Templeton Strong*, vol. 4: *Post-War Years, 1865–1875*, ed. Allan Nevins and Milton H. Thomas (Macmillan, 1952), 493 ("general smash" and "had closed"); and "The Epidemic," *Holt County Sentinel* (Oregon, MO), October 3, 1873 ("has raged"). My interpretation here and below draws on Rendigs Fels, *American Business Cycles, 1865–1897* (University of North Carolina Press, 1959), 99; M. John Lubetkin, *Jay Cooke's Gamble: The Northern Pacific Railroad, the Sioux, and the Panic of 1873* (University of Oklahoma Press, 2006), 276–82; and Christoph Nitschke, "Theory and History of Financial Crises: Explaining the Panic of 1873," *Journal of the Gilded Age and Progressive Era* 17 (2018): 222–29.

40. "Notes and Notions," *Clinton (IL) Register*, October 17, 1873 ("horsemen"); "The Epidemic," *Holt County Sentinel* (Oregon, MO), October 3, 1873 ("disease broke out"); *Bristol (TN) News*, September 30, 1873 ("suspension"); CT, October 5, 1873 ("paralyzed business"); "Personal," *Holt County Sentinel* (Oregon, MO), October 3, 1873 ("great bank"). For other invocations of the epizootic in narrating the panic, see "Faster," *Cedar Falls (IA) Gazette*, October 3, 1873; *Bucyrus (OH) Telegraph-Forum*, October 7, 1873; "Sparks and Flashes," *Northumberland County Democrat* (Sunbury, PA), October 10, 1873; and "Not Felt Here," *Wheeling (WV) Register*, November 8, 1873.

41. Hannah Catherine Davies, *Transatlantic Speculations: Globalization and the Panics of 1873* (Columbia University Press, 2018), 63; Nitschke, "Theory and History of Financial Crises," 221–35; Fels, *American Business Cycles*, 101. There is an underwhelming discussion of a few of these factors in Milton Friedman and Anna Jacobson Schwartz, *A Monetary History of the United States 1867–1960* (Princeton University Press, 1963), chap. 2. The 1873 changes to silver, often decried as the "crime" or "fraud" of '73, served as a pivotal organizing factor for political insurgencies in the decades that followed. See, e.g., Samuel Leavitt, *Our Money Wars: The Example and Warning* (Boston: Arena, 1894), 154–77. For a masterful articulation of cycles in this context, see William J. Cronon, *Nature's Metropolis: Chicago and the Great West* (W. W. Norton, 1991).

42. "From Wichita," *Junction City (KS) Weekly Union*, November 8, 1873.

43. Carlos Marichal, *A Century of Debt Crises in Latin America: From Independence to the Great Depression, 1820–1930* (Princeton University Press, 1989), 82 ("world depression"); Louis A. Pérez, "Toward Dependency and Revolution: The Political Economy of Cuba Between Wars, 1878–1895," *Latin American Research Review* 18 (1983): 127 ("its economy"); and R. T. Naylor, *History of Canadian Business* (1975; repr., McGill-Queen's University Press, 2006), 8 ("period 1873–1879"). The precise timing of Mexico's recovery remains somewhat elusive; John H. Coatsworth, "Obstacles to Economic Growth in Nineteenth-Century Mexico," *American Historical Review* 83 (1978): 81. Much of the rest of the world, meanwhile, remained mired in a so-called long depression until the late 1890s; Rendigs Fels, "The Long-Wave Depression, 1873–97," *Review of Economics and Statistics* 31 (1949): 69–73. My take on the panic and depression draws on Nicolas Barreyre, "The Politics of Economic Crises: The Panic of 1873, the End of Reconstruction, and the Realignment of American Politics," *Journal of the Gilded Age and Progressive Era* 10 (2011): 408; Richard White, *Republic for Which It Stands: The United States During Reconstruction and the Gilded Age, 1865–1896* (Oxford University Press, 2017), 267; Fred Moseley, "Depression of 1873–1879," in *Business Cycles and Depressions: An Encyclopedia*, ed. David Glasner (Routledge, 1997), 148–49; Kieran Furlong, "Economic Fluctuations in Canada, 1867–1897" (PhD diss., University of Toronto, 1997), 72–78. Roeliff Morton Breckenridge emphasizes that "no panic, in the accepted sense of the term, occurred in Canada in 1873"; instead, "relaxation from the tense activity of the preceding period began in the fall of 1873, and continued through 1874"; Roeliff Morton Breckenridge, *The Canadian Banking System 1817–1890* (New York: Macmillan, 1895), 272–78. Traditionally, economists identified 1879 as the depression's end. More recently, though, scholars have adjusted key statistics, suggesting that this downturn lasted only until 1875. Joseph H. Davis, "An Improved Chronology of US Business Cycles Since the 1790s," *Journal of Economic History* 66 (2006): 103–21. This interpretation, however, ignores the widespread economic suffering that continued to roil for several additional years.

44. "From Chicago," *Rocky Mountain News*, December 17, 1873; "The Panic of 1873," *Chicago Inter Ocean*, November 8, 1875.

45. Mark Wahlgren Summers, *Ordeal of Reunion: A New History of Reconstruction* (University of North Carolina Press, 2014), 347 (quoted); Foner, *Reconstruction*, 461; Barreyre, "Politics of Economic Crises," 405; Nicolas Barreyre, *Gold and Freedom: The Political Economy of Reconstruction*, trans. Arthur Goldhammer (University of Virginia Press, 2015), 234.

46. John Hope Franklin, *Reconstruction After the Civil War* (1961; repr., University of Chicago Press, 2013), 219 (quoted); Foner, *Reconstruction*, 535; Sean Dennis Cashman, *America in the Gilded Age: From the Death of Lincoln to the Rise of Roosevelt*, 3rd ed. (New York University

Press, 1993); Charles W. Calhoun, ed., *The Gilded Age: Essays on the Origins of Modern America* (Scholar Resources, 1996); White, *Republic for Which It Stands*; Christopher McKnight Nichols and Nancy Unger, eds., *A Companion to the Gilded Age and Progressive Era* (Wiley Blackwell, 2017); Charles Postel, *Equality: An American Dilemma 1866–1896* (Farrar, Straus and Giroux, 2019); Jefferson Cowie, *Freedom's Dominion: A Saga of White Resistance to Federal Power* (Basic Books, 2022), chaps. 8–10.

EPILOGUE

1. My thinking here has been shaped by Erica Charters and Kristin Heitman, "How Epidemics End," *Centaurus* 63 (2021): 210–24.

2. John M. Woodworth, *The Cholera Epidemic of 1873 in the United States* (GPO, 1875); "Pestilence and Sanitary Reform," *Shreveport Times*, September 6, 1873; "Terrible Fatality," *Montgomery Advertiser*, October 29, 1873; "America," *The American Annual Cyclopedia and Register of Important Events of the Year* 13 (1874): 20; "Indiana," CEP, November 21, 1872; "Taunton," *Fall River Evening News*, April 8, 1873.

3. The literature on these subjects is too vast to usefully cite here.

4. George A. Gipe, "The First Energy Crisis: When Horses Failed," *BS Sunday Magazine*, February 3, 1974.

5. Patrick Berche, "The Enigma of the 1889 Russian Flu Pandemic: A Coronavirus?," *La Presse Médicale* 51 (2022): 104111. The 2008 figure is from Kate E. Jones et al., "Global Trends in Emerging Infectious Diseases," *Nature* 451 (2008): 990–94. On avian flu culling, see Susanne Rust and Karen Kaplan, "Killing 166 Million Birds Hasn't Helped Poultry Farmers Stop H5N1," *Los Angeles Times*, February 26, 2025.

6. I. W. Fong and Ken Alibek, eds., *New and Evolving Infections of the 21st Century* (Springer, 2007); I. W. Fong, *Emerging Zoonoses: A Worldwide Perspective* (Springer, 2017). For a recent attempt to capture the contours of this "polycrisis," see Peter Sogaard Jorgenson et al., "Evolution of the Polycrisis: Anthropocene Traps That Challenge Global Sustainability," *Philosophical Transactions of the Royal Society B-Biological Sciences* 379 (2024): 20220261. On climate change, see Colin J. Carlson et al., "Climate Change Increases Cross-Species Viral Transmission Risk," *Nature* 607 (2022): 555–62. For statistical evidence suggesting that "the yearly probability of occurrence of extreme epidemics can increase up to three fold in the coming decades," see Marco Marani et al., "Intensity and Frequency of Extreme Novel Epidemics," *Proceedings of the National Academy of Sciences* 118 (2021): e2105482118. On biodiversity, see Felicia Keesing and Richard S. Ostfeld, "Impacts of Biodiversity and Biodiversity Loss on Zoonotic Diseases," *Proceedings of the National Academy of Sciences of the United States of America* 118 (2021): e2023540118.

7. Stephen Olaide Aremu et al., "The United States Withdrawal from the World Health Organization (WHO), Its Implications for Global Health Governance," *Global Health* 21 (2025): article 48.

INDEX

GHF refers to the Great Horse Flu.